D1534722

A Woman's Guide to Good Health After 50

Marie Feltin, M.D.

With the editorial assistance of
Joyce G. Moss and Barbara B. Whitesides

An AARP Book
published by
American Association of Retired Persons, Washington, D.C.
Scott, Foresman and Company, Lifelong Learning Division,
Glenview, Illinois

Library of Congress Cataloging-in-Publication Data

Feltin, Marie, 1944–
  A woman's guide to good health after 50.

  Includes index.
  1. Aged women—Health and hygiene. 2. Middle aged women—Health and hygiene. I.
Moss, Joyce G. II. Whitesides, Barbara B. III. Title. [DNLM: 1. Geriatrics— popular works. 2.
Health. 3. Women—popular works. WT 120 F315w]
RA778.F43 1987   613'.043   86–17866
ISBN 0–673–24815–1

ABCDs of melanoma (pages 12–13) courtesy of American Academy of Dermatology, Inc.

Age-Specific Height-Weight Table (page 150) excerpted from *Impact of Age on Weight Goals* by Reubin Andres, M.D., Annals of Internal Medicine, 1985, Table 2.

Causes of Vaginal Bleeding at Different Phases of Reproductive Life (page 205) adapted from "Some Important Causes of Vaginal Bleeding" from *Harrison's Principles of Internal Medicine,* 6th ed. Copyright © 1970 by McGraw-Hill, Inc. Reprinted by permission.

Complete Natural Breathing (page 273) adapted from *The Relaxation & Stress Reduction Workbook* by Martha Davis, Elizabeth Robbins Eshelman, and Matthew McKay. Copyright © 1980 by New Harbinger Publications, Oakland, California. Reprinted by permission.

Adaptation of "The Relaxation Response" (page 275) from *The Relaxation Response* by Herbert Benson, M.D., with Miriam Z. Klipper. Copyright © 1975 by William Morrow and Company, Inc. Adapted by permission of the publisher and by permission of Bill Adler Books.

A Model Patients' Bill of Rights (pages 349–351) from *The Rights of Doctors, Nurses, and Allied Health Professionals: A Health Law Primer* by G. J. Annas, L. H. Glantz, and B. F. Katz. Reprinted by permission.

AARP Books is an educational and public service project of the American Association of Retired Persons, which, with a membership of more than 23 million, is the largest association of persons fifty and over in the world today. Founded in 1958, AARP provides older Americans with a wide range of membership programs and services, including legislative representation at both federal and state levels. For further information about additional association activities, write to AARP, 1909 K Street, N.W., Washington, DC 20049.

Publisher's Note

Contents

Acknowledgments

M any medical and life experiences and many people have inspired me in both professional and personal ways in the writing of this book. I wish to thank all my patients, especially older women patients, who shared important parts of their lives with me during my training in San Francisco and in my work at Urban Medical Group, the East Boston Neighborhood Health Center, and Beth Israel Hospital. My colleagues and students at Boston University School of Public Health and the Channing Laboratory at Harvard Medical School helped me to always view medicine in its broader social context, to be mindful of good research, and to be critical of public policy and pursue its change.

There are certain people whom I would like to name in particular. Joyce Moss and Barbara Whitesides gave enthusiastically, often unconditionally, and unrelentingly of their time, expertise, wisdom, creativity, and humor in vigorous editing of this book. The process of working with them added fun, laughter, and a sharing of burdens and gave me the rich gift of two new friendships with women I enjoy and admire.

Barb Quaintance of the American Association of Retired Persons and Dr. William Bicknell helped initiate the project. Dr. Norman Scotch, an author himself, taught me the discipline of writing. Elaine Goldberg of Scott, Foresman and Company was most valuable in helping me keep an appropriate focus, clarity, and style in the book. Several women—my mother, Jeannette Feltin; my aunt, Annette Epstein; Edna Homa Hunt; Freda Scotch; Molly Masland; Faina Ostrovsky; and Galina Krivoy—were important role models and critical advisors in the project. Certain men, and especially my spouse, Dr. Robert Master, and my father, Francois Feltin, gave me valuable insights and, in the case of Robert, contributed many ideas to the work.

Certain colleagues at Beth Israel Hospital and other medical professionals deserve many thanks for critically reviewing chapters in their area of expertise. Kenneth Arndt, M.D.; Frank Berson,

M.D.; Ruth S. Campanella, M.D.; Leon Carrow, M.D.; Alice B. Daniels, M.D.; Marilyn Ehline, M.S.W., A.C.S.W.; Marvin Freed, M.D.; Peggy Howrigan, M.D.; Fred Kantrowitz, M.D.; William Kavesh, M.D.; Martita Lopez, Ph.D.; Susan Love, M.D.; Kenneth Minaker, M.D.; Amy S. Paller, M.D.; Kathy Parsonnette, R.N.; Marcie Richardson, M.D.; Aaron G. Rosenberg, M.D.; Alice Rothchild, M.D.; Robert Russell, M.D.; Carol Stollar, M.Ed., R.D.; Nadine Sahyoum; Kathleen M. Taylor, M.S., R.D.; William A. Tisdale, M.D.; Sonia Vorotnitsky, M.D.; Steve Weinberger, M.D.; and Lois Young all gave freely of their time and experience. I greatly appreciate their comments; the final responsibility for the writing, however, is my own.

My family and friends thought up titles and jokes and were helpful, tolerant, sympathetic, kind, critical, and inspirational. They baby-sat my youngest children for countless hours. Words fail to praise their patience and contributions appropriately. I especially want to thank my parents, Jeannette and Francois Feltin, for being the greatest grandparents; Bob Master for helping me keep perspective on the important things in life; our children and my stepchildren—Daniel, Johanne, Steven, Jonas, and Sarina—for being themselves; my dog, Pitou, for ever being faithful; my father-in-law, Nathan Master, for his endless supply of chicken soup; Jacques Weissgerber, George Feltin, Pamela and Gregory Palmer, Michael Weinberger, and Eric Prahl for support, humor, and baby-sitting; Marguerite Collins, SBA, Trevor Daniels, George, and Jacques for the great conga music sessions; Jean Nesbitt, Christine Chamberlain, James Miller, Annette Furst, Phillippe Jacob, and Rose Ellen Morrell for being friends despite the fact that I hardly ever saw them; and George, George T., and Ben Whitesides and Guy, Jason, and David Moss for bearing with their mothers' (or wives') crazy work schedules during the extensive times they were helping me with the manuscript.

Introduction

Nobody grows old by merely living a number of
years. People grow old only by deserting their
ideals. Years wrinkle the face, but to give up
enthusiasm wrinkles the soul. Worry, doubt, self-
interest, fear, despair—these are the long, long
years that bow the head and turn the growing
spirit back to dust.

—*Cicero*

OLDER women have never been so young. A fifty-year-old attending a rock concert is astonished to overhear teenagers call
her "old." A grandmother is still surprised when movie attendants
automatically offer her a senior citizen's discount without asking to
see her card. A diminutive eighty-year-old winks and defines old age
as "ten years older than you are now." As Simone de Beauvoir
wrote, "So long as the inner feeling of youth remains alive . . . the
objective truth of age . . . is fallacious."

I was pushing my grandson in a stroller, and
people who came to admire asked me, "Are you
the grandma?" Do I look like a grandmother,
and not the mama?

—*Jeannette Q., sixty-five*

AGES AND AGING

Aging has no simple, single measure. The number of years we have
lived pinpoints our chronological age; the way we feel we have lived
gives a clue to our psychological age; the condition of our bodies
provides a measure of our biological age. These ages may not be
remotely the same. But time and events transfigure us, helping us
come to terms with their meaning and ultimately with ourselves.

1

I have everything now that I had twenty years
ago except it's all lower.

—*Gypsy Rose Lee*

One American gerontologist compares aging to a flight of irregular
stairs down which some journey more quickly than others. Gerontologists define aging, or senescence, as the gradual and progressive inability
of an organism to adapt biologically to the environment, culminating in
death. In other words, the cells and organs of the body, and eventually
the body as a whole, gradually perform their functions less and less well,
and finally not at all. Disease can accelerate the aging process, but
absence of disease does not prevent it.

If a woman's body is viewed as a biological machine, we would
have to agree that its peak performance occurs in the late teens and
declines slowly thereafter. Certain biological functions diminish
gradually with age for both women and men: the ability of the heart
to pump blood, the ability of the kidneys to excrete wastes, the
ability of the pancreas to direct the body to metabolize sugar. Our
total muscle mass grows smaller, our skin becomes less elastic, and
our defense system against disease weakens. Other functions, such
as those of the liver and the lungs, stay about the same. Only the
ability to reproduce is lost to women as we age.

If we could suddenly eradicate the ten leading causes of death in
the United States, American women would live about 88
years—rather than 78 years, the current average. If we could unlock
as yet unknown secrets of aging, our maximum human life span
might be about 115 years. No doubt research on aging in the next
decade may bring us closer to our maximum life span.

We wonder how long we will be able to choose the road we
want to travel. We wonder how long it will be mind over matter
before our bodies put us in our place. We are eager to learn about
further changes we can make in our health, living habits, and environment that will reduce age-related disorders and improve our
fitness, our looks, and our sense of well-being.

THEORIES OF AGING

The imminence of mortality has goaded humans to study the process of aging. It is easy to observe that longevity, like hair color,
runs in families. But explanations of longevity based on genetics
alone are not comprehensive enough to account for the way all peo-

ple age. Additional theories of aging point to the importance of the way you live and the environment in which you live.

There is some evidence that aging can result from random damage to your body's cells and tissues. This damage can take the form of mutations, that is, accidental changes in the genetic code of your cells; accumulated wastes in cells and tissues; or the effects of a class of particularly reactive molecules (known as "free radicals") produced in the body. Scientists have also found evidence for an immune theory of aging, which suggests that your body may, in later years, view various parts of itself as foreign material and attack its own cells and tissues.

A NEW "CHANGE OF LIFE"

Historically, woman was valued for her fertility. She was felt to be akin to wild animals—intuitive, ruled by her biology. Myths developed about her link to the moon, about menstruation as a sign of sinfulness, about barrenness as a punishment from God, and about hysteria as the wandering of the womb through the body. The female mystique was bound to the stages of a woman's reproductive life—whether virginity, fertility, or maternity.

Nineteenth-century European physicians thought women decayed at menopause and that all manner of illnesses in women after menopause were therefore futile to treat. Menopause was seen as the end of life rather than the change of life.

The Victorian medical attitude toward postmenopausal women might have persevered were it not for several things: the movement for women's rights, demands for equal educational opportunities, improved life expectancy for women once they stopped dying in childbirth, and the invention of the birth control pill. In the early 1900s, women lived on the average fifty years, or to the age of menopause.

Women now live approximately thirty years beyond menopause. These years are a gift of time in which to live and grow and celebrate the understanding that decades of experience confer.

AGING GRACEFULLY IN THE BEST OF HEALTH

How can we enjoy the best of health in these later years? The following chapters cover the common health questions and concerns of older women. Our physical health, like our spirit, is something over which we have a measure of control. By becoming more knowledgeable about the normal aging process and by learning to assess our symptoms in health and disease, we can bolster our strength and peace of mind. We can learn to modify our diets and living habits to feel and appear our best and to retard the development of diseases that accompany aging. We can learn to differentiate between those problems that we can monitor ourselves and those that are potentially serious and merit immediate medical attention. We can identify specialized resources and support services to help ourselves remain independent and vigorous.

On these pages you will realize how much you have in common with other women—how much their concerns are your concerns and how much support you can lend one another.

Older women live on the average seven years longer than men and eventually outnumber men two to one. But women use more drugs and more medical services than men. Women have relinquished much control of their medical problems to doctors and to a complex medical care system and have relied too little on their own innate resources and on the wisdom of their bodies.

This book helps you take control over forces that affect your health. You need to be a sophisticated consumer of medical services to get the best of care. You need to be an active partner with your physician. This book gives you the tools to enter that partnership.

You can develop the confidence and competence to maintain your independence, thrive, and savor the second half of your life. Prize older age for what it is—a badge of strength and a proof of survival. You can age gracefully and in the best of health.

> My enthusiasm for all facets of life is greater than ever, as I realize that these are my golden years, the best of my whole life. I am appreciating every minute of them. I am gathering my strength and concentrating on myself.
> —*Annette L., eighty-one*

One

Your Skin, Face, and Hair

No Spring, nor Summer beauty hath such grace
As I have seen in one Autumnal face.
                                   —*John Donne, Elegy 9*
                                   "The Autumnal"

They aren't making mirrors the way they used to.
                                   —*Tallulah Bankhead*

F EW of us do not take some pride in our years. We relish time's
seasoning while we grant youth's inexperience. Yet we stand in
awe of youth's beauty and fear that what we naturally look like as
we age is less desirable. Most of us will not ignore our wrinkles, but
we do well to look beyond them. Beauty is better reflected by our
state of health and our vitality than by our age. There is much we
can do to improve the condition of our skin, face, and hair and to
put our best face forward.

YOUR SKIN

The skin is composed of several layers (see figure 1). The outermost
layer, or epidermis, has flat, dead cells on its surface. These cells accumulate in the sun-exposed areas, giving older skin a coarser,
duller appearance. Oil glands and sweat glands are embedded in the
skin, lubricating it and controlling the release of moisture and heat
from the body. Aging oil glands produce less oil, making the skin
drier. This drying trend is very slow in women until after
menopause and is dependent on hormone levels. Taking estrogen
after menopause slows some of these skin changes.

Sweat glands allow excess heat to evaporate from the body.
With age, these glands produce less sweat, and only at higher body

temperatures, so the skin becomes less efficient at dispersing heat, making you more prone to getting overheated.

The dermis, beneath the epidermis, contains a network of collagen, which provides the main support and strength for skin. The suppleness of skin is dependent on elastic tissue, also found in the dermis. Age brings a decrease in the amount of collagen as well as a sunlight-induced disorganization and decrease in the elastic tissue in sun-exposed areas, which makes your skin thinner and less able to stretch. When you pinch young skin on the back of the hand and then let go, the skin flattens right away. When you pinch aged skin in the same spot and let go, it stays pinched for a while. This diminished elasticity and stretching is what causes wrinkles, the deep frown lines on your forehead and the grooves from your nose to the corners of your mouth. Loss of the third component of the dermis, called the ground substance, results in the smaller wrinkles known as crepe-paper wrinkles above and below the mouth and on the neck and the "crow's feet" around the eyes.

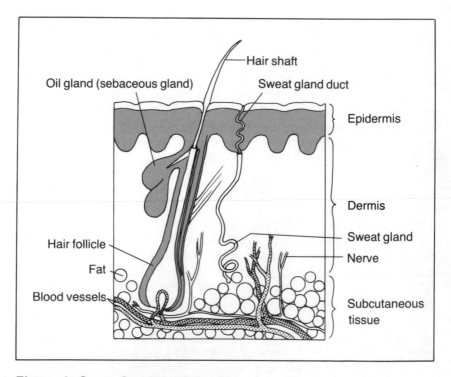

Figure 1. Cross Section of the Skin

Everyone gets wrinkles with age. The speed with which your skin forms wrinkles depends on the amount of your sun exposure and, to a lesser degree, on your heredity (fair skins wrinkle faster). Look at your parents and their siblings; their inventory of wrinkles suggests how your skin may look at their age. Other influences are losing estrogen at menopause, smoking cigarettes, breathing polluted air, and drinking alcohol.

The dermis also contains small blood vessels, which diminish in number with age. Changes in some of the remaining blood vessels result in the common but not serious marks you may see on your skin: small red dots, called cherry angiomas, found mostly on your trunk; little red threadlike areas, called spider angiomas; somewhat larger blue swellings; and thin visible, dilated blood vessels, found on the lips, ears, face, and neck. These marks can be removed by a dermatologist, or skin specialist, or by a plastic surgeon with an electric pencil that cauterizes (burns and closes off) the small vessels. The elastic tissue of blood vessels is also altered by age and sunlight. As a result, you can get purple patches, called purpura, after minimal trauma to the skin because blood cells leak easily through the damaged blood vessels.

Pigmentary changes, or changes in the color of the skin, in older age result in some common blemishes. The brown spots—also known as age spots, liver spots, or, technically, as senile lentigos—are small flat areas on the skin that are darker than the surrounding skin and are found most commonly on the hands, arms, and face. Sun exposure darkens them. Raised, scaly, darker areas that are often oily and thick to the touch and are found mostly on the chest or back are called seborrheic keratoses. The color of keratoses fades somewhat when you decrease their exposure to sunshine or when you gently rub on them with a wet facecloth or apply a vitamin A cream. Generally, creams containing hydroquinone that are advertised to bleach pigmented spots do not work for either lentigos or keratoses. Seborrheic keratoses may be easily removed by a physician by freezing them with liquid nitrogen.

Aging and Sunlight

Your skin is the largest organ of your body, and the one most exposed to the environment. Sunlight damages and ages the skin more than any other environmental factor. The extent of damage depends on your inherited susceptibility to ultraviolet light damage and how much you expose your skin to the sun. Exposure depends on your habits, the climate you live in, your occupation, and the way you dress and otherwise protect your skin. By minimizing sun exposure, you offer your skin its greatest protection from wrinkles, not to mention skin cancer.

Styles change. Until the 1920s, the porcelain-pale woman was considered beautiful. Women protected their faces from sunlight with broad-rimmed hats and powdered their faces with ivory colors. Since then, people have prized the tanned, healthy look. The hatless, tanned woman became fashionable, and Americans are still under her spell.

How does sunlight damage the skin? The shorter ultraviolet waves of light tan, burn, and thicken the top layer of skin. These light waves do not pass through window glass, but they do penetrate most clouds. Their harmful effects accumulate through repeated exposure to the sun. Ultraviolet light damages the DNA, or genetic material, of skin cells. Scientists suspect that as you age, your skin's repair mechanisms grow less efficient, so occasionally a damaged cell suddenly wildly multiplies and forms a cancer. The incidence of skin cancer has doubled in the past thirty years, as people have pursued the perfect tan.

People vary in their sensitivity to the harmful effects of sunshine. Blonds, redheads, and freckled women find that they rarely tan but easily burn. These are the women most at risk for developing skin cancer because their skin has the least natural protection from ultraviolet rays.

Tanning is actually the result of your skin protecting itself from the sun's harmful ultraviolet rays. Small cells in the lower layer of the skin, called melanocytes, are activated by sunlight to produce their pigment, melanin—a protein that absorbs ultraviolet energy and protects the skin from damage. Very fair women who lack large quantities of these melanocytes cannot adequately tan before their skin burns unless they use sunscreen creams. Even black women, who have greater natural protection, can be sunburned from too intense sun exposure. It takes about fifteen to forty years of sun exposure to cause skin cancer, but lesser exposures also damage skin.

Photosensitivity

Certain substances taken internally or applied to the skin can seriously alter or accelerate the effects of sunlight. These substances are photosensitizers, and a person's reaction to them is called photosensitivity. Women taking them are more than usually sensitive to sunlight and hence get sunburned more quickly than usual. They must use extra protection from either clothing or sunscreen cream. Substances causing photosensitivity include these:

Drugs
> tetracycline (antibiotic)
> sulfa drugs (antibiotics), such as Gantrisin and Bactrim
> nalidixic acid (antibiotic), such as NegGram
> phenothiazines (tranquilizers), such as Thorazine and Stelazine
> thiazides (diuretics), such as Diuril and HydroDIURIL

Topical Sensitizers
> furocoumarin (contained in parsley, limes, carrots, and oil of bergamot and found in certain perfumes or after-shave lotions)
> coal tars, wood tars (contained in shampoos)

Protection from the Sun

The key to protecting your skin is to enjoy the sun wisely—to tan gradually and *not burn*. Keep the following in mind:

- The closer you are to the equator (which, in the United States, means the closer you live to our southern border) or the higher you are above sea level, the more intense are the sun's ultraviolet rays.

- The closer to midday you sun yourself, the more intense is your exposure to ultraviolet rays. The worst hours for getting sunburn are from 10:00 A.M. to 2:00 P.M.

- The chances for sunburn are increased if you are in or near water, since water reflects sunlight.

- Dark clothes absorb heat; light-colored clothes reflect light away from the body. It is best, therefore, to wear light colors in the summertime.

- Liberal doses of maximum-protection sunscreens used before and as your tan develops can prevent skin damage. (This is especially important if you are fair-skinned, blond, or red-haired.)

Since 1980, sunscreen products have had to advertise a numerical rating called the SPF, or sun protection factor, on the package. The SPF is the ratio of the length of time it takes for untanned skin protected by the product to turn red, to the length of time it takes for untanned, unprotected skin to turn red. The numbers vary from 2 (which is almost no protection) to 15 or higher (which offers much greater protection). The lower the SPF, the less protection from ultraviolet rays. Products in the middle range, such as those with an SPF of 6 or 8, offer some protection as well as some tanning; but keep in mind that sunscreens are not sun blocks, and you can burn in mid-day even with a sunscreen containing an SPF of 15.

When you apply sunscreens, do not forget your lips. Some products for chapped lips contain a sunscreen (Chap Stick Lip Balm, for example), and some are specific lip sunscreens, such as PreSun or Chap Stick Sunblock 15 lip protectants. If you are especially sun-sensitive, use an opaque sunscreen, containing titanium dioxide, or use zinc oxide, on areas like lips and nose, which are very vulnerable to burn.

The most common and most protective sunscreen chemicals are para-aminobenzoic acid, or PABA, and PABA derivatives. About fifty such products are available on the market, including Eclipse Sunscreen Lotion, Paba film, PreSun, Sea and Ski, and Sundown Sunscreen—all excellent sunscreens. Products containing salicylate sunscreens or other chemicals are not as effective. The ben-zophenones (such as oxybenzone) that are contained in products such as PreSun and Shade Sunscreen Lotion, while very good, do not offer complete protection when used alone.

Sun lotions differ in the concentration of the chemicals they contain and in their bases. Most have an alcohol base, which allows easier spreading and is not greasy. The problem with these lotions is that they are drying to the skin, and they drip off when you are wet. Therefore, they need to be applied frequently, especially if you have been swimming or perspiring. Lotions with oil or cream bases, while greasier and messier, stay on much better and resist perspira-tion and water.

Treatment of Sunburn

You can best treat mild sunburn by applying cold compresses three or four times a day. While nonprescription creams that con-tain a mild anesthetic such as benzocaine provide relief, they can cause an allergic reaction. Creams such as Nivea or Eucerin, creams containing aloe vera, or Vaseline can help counteract dryness, and aspirin (if taken soon enough) can reduce the intensity of the in-flammatory reaction.

In severe sunburn cases, a physician may prescribe oral cortisone tablets for a week to relieve some of the severe swelling, blistering, and redness of sunburned skin.

Skin Cancers Related to Sun Exposure

Precancerous areas of skin are known as actinic keratoses. These areas are generally found on the face, neck, or back of hand and ap-pear as small red patches, with a few visible blood vessels, that develop a rough, yellow-brown surface. If you avoid exposing these patches to sunlight, many of them may totally disappear. If you continue to expose such areas to the sun, they may eventually change into skin cancers, usually in about ten years.

Protecting actinic keratoses from the sun through constant use of sunscreens is essential. A dermatologist will decide whether some areas need more vigorous treatment, such as freezing (cryosurgery), burning (electrosurgery), or application of a powerful cream called Fluoroplex (fluorouracil).

Basal cell epithelioma, or basal cell cancer, is the most common skin cancer in Caucasians. It appears as a pink, hairless, waxy-looking growth on the head and neck. In later stages, it may be a small cluster of tiny, pearly pimples or a crusted sore surrounded by a craterlike rim. These tumors spread by enlarging into the surrounding area and rarely travel to other parts of the body. If untreated, they can erode normal tissue.

Small skin tumors are easily removed by a dermatologist by scraping, cauterizing, or excision, under local anesthesia, or by freezing. These treatments leave inconspicuous scars. If the tumors have been allowed to grow very large, they may require radiation treatments or more extensive surgery and, occasionally, both surgery and subsequent radiation treatments. In about 5 percent of cases, the cancer may recur, and new basal cell cancers may develop. If you have ever had a basal cell cancer, you should see a dermatologist annually.

It is important to remember that noninvasive skin cancer, though not usually dangerous, will not just disappear if ignored. In fact, it will grow larger and require more extensive surgery for its removal. If extensive surgery is required, the skill of a plastic surgeon may be needed to minimize the scars.

Squamous cell cancer is a more dangerous skin cancer because it can spread both locally and to other parts of the body. It occurs most commonly on the lower lip, other parts of the face, and the hands. At first, a squamous cell cancer may be a small, hard, red pimple that soon forms a sore that will not heal—a sore with a crust and an irregular rim. It should be removed by a doctor as soon as possible by excision, scraping, or burning, depending on the size, location, and history of the cancer. Tumors on the ears spread quickly and should be attended to as soon as they are seen.

Malignant melanoma, the most deadly form of skin cancer, used to be rare but is now significantly on the rise. In 1985, the American Cancer Society estimated that one in every 150 people in the United States will eventually develop melanoma and that by the year 2000 the figure will be one in 100. It occurs most often on the sun-exposed skin of populations of European descent. This cancer usually is first noticed as a slightly raised or bumpy, dark brown, black, or blue area of skin that begins to change in color, shape, and size, and which may suddenly start to itch or feel sore. Older people are especially prone to a particular type of melanoma, fortunately less harmful, called lentigo maligna melanoma, in which the dark area of skin has irregular borders and patchy coloration, mixing areas of black, dark brown, and pale brown. Noncancerous moles or warts containing blood clots may look similar, so show any such suspicious area to an internist or dermatologist. If the internist or dermatologist suspects melanoma, he or she will perform an excisional biopsy, in which the entire suspicious area is removed and examined under a microscope for diagnosis. The procedure is performed under local anesthesia, with minimal discomfort. Malignant melanomas require complete removal of skin at and around the site. Left untreated, or treated late, malignant melanomas may spread to many parts of the body and can cause death.

Detecting Skin Cancer

In the American Cancer Society's journal, *CA—A Journal for Clinicians,* doctors recently advised that people check their bodies monthly for signs of melanoma (see figure 2). They recommend ex-

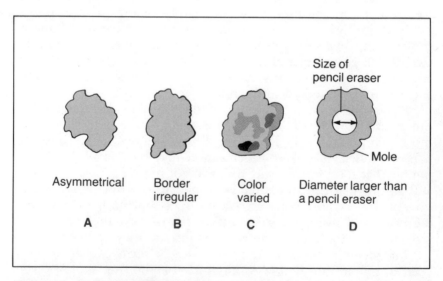

Figure 2. Malignant Melanoma   Malignant melanoma begins with moles that are asymmetrical (**A**), have irregular borders (**B**), include various colors (**C**), and have a diameter larger than a pencil eraser (**D**).

amining the entire body in front of a full-length mirror, using a hand mirror to look at the back of the body. The doctors suggest studying pigmented areas for the "ABCD" signs:

A. Asymmetrical shape (pointed, or elliptic, since benign areas are usually round)

B. Border irregularity (since benign areas have smooth borders)

C. Color variability within the mole (brown, black, white, red, or mixed, since benign moles are usually one color)

D. Diameter larger than a pencil eraser (since benign moles are usually smaller)

Any moles or "spots" that change in color, size, shape, or consistency should be examined right away by your doctor or a dermatologist. Areas that are red and scaly or that bleed, get crusted, or scab but do not heal also should be checked.

PUTTING YOUR BEST FACE FORWARD

Artists divide the human face into three horizontal regions: the forehead, the nose and cheekbones, and the mouth and chin. These three areas are about equal in size in youth and early adulthood. In older age, the forehead broadens if the hairline recedes; the nose appears somewhat longer and wider and the cheekbones more prominent; and the mouth and the chin area become smaller.

The contours of the face depend upon three muscle groups. One group encircles the eyes; another encircles the mouth, with a branch to the cheekbones; a third includes the muscles of the cheeks and jaw. A sheet of muscle below the face covers the neck. Overlying the muscle layers is fat, distributed in a pattern that varies from woman to woman. This pattern is dependent upon heredity, hormones, and age.

All our muscles diminish in volume and tone with age. Our facial muscles are no exception. The causes are several:

1. We use our muscles less with age, so they become weaker and slowly decrease in number as they are unused.

2. The nerves that command muscles to contract or relax may also diminish with age, and their corresponding muscle fibers wither.

3. Some of the chemical packets at the ends of nerves that instruct muscles in what to do decrease as the body ages.

The overall effect is that the face subtly changes shape, and the overlying skin begins to sag.

Age and the postmenopausal gradual decrease of the female hormone estrogen cause a slow loss in the size of the fat pads of a woman's face. The skin loses its elastic tone, causing bones to become more prominent in some places and the skin more lax in others.

The jawbone recedes with age, especially if teeth have been lost. Women who regularly wear their dentures can greatly slow this process.

Some doctors advocate facial exercises to retard the loss of facial muscle tone. While there is no good evidence that such exercise achieves that goal, the exercises relax facial muscles, which can make you feel better, and if you feel better, you will look better.

Here is a simple series of facial exercises, which takes under three minutes to perform. By the end of the exercises, you may feel silly, but your face should feel better and its muscle tone less slack.

1. Say "Meow," accentuating each syllable. Say it slowly three times and rapidly five times.

2. Say "Bow!" (like a dog). Say it slowly three times and rapidly five times.

3. Say "Quack," accentuating each sound. Say it slowly three times and rapidly five times.

4. Say "Moo." Say it slowly three times and rapidly five times.

5. Close your eyes tight; suddenly open them at the count of three. Tightly close and rapidly open your eyes five times.

6. Stretch your lower jaw toward your ears, sliding the jaw toward one ear at a time. This exercise stretches your neck. Try it three times slowly and five times fast.

Care of the Face and Skin

After avoiding the sun, the next great protection for your face is cleaning and moisturizing.

Clean your face daily, preferably at night, to remove the accumulation of dirt, pollutants, and oils. Cleansing creams (which are a combination of detergent, wetting agent, beeswax, alcohol, water, oil, and borax) and soaps (which are made from alkali and fats) are both good; either can be used. They should rinse off completely with water. All kinds of expensive soaps are offered on the market: heavily fatted soaps, glycerin soaps, and soaps with organic acids. Each promises to give more moisture than the next one, maintain the skin's acid balance, and soften the skin. Basically, the extra money goes down the drain with all the expensive components. An inexpensive superfatted soap—such as Dove or Nivea—used sparingly, and thoroughly rinsed off with warm or cool water, is all that is needed. Washing with soap removes oils. Since the older skin makes less oil, you may want to consider just rinsing your face with cool water or using a cleansing cream.

To reduce dryness of the skin, use warm or cool water rather than hot water, which removes natural oils. You need not use a washcloth. You can simply use your fingers, or one of the gentle natural or artificial face sponges. After rinsing with cold water, which is a good astringent (that is, it closes the pores), you should dry your face delicately—patting, not rubbing, it.

Next, you need to moisturize your face, to replace the natural oils lost in washing. Hundreds of moisturizing creams are available, from the banal to the exotic. They usually have oil bases to reduce the evaporation of moisture from your skin, and most are suspended in water to minimize greasiness. Some of the more unusual creams contain mink, chinchilla, or caviar oil; others contain royal jelly (from queen bees); still others contain ginseng root. Although they sound more effective than cheaper preparations, and their prices tempt you to believe it, their effectiveness may be determined only by how good they make you feel. What counts is how regularly you use your moisturizer.

Some moisturizers contain female hormones. Advertisements for these creams imply that they can retard the effects of aging in postmenopausal women. Because these hormones are absorbed by the body and, consequently, could stimulate cancer, the Food and Drug Administration (FDA) has restricted the levels of hormones in such creams to ineffective amounts. Thus these creams do little other than moisturize.

You can best moisturize the rest of your body with lotion or bath oil or with such products as Alpha Keri, applied to your body immediately after a bath or shower. (Be sure to use a rubber mat in the tub, *especially* when you've added bath oil to the water; the oil can make the tub very slippery.)

Protecting, cleansing, and moisturizing your skin will keep it in the best possible shape.

Facial Rejuvenation

> For years I had looked at myself in the mirror,
> wondering what I would look like with a face-lift.
> Finally I got up the courage to have one, and I
> feel so much better.
>
> —*Connie R., sixty-seven*

> I was ashamed of wanting to have my good looks
> back, and for not being able to cope with the
> signs of age on my face. All my family thought I
> was crazy for wanting a face-lift.
>
> —*Dorothy P., fifty-eight*

When Betty Ford, then First Lady, publicly announced that she had had a face-lift and explained why, she made front-page news and created a dramatic surge in the face-lift business: "I'm sixty years old, and I wanted a new face to go with my beautiful life." She suddenly legitimized for the average woman what had previously been associated only with actresses and socialites.

Americans are more occupied with sculpting their bodies now than ever before, and cosmetic surgery is becoming more acceptable, but we still suspect vanity. If you are contemplating cosmetic surgery, you may find your family nonsupportive, or even hostile. You may feel guilty about being "frivolous" and narcissistic because you want to retard the course of nature. Even your family doctor may express outright disapproval, leaving you feeling very alone.

To make an intelligent decision about plastic surgery, you have to know what the surgery can accomplish. Plastic surgery will not make you look twenty years old again, but it can improve baggy eyelids, jowls, and "turkey gobbler" neck.

What to Expect from Plastic Surgery

> I'm disappointed about the results [of my face-
> lift]. I fantasized that I would actually get
> younger, but I still look and feel like the older
> generation. Is it me or the doctor who messed
> up?
>
> —*Donna F., sixty-five*

As Gertrude Stein put it, "A difference to be a difference must be a difference." Women expect to look significantly better after a face-lift than before, and they usually do. The majority of women are happy with the results of the procedure and are pleased that they went through with it. Some women, however, find that few people notice anything new about them afterward, or they find that their new appearance does not translate into the social or business success that they had expected.

Face-Lift

A face-lift, or rhytidectomy (Greek for "removal of wrinkle"), should be thought of as a procedure to reduce the amount and improve the distribution of skin on the face and neck. It can diminish jowls, baggy skin, "turkey gobbler" skin of the neck, and excess fatty tissue in the neck. It can give you a cleaner jawline and your face a rested appearance. A face-lift will improve the creases at the junction of the cheek and nose, but it will not eliminate them. Nor will a face-lift eliminate the fine wrinkles that develop around the mouth and eyes—a chemical peel is required to do this.

Women frequently ask whether their faces will "fall" at some point after the face-lift. The answer is no. The clock does not speed up following a face-lift; but the process of aging continues in the face, just as it does in the rest of the body. Skin ages differently with different people. Weight loss after the procedure can hasten the need to repeat it. Your skin will relax if you lose a substantial amount of weight after your surgery. Therefore, if you are contemplating losing weight, do so prior to having a face-lift.

Often subjective judgment determines whether, or when, a face-lift needs to be done initially or repeated. One woman might seek a face-lift when there are substantial age-related changes in her face and neck. She may be happy with the improvement brought about by her face-lift and not desire any further surgery. Another woman might consider plastic surgery at the first sign of a wrinkle. This woman will not be any more accepting of age-related changes in the years following her face-lift than she was before the face-lift and will seek repeated face-lifting or other procedures.

A face-lift is frequently an outpatient procedure, in which case the patient has surgery, recovers from sedation, and goes home all in the same day. The surgery can be performed under local anesthesia with sedation or under general anesthesia. Incisions are made in the hair-bearing scalp and at the base of the ear (see figure 3). The underlying tissues are plicated, or tucked, to tighten them. Excess fat may be removed from the neck, and excess skin is trimmed. Then the incisions are closed. A bulky dressing is applied. There is moderate discomfort following the surgery, for which pain medication is

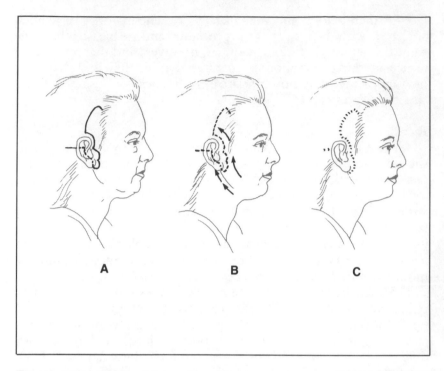

Figure 3. Face-Lift   For a face-lift, the surgeon makes incisions in the scalp and around the ear (**A**); tissues are pulled up and back; excess skin and fat are trimmed away (**B**); and the incision is closed (**C**).

prescribed. The patient is instructed to rest for twenty-four hours with her head elevated.

At subsequent office visits, the dressing and stitches are removed. The patient will have some bruising of the skin, swelling, and areas of temporary numbness. These conditions improve with time. For instance, the bruising lasts approximately ten days but may be camouflaged with makeup.

Eye-Lift

A blepharoplasty, or eye-lift, removes the pouches and wrinkled skin above and below the eyes. This procedure will not remove "laugh" lines. The surgeon makes careful incisions close to the edge of the eyelids and trims off fat and excess skin (see figure 4). The surgical scar is usually not visible, or it may resemble a laugh line. This operation rarely needs to be repeated.

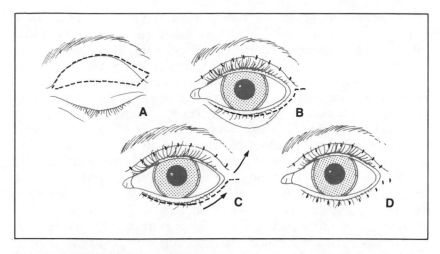

Figure 4. Eye-Lift   An eye-lift may involve surgery on both the upper and lower eyelids. To tighten the upper lid, the surgeon makes an incision along the natural fold lines (**A**). Excess fatty tissue and loose skin are removed, and the incision is stitched closed; then another incision is made beneath the lower lashes (**B**). To tighten the lower eyelid, skin is shifted to the side (**C**), and the incision is closed (**D**).

Neck-Lift

A neck-lift is often done as part of a full or partial face-lift. The incision behind the ear is extended down the hairline and partway down the neck. Skin is removed from the tissues and pulled back. A cut may be made below the chin to remove a "double chin."

Risks of Plastic Surgery

All surgery involves the risk of bleeding, the risk of infection, and the risk of not tolerating anesthesia. Surgeons are trained to minimize these risks. They make sure there is no active bleeding at the completion of surgery. If a hematoma, or swelling containing blood, should occur following surgery, it requires drainage. Antibiotics are given to minimize the risk of infection and to treat infection if it occurs. Local anesthesia with sedation is, on the whole, safer than general anesthesia.

In rare cases, women who undergo an extensive face-lift procedure end up with an overly tight face or a staring expression.

Any excess pain, swelling with redness, or fever after a face-lift operation should be reported to the doctor immediately.

After consulting with a plastic surgeon, go home and mull over what you have discussed. If you have other questions or concerns, either make a second appointment or call back. If you are unsure whether to proceed with the surgery, don't. It is not something to hurry into. Give it more thought. Should you still be undecided, it is best to try some other changes in your life first: a more flattering hairstyle, some new clothes, new makeup, a vacation, a new job, a plan to lose weight—even massages.

There are certain vulnerable times in an older woman's life when it is not so much her face as her spirits that need lifting. The death of a spouse or sibling, a recent divorce, a breakup with a lover, gynecologic or breast surgery—all are events that can leave you feeling acutely dissatisfied and depressed. You may hope that changing your appearance will ease the pain in your life. Women in such crises need reassurance that their discouragement and their need for change are perfectly normal and that it is best not to do anything drastic until the crisis has faded.

If you do decide to proceed with plastic surgery, have reasonable expectations, and have the surgery performed by a well-trained, competent doctor, you should be happy with the result.

Costs of Plastic Surgery

A complete face-lift will cost from $3,000 to $6,000, depending on the surgeon and location. In cities such as New York or Los Angeles, surgery is more expensive. Partial face-lifts cost from $1,000 to $2,000, and an eyelid operation costs from $1,000 to $3,000. Almost all plastic surgeons expect payment in advance. Insurance very rarely covers any cosmetic procedure unless it is performed, in part, for medical reasons. (Sometimes it can be documented that the condition existing before eye-lift surgery interfered with normal vision.) Recently, the Internal Revenue Service has allowed cosmetic surgery as a legitimate deductible expense; hence, some of the costs may be recovered.

How to Choose a Good Plastic Surgeon

Choosing a good plastic surgeon can make all the difference in the result of your face-lift. While there is an abundance of good plastic surgeons in New York City and Los Angeles, most large cities in the United States have a number of surgeons trained in cosmetic surgery.

Sometimes your family doctor can refer you to a qualified surgeon. If not, you can consult the American Society of Plastic and Reconstructive Surgeons (ASPRS) for the names of several plastic surgeons in your area. Although most states have their own branch, the ASPRS's main office is in Chicago. A referral by the ASPRS will mean that the surgeon has completed postmedical training in plastic surgery and has passed board examinations.

If a surgeon does not have these qualifications, he or she may not have had specific training in cosmetic surgery. Plan to investigate the individual surgeon's credentials and competence. The specialists who offer to make a woman's face look younger range from the medically responsible to the racketeer.

When you consult a plastic surgeon, he or she will evaluate the feature that you wish to change and make a recommendation. This recommendation may be different from or more or less extensive than the procedure you have requested. As one woman put it, "I went to the plastic surgeon to see about pulling the sag out of my cheeks. He went on to criticize the shape of my nose, the sagging around my eyes, the shape of my chin, and my neck. I had never seen anything wrong with all those parts!" It is good to keep in mind that the eyes as well as the hands of plastic surgeons have been trained. The surgeons see things differently from their patients and may wish to present all the available possibilities. These can be overwhelming. Keep in mind that they are merely suggestions for highly elective procedures; you are not obliged to change any more of your face than you wish.

You may be very impressed with the results of a friend's face-lift. You may decide on the spot that her doctor is the only doctor for you. While it is hard to argue with success, it is wise to keep in mind that each face is different and poses different problems for the surgeon.

It may be necessary to visit several surgeons until you find one with whom you are completely satisfied, but it is better to be cautious beforehand than sorry afterward. Ask questions and be sure all have been answered to your satisfaction before making a decision.

Other Facial Rejuvenation Procedures

In addition to partial or full face-lifting, there are other procedures that produce a more youthful face. Chemical face-peeling is especially useful for treating the fine wrinkles about the mouth and eyes. It is a serious procedure that should only be done by board-certified dermatologists or plastic surgeons, since it can cause permanent scarring or pigment changes. It should not be performed on black women, as they are particularly susceptible to scarring and irregular pigmentation.

The procedure may be done in a doctor's office or in a hospital, depending on the extent of the peeling. The patient receives sedation before a solution of a strong chemical, usually trichloroacetic acid, is applied to parts of her face. Her face is then covered with waterproof adhesive tape for about forty-eight hours, leaving eyes, nostrils, and mouth uncovered. The acid burns most of the top layer of the skin, and the removal of the tape peels this burned skin layer off. The freshly peeled skin is covered with thymol iodide powder for about five days, to keep the skin dry and allow healing. After the mask of powder is removed, the skin appears fresh, pink, and unwrinkled—much like a baby's skin. Over a few weeks, the skin's mild swelling subsides, and, over about three months, the pink color fades.

If you have had a chemical peel, you should stay out of the sunlight for about a year, since the new skin is very delicate and may pigment unevenly. You should wear a sun block or sunscreen with an SPF of 15 if you do go out in the sun; also wear a hat.

Dermabrasion removes the top layer of skin by the grating movement of a wheel or flat surface and is much like using delicate sandpaper. It is useful in removing blemishes and acne scars but not too useful for removing wrinkles. The likelihood of scarring and pigment changes limits the success of this procedure in older women. Dermatologists or plastic surgeons usually perform this procedure in the office. After dermabrasion, patients must protect themselves from sunlight.

In another procedure, liquid collagen can be injected into specific facial areas to fill out wrinkles. The effect is considered temporary and lasts only six to twelve months. This technique is performed by dermatologists or plastic surgeons.

Facial masks—of wax, clay, or plastic—adhere to the skin and, after drying, are supposed to peel off dead surface skin cells. Some masks, however, can damage the elastic fibers of the skin and actually cause further loosening of the skin. Masks usually are applied by cosmetologists.

YOUR HAIR

Every square inch of the skin, except for the palms of the hands and the soles of the feet, grows some hair. Most of a woman's body is covered by fine, delicate hair that sometimes can be seen only in particularly good light or with the aid of a magnifying glass. During and after puberty, coarser, thicker, and longer hair replaces the fine hair in the armpit and pubic areas. This coarse hair does not turn gray as early as the hair on the head.

Each hair follicle goes through a normal life cycle of three phases. The first is a phase of hair growth. During the second, or resting, phase, no hair growth occurs, but the hair remains firmly attached to its follicle. During the final phase, the hair falls out, and the cycle starts again.

Scalp hair has a longer growth phase than hair on other parts of the body. Depending on the individual, scalp hair grows about 0.3 millimeters per day, for three to six years, which explains why this hair can grow so long. This growth period is rarely long enough, however, to produce hair reaching to the ground.

Hair Color

The color of hair—brown, red, blond, black, or gray—depends on the concentrations of melanin granules and iron in the hair shaft. Hair turns gray when the pigment cells no longer produce melanin. Even in your early twenties, you probably saw among your female friends at least one or two whose hair was noticeably sprinkled with "salt," or gray. By the age of fifty, these prematurely gray-haired women have plenty of company, for by then at least 50 percent of women have watched 50 percent or more of their scalp hair turn gray. Or they would have if they had given it half a chance.

> I used to pull out each of my gray hairs as they
> appeared. But gradually the gray hair became so
> plentiful that I gave up fighting it.
> —*Sarah M., fifty-two*

When you spot your first gray hair, it may give you only a small turn, for it is such an easily removable sign of age. When its companions appear and multiply, you may be less blithe about them. Your attitude toward your graying head may change back and forth as you get older and as you weigh these factors:

- how attractive you find the gray hair
- how attractive you find your hair when it is rinsed or dyed
- how much time and money you're willing to spend on rinsing or dyeing your hair
- how attractive your spouse, friends, and/or children find your hair

- how your gray hair affects your success at work (many working women find that they must look as young as possible to keep their jobs or to get promoted)
- what your whims are at the time

Long-Term Hair Coloring

Women whose skin is sensitive to the oxidants used in hair rinses and dyes and who develop rashes or painful scalp from them should avoid hair colorants. (It is always best to do a patch skin test before using a new hair rinse or dye.) The FDA has raised questions about diaminazole, a common ingredient in hair dyes that has been shown to cause cancer when fed to rats. Some manufacturers have developed dyes without diaminazole. An alternative dye that is natural and safe, but not good at concealing a large quantity of gray hair, is henna. It is available in red, brown, and black, with additional possible mixtures. Henna adds luster to your hair; it must be applied every month or so. Nonorganic hair rinses color the outside of the hair shaft and must be applied every five to six washes. If you sit under a hooded hair dryer and "bake" the hair rinse or henna in, it may last several months.

Before having your hair dyed, find out what chemicals are present in the dye your hairdresser uses. Call or write your local FDA office to learn whether the dye contains any potential cancerous substances.

Too Little Hair

Men are not the only people plagued by hair loss. Many women notice their hair thinning for some time after having a baby. Generally, the hair, or most of it, will grow back. Some women with very low iron reserves may find that their hair continues to fall out after the postpartum period. This condition is verifiable by tests and can be treated by a doctor.

Hair loss is becoming a more widespread problem among younger women as dieting has become more extreme. Anorexic women often find their hair falling out by the handful, but even women who diet conservatively and lose weight very gradually may lose a significant amount of hair as well as excess poundage. Usually the hair grows back after women cease dieting or after their bodies have readjusted following a considerable loss of weight.

Women's hair can also grow thinner as they age. This process is especially evident in women who have a strong family history of baldness. Usually, the hair around the temples begins to thin after age thirty. Gradually all scalp hair develops a shorter growth phase. Some of the older follicles do not restart another normal hair cycle but produce instead a tiny, thin hair of the kind that was present before birth.

About 60 percent of women between forty and seventy years of age show some thinning and recession of the hair in the temple areas, and 20 percent of these women also have some thinning on top of the head. More commonly, hair thinning starts after menopause, since the estrogen hormone that stimulates hair follicles is in much lower supply. In addition, the adrenal gland continues to produce small amounts of male hormones, or androgens, which stimulate loss of scalp hair. After age fifty, the amount of hair slowly decreases in the armpit and pubic areas as well, and some 30 percent of women over sixty may have barely any armpit hair left.

> My hair used to be one of my best features. Now that I'm sixty-three, it has become all thinned out. My father was totally bald, and my mother had very little hair left when she died in her eighties. I guess I'm destined to do the same. But isn't there anything I can do to stop it?
> —*Helen G.*

There is nothing you can do to stop the aging of your hair follicles. Taking estrogen by mouth does not seem to slow hair loss. What you *can* do is make certain that your hair is not falling out for other, treatable reasons such as these:

- Iron shortage and severe anemia, dramatic weight loss, or high fever. These conditions are temporary, and the hair grows back in months.

- Hypothyroidism. Low levels of thyroid hormone can cause hair loss as well as other problems. This condition can be diagnosed by a blood test and treated with thyroid hormone.

- Certain drugs. Cortisone (prednisone), diet pills, antithyroid pills (Propylthiouracil), and anticancer drugs can produce temporary hair loss.

- Too many permanent waves and too frequent straightening or bleaching of the hair. These processes involve a temporary, reversible chemical softening of the hair and, if overdone, can damage the hair shaft near the scalp, causing the hair to break and fall out. Conditioners may help somewhat, but the best remedy is to give your hair more rest between chemical treatments and be sure to protect it from the sun, which dries and splits hair.

• Too much heat applied to the hair. Heat damages hair, causing it to weaken and break. Try not to blow-dry your hair with hot air; use warm or cool air and hold the dryer at least a foot from your hair. Do not use electric curlers and hot combs every day.

Too Much Hair

> I never thought I was old until, one day, I
> noticed I was developing whiskers!
> —*Nancy A., fifty-four*

In the teens and early twenties, the changing hormonal balance of some women transforms some of the fine facial hair to a fine moustache, beard, or whiskers. Such women, particularly Caucasian women of Mediterranean ancestry, may have longer, coarser hairs on the chin and above the upper lip. Usually these women have slightly higher than normal levels of testosterone, the male hormone that is produced in small quantities in all women and that produces facial beards in men.

By their thirties and early forties, many women will notice a slight increase in quantity and thickness of facial hair. The condition, though a nuisance, is totally benign and can be treated by tweezing or with electrolysis.

Obese women tend to have more facial hair than thinner women; they may have mild problems metabolizing testosterone in the liver, thus giving it a chance to build up in their blood.

Certain drugs can produce excessive facial hair in women. These drugs include a blood pressure pill, minoxidil (Loniten); a diuretic, diazoxide (Proglycem); antidepressants doxepin hydrochloride (Sinequan) and imipramine (Tofranil); the tranquilizer meprobamate (Miltown); phenothiazines (Thorazine, Stelazine); an antiseizure drug, Dilantin; the anti-breast-cancer drug, tamoxifen; and cortisone.

In rare cases, the increase of facial hair can suggest a serious medical problem, such as a tumor of the ovary or adrenal gland. In these cases, the hair growth increases rapidly and may be accompanied by a deepening of the voice. Women who notice rapid new growth of facial hair must be checked out by their internist or gynecologist.

Treatment of Unwanted Facial Hair

If your facial hairs are few, you can tweeze them. Check for them regularly while standing near a good strong light and holding a mirror close to your face. That way you will save yourself the disgruntlement of discovering that you've been displaying some healthy facial hair for several days. Tweezing, however, sometimes renders future electrolysis less effective by distorting the hair roots.

Special facial bleaches can dye your facial hair, making it much less conspicuous. A waxing procedure, which uses either hot or cold wax, removes hair closer to the root. (Be careful not to burn yourself with hot wax by doing it yourself at home rather than going to a cosmetic salon.) Facial depilatories also remove facial hair effectively. Be sure your skin is not overly sensitive to the chemicals, since this treatment must be repeated about once a week.

The most permanent treatment for the growth of facial hair is electrolysis. This treatment involves passing an electric current to the hair follicle and, if well performed, permanently destroys the root. A certain amount of new growth will occur, even after treatment by the best hands. Look up Electrolysis in the Yellow Pages and find a licensed electrologist or dermatologist, since improperly practiced techniques can lead to scarring.

Other treatments should be reserved for women who have significant unwanted hair growth and who are closely monitored by their doctors. These include the following:

1. *Estrogen.* Moderate doses of estrogen can diminish the hair growth and should be prescribed with progesterone to decrease the risk of endometrial cancer (see chapter 9).

2. *Spironolactone* (Aldactone). This pill, which is an antiandrogen, can help when taken in doses of 100 milligrams twice a day. It takes about three to four months to show an effect.

General Tips for Healthy Hair

The following suggestions should prove helpful in maintaining a healthy head of hair:

1. Eat a well-balanced diet. Hair growth requires protein, vitamins, and minerals.

2. Use shampoo that is not too concentrated—such as baby shampoo, Nature's Gate Raindrops shampoo, or L'Oreal sham-

poo—for normal or dry hair. Strong shampoo is very drying to the hair.

3. Use a natural bristle brush on your hair, and do not brush the 100 strokes a day that you were taught in childhood. Avoid vigorous brushing or toweling, which can injure hair shafts.

4. Use a conditioner if your hair is dry or brittle; it coats the hair shaft and prevents breakage.

5. Protect your hair from the sun during hot months, since sunlight dries hair and makes it brittle. Wear a hat, a scarf, or a bandanna when the sun is hottest. Use a hair conditioner after swimming.

SUGGESTED READINGS

Cirillo, Dennis P., M.D., and Rubinstein, Mark, M.D. *The Complete Book of Cosmetic Facial Surgery: A Step-by-Step Guide to the Physical and Psychological Process*. New York: Simon & Schuster, 1984.

Morrison, Maggie, and *Glamour* magazine editors. *Glamour Guide to Hair*. New York: Fawcett, 1986.

Two

Your Musculoskeletal System

T HROUGHOUT life, your figure changes. Stomach muscles weaken in most women from lack of exercise, stretching during pregnancy, and normal aging changes in skin and elastic tissue. Shoulders become more rounded and slope more because of changing fat placement and a decrease in the muscle and skeletal mass; breasts sag from decreased skin tone and decreased glandular tissue. Successive pregnancies loosen joints, broaden hips, widen the rib cage, and thicken the waistline. Slowly we become softer and broader all over.

The ideal American female figure, however, seems to grow leaner each year. Popular magazines, TV shows, and the entire advertising industry trumpet the message that we can never be too thin and that we should never give up hope of being able to starve, stretch, or sweat ourselves into the perfect shape.

The image of supple slimness is hard to resist. If we let ourselves go, we suspect that we are engaging in an act of moral turpitude. We know that a sedentary lifestyle is unhealthful. A well-toned slender body is, indeed, attractive and youthful. Weight is aging. But for the woman over fifty, the question of fitness and shape is one of balance. What should we do? How do we know when we've overdone it? Can we still reshape our figure, or will our aging flesh and bones betray us?

YOUR BONES

Every body part or organ, however soft or hard, is composed of tissues or specialized cells. Bones and flesh both are composed of

29

thousands of cells that are constantly changing; some cells are living and multiplying, while some are dying and disappearing.

Bones form the skeleton, or frame, of the body, providing support and protection for all the organs (see figure 5). Bone is a hardened spongy structure, a mixture of living cells and deposited minerals, much like limestone from the earth.

Bone loses its very hard mineral accumulation as it ages. The inside of the bone gradually erodes, while the outside thickens. The result is a net loss of bone tissue. After menopause, women experience a dramatic loss of bone tissue because of the sudden waning of their estrogen, and their bones become more fragile. An eighty-year-old woman has one chance in five of suffering a hip fracture.

YOUR FLESH

Flesh is composed of three kinds of tissue: connective, muscle, and fat. Connective tissue comes in many forms. As tough, sinewy fibers (ligaments and tendons), it connects bones at joints, allowing the bones to support weight and move while resisting dislocation. As sheets of strong material, it covers muscles and large organs, giving them protection and form. As cartilage, or white rubbery material, it coats the joint ends of bone, providing a smooth, lubricated area (the synovial membrane) that permits the flexible motions of joints.

The connective and supportive tissues of the body lose some of their water and elasticity with age, becoming more dense. Skin loses its elasticity and begins to wrinkle and sag. Joints become stiffer because the tendons, ligaments, and denser fibers grow less flexible. The spine shortens as the discs between vertebrae lose water and shrink. The arterial walls lose some of their elasticity, and blood pressure increases.

Attached to the bony skeleton is the flexible, powerful muscle tissue (see figure 6). Each muscle is composed of many bundles of muscle fibers enclosed by a membranous sheath. The fibers and sheath terminate at each end in a glistening white, hard cord that attaches to bone, called a tendon.

Most of the muscles familiar to us relax and contract at our pleasure, under our voluntary control. These are the muscles with which we smile, frown, speak, eat, and move. Many muscles in our body are not under our voluntary control, however, but are influenced instead by the autonomic nervous system. These muscles maintain our life-sustaining processes, such as respiration, circulation, and digestion.

Muscle tissue diminishes by about 30 percent between the ages of thirty and eighty. Without an effort to stay fit, your muscles grow less powerful. It becomes harder to move, and even when you do, your range of muscle expansion and contraction grows smaller than it was.

Fat, or adipose, tissue, a collection of fat-storage cells with highly specialized chemical abilities, is the third component of human flesh. Eighty to 90 percent of your total body fat lies just under the skin and serves as a thermal blanket and as padding. Fat surrounds many abdominal organs; fat cells are also found in the liver and breasts. There are two types of fat tissue: brown and white. Brown adipose tissue regulates heat in the newborn and changes into white adipose tissue as the infant grows. White adipose tissue acts as the body's insulation and cushioning; in addition, it stores energy when you eat too much food and releases energy when you eat too little.

Women's fat cells are larger than men's, probably because of hormonal differences. At birth, about 15 percent of body weight is fat. That proportion stays about the same for men but in adult women grows to 22 percent to 30 percent of body weight.

The distribution of fat is determined in large measure by heredity. Women whose mothers, aunts, and grandmothers were buxom or callipygian are likely to be equally endowed.

Your body never loses the capacity to form fat tissue. The vast majority of women and men increase their fat tissue as they age. Not only do you never lose the fat cells you had in childhood, but your body adds new fat cells that remain on board for life every time you gain a significant amount of weight. Pound for pound, fat is bulkier than muscle. These facts mean that to lose some fat, you must exercise and diet intensely to decrease the size of the fat cells to below the normal size, since you cannot diminish their numbers. While heredity influences your amount of fat, your lifestyle can help you shrink or expand it.

MAKING FRIENDS WITH YOUR BODY

While we all have to deal with physical changes in our bodies, not all of us wage the battle of the bulge. Like Alice in Wonderland drinking the contents of the magic bottle, some of us feel that we're growing smaller and smaller or thinner and thinner. But one way or another, almost all of us have a long history of fighting our bodies. We were not brought up to "let it all hang out," and we often

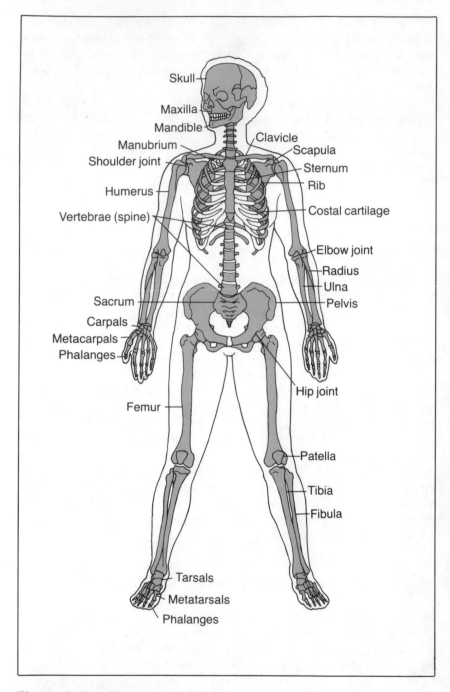

Figure 5. The Skeletal System

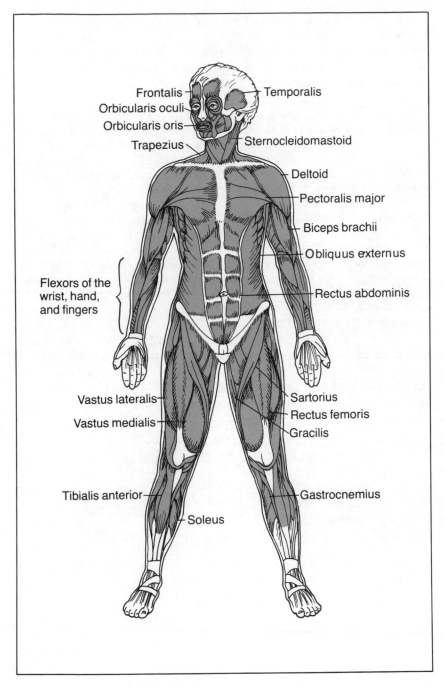

Figure 6. The Muscular System

regret our physical unease. As one robust seventy-five-year-old declared, "If I had a chance to come back to this earth, I wish I could come back without my corsets." People over fifty should finally learn to make friends with their bodies and be good to themselves at the same time.

Beatrice P., fifty-two, decided that she had let her weight creep up long enough and that it was time to take some off. She went to a local diet center, where the staff designed a weight-reduction and exercise plan for her. Beatrice had no trouble sticking to the required menus. And she loved working out on her stationary exercise bicycle because its attached reading stand allowed her to pedal her way through many a novel.

In no time, it seemed, she had lost fifteen pounds. The people at the diet clinic felt that she could do even better and pressured her to lose ten more pounds. Beatrice resisted. "I felt I looked fine, " she explained. The staff pressure continued at her maintenance weigh-ins. Finally, she became very annoyed. "I told them that I was fifty-two, not twenty-two, and that it was all right for me to weigh 140 pounds, that I was pleased even if I wasn't perfect. I couldn't believe that I had to fight to get out of there without an ideal figure."

It is often difficult to hear your own voice amidst the din of other people's opinions. It makes sense to watch your weight and be fit. Diet and exercise, even if begun in middle age, can cause musculoskeletal changes to be less than they would otherwise be. But, most of all, it is important to exercise your common sense.

EXERCISE AND FITNESS

> It is fascinating to know that one can grow healthier as one grows older. Not necessarily the reverse.
>
> —*Paul Dudley White, M.D.*

Your body was made for motion, yet most aspects of industrialized civilization spare you from moving. Cars take you around outdoors; elevators carry you upstairs; food processors prepare your meals; machines scrub and dry your clothes; grain refineries even take the effort out of chewing. The list of reasons you needn't use your muscles could go on and on. The work you have been saved gives you invaluable leisure; ironically, now you have to "work" to exercise enough for good health.

By giving attention to your body each day, you can feel

healthier and more limber as you age. Exercise not only oils your joints and tones your muscles, but it also increases your endurance, helps bowel elimination, improves circulation, raises your spirits, and relieves stress. Put more simply, it makes you feel better and more attractive.

Saundra M., sixty-three, had been in a slump since her divorce three years before. Not only had she left her job, but she had also managed to put on twenty-three pounds while sitting at home night after night, having no energy to make a change. One day she was put to shame at a family picnic, when her older sister by eight years outlasted her on a walk. She decided to become more fit.

Saundra started a diet, joined the YWCA exercise classes, and even began to exercise by herself at home in the morning. Even before she lost much weight, she had begun to discover her own inner strength. Her face radiated pride, and she found herself telling friends that she was interested in getting a job again.

Starting a Fitness Program

It is never too late to start exercising on a regular basis. The type and amount of safe exercise to begin with vary from woman to woman, depending on individual medical condition and overall fitness.

Before you start a new pattern of exercise, you owe your body a checkup. Some of your medical problems might need to be attended to or more closely monitored to allow you to participate at your best. You may need to know what activities can be built up to gradually and what types of exercises might be too stressful for your system.

Tell your doctor the kind of fitness program you are planning and how much or how little exercise you have had until now. Describe your various aches and pains, paying particular attention to any chest symptoms (such as pressure or shortness of breath) that you experience when you exert yourself (for example, climb stairs or carry bundles).

Your doctor will examine your blood pressure, heart, lungs, spine, muscles, and joints. If you have not had an electrocardiogram in several years, he or she should order one done. You may also get a blood test and a urine test.

After the examination, your doctor may advise further tests or some treatments before you embark on your exercise program; more likely, he or she will give you a clear go-ahead.

Ask your doctor whether there are certain exercises—such as isometric ones, that is, exercises that increase pressure on joints and tighten muscles—that you should avoid because of a heart condition. Are there certain movements that would aggravate your back problem or osteoarthritis of the knee? If you are a diabetic, exercise may reduce your need for insulin, and you must know how to monitor your insulin needs on a daily basis.

Find out the safe and healthful boundaries of your exercise program before you start.

Realistic Expectations

Clare F., fifty-one, looked in the mirror one day and felt absolutely disgusted. Bulging flab everywhere. None of her clothes fit properly. Next day, she came across a discount coupon for a local health spa and went out to sign up for a six-week membership.

The health spa's exercise program was vigorous, and she found herself huffing and puffing to keep up with the twenty-five-year-old teacher. Energized by her original disgust with her appearance, Clare tried to follow every exercise to the letter. One day, while arching her back in class, she heard a snap and found that she was unable to straighten up.

Her doctor diagnosed a lumbar strain with muscle spasm and, in addition, a low potassium level from the diuretic pills she was taking for hypertension. The low potassium had probably increased her tendency to have muscle spasms.

Clare spent ten days lying flat in bed, taking pain pills and potassium. When her back finally got better, she said to herself, "I'm definitely not going back to exercise. Look at what it did to me!"

Nothing will turn you off exercise as easily as something going wrong with your body at the beginning. If you crave instant results, you may sabotage yourself by attempting too much too soon. Crash exercise programs are even less successful over the long term than are crash diets, as well as being more dangerous. It is hard to will yourself to begin gently. It is hard to begin at all. You may be tempted to think up excuses instead: your arthritis, your bad veins, your high blood pressure, your heart condition. But if you talk yourself into believing that exercise will harm you, it behooves you to remind yourself that you will harm yourself more by *not* exercising, especially when you are over fifty.

Your Daily Routine

The easiest way to grow physically fit is to incorporate exercise into your daily routine.

- The simplest road to exercise is the one at your front door—begin walking instead of driving or riding every time you leave home.

There is no exercise safer, more wholesome, and less expensive than walking. Studies consistently show that walking improves your cardiovascular condition. Your steps should be brisk to build up your endurance as well as to limber and strengthen joints and muscles. Weight-bearing exercise like walking is the best way for you to keep your bones strong.

- Instead of taking elevators, try walking up one or two flights of stairs, stopping if you get out of breath. Walk downstairs too.
- When you do housework, give it a little bit extra. Sweep a bit more vigorously; bend over more to get into corners; put more elbow grease into your dusting and polishing.

Yoga

Yoga teaches you to move slowly and concentrate completely on the specific section of the body you are exercising. There is much value in this gradual approach. First, by moving slowly and without strain, you can feel the stretch and pull in muscles and ligaments and know when you have gone far enough.

Yoga's other virtue is that when you concentrate on the particular part of your body being exercised, you clear your mind of other thoughts. In addition to relaxing you and relieving stress, this new focus makes you feel much more in harmony with your body than before.

Most of us have heard the claim "It has to hurt to do you good." This is not true. Straining yourself beyond your limits will cause pain and injury that will retard your progress. Build your strength gradually. Help yourself enjoy your exercise rather than make it painful work.

Exercise Classes

There are plenty of exercise classes to join, whether on television or away from home. Follow the movements that you can at your own pace. Do not worry if you cannot keep up with a limber twenty-five-year-old teacher. Many exercise clubs offer exercise classes, aerobics, and Nautilus (see page 38). You can join a dance class—in ballroom dancing, swing, jazz, tap, modern dance, or ballet. Joining a class gives you that little extra motivation, since people expect you to show up and will note your absence.

Swimming

Although swimming is not a weight-bearing exercise like walking, it allows you to tone your muscles and increase endurance.

Practice stretching and balance exercises in the water before swimming laps. You will not hurt yourself in the water.

Aerobics

Aerobic exercise is any strenuous exercise that increases your pulse but does not get you badly out of breath—in physiological terms, does not incur oxygen deficit. Aerobics are a series of exercises devised to improve the condition of your heart, circulation, and respiration. During these exercises, your heartbeat will speed up, your breathing will grow short and rapid, and your circulation will improve. You will get hot and perspire; in the beginning, you may huff and puff and feel your heart racing in your chest. When you stop the exercises, all systems will return to normal; the more fit you are, the quicker your heart and lungs will return to their resting pace, and the lower your resting pulse will be.

Women with heart or respiratory conditions should not begin aerobic exercises before discussing the prospect with their doctors. Women with severe arthritis may not be able to do many of the exercises because of joint pains.

Nautilus

Nautilus is a body-building technique that exercises specific parts of your body on specific machines so as to build up strength. Exercise salons with Nautilus equipment have trained staffs, who will instruct you in the kinds and amounts of exercise you should do and will supervise your movements. Be sure not to overdo Nautilus exercises, since you can injure muscles and damage joints. If you have a heart condition, discuss the possible range of arm and shoulder exercises with your physician in case certain motions or weight loads are not advisable.

Treating Muscle Strains

If you are unaccustomed to exercising, you may feel stiff and sore after several days. Despite precautions you may have taken not to overdo your movements, you may have overstretched and mildly injured your muscles. When muscles are overworked, they outstrip their supply of blood and oxygen, and you experience mild inflammation, pain, and tightening.

The best way to treat these strains is rest. Stop any vigorous exercises of the injured area, but continue some very light and gentle movements. On days when your thighs are stiff and sore, you can sit on a chair and raise your foot off the floor until just the ball of the foot touches the floor and then let it down, alternating feet. If your shoulder is sore, do gentle rotary motions forward and back. If your neck is stiff, gently roll your head to one side and the next, if it is not too painful.

Gentle massaging of the stiff muscles will gradually loosen them up. The best time to do this is when you are soaking in a warm bath. The warmth relaxes your muscles and improves circulation; as a result, any inflammation will disappear faster. Usually all signs of stiffness and soreness disappear within a week, and you can resume a more vigorous exercise program, this time taking care to work your muscles a little more gradually. Remember, there is no rush.

General Tips for Better Exercising

If you make your exercise sessions as comfortable and pleasant as possible, you are more likely to continue with them. Consider these hints:

1. Wait about an hour and a half after a meal before starting to exercise.

2. Choose a time when you are not likely to be interrupted—early in the morning, during lunch break, or before bedtime.

3. Practice in a well-ventilated room, or out of doors if you prefer.

4. Wear comfortable clothes. Loose slacks or sweatpants allow easy movement.

5. Before beginning to exercise and at the end of your exercise session, take five slow, deep breaths with your eyes closed and your legs slightly apart. As you exhale, concentrate on relaxing all your muscles, starting with face, head, neck, and shoulders and progressing to arms, back, chest, abdomen, hips, thighs, legs, feet, and hands. As a warm-up exercise before you start your program, walk in place for three to five minutes, slowly swinging your arms, moving your shoulders, and swaying your head slightly.

6. Start slowly, gradually building up the time you spend and your speed.

7. Use music to accompany your exercise; it will improve your grace and make the time more pleasurable. Many people enjoy walking while wearing a radio or cassette player with earphones.

8. Be creative in your exercise program. You might invite friends to join you, start a walking group or club, or bicycle in the park.

BODY REJUVENATION PROCEDURES

You can work out in every health spa in the country, but you cannot exercise away an abdomen that has been slackened from repeated pregnancies nor raise flattened and heavy breasts nor jog away very heavy thighs. Probably you are willing to live with your figure problems. If you do not choose to, you might seek the help of a plastic surgeon.

Be prepared for a chorus of contrary opinions about your desired plans. People may only raise their eyebrows about face-lifts these days, but they still hoot and snort over the idea of a tummy tuck. Examining your motivations for undergoing plastic surgery may mean scrutinizing a messy can of worms. But that is no reason to recoil from the prospect. There are many compelling reasons you might want to change your body contours.

Any given procedure you may be considering means weighing pluses and minuses. The majority of women who undergo plastic surgery are happy with the results, and suffer no complications. They embrace their revised body with joy and often wonder why they did not have their surgery earlier.

Breast-Lift

Kate O., a fifty-five-year-old, had a charming, attractive face and a very youthful body—except for her breasts, which were very thin and flabby. Whether it was due to four pregnancies and nursing four babies or to the normal aging of tissue, Kate didn't know. Before middle age, she had always shrunk from the idea of cosmetic surgery, but now, after much thought and consultation with her husband and with doctors, she made up her mind to have plastic surgery on her breasts. The surgeon made her breasts firmer, fuller, and less saggy. "My body parts belong together again," she explained proudly to a friend. "I've traded in my hundred-year-old breasts for ones that fit my body."

The breast-lift procedure, called mastopexy, raises sagging breasts and relocates the nipples on the reshaped breasts. The volume of the breast tissue does not change with mastopexy, but the procedure lifts and tightens the breasts. Mastopexy may be done either under general anesthesia or under local anesthesia with sedation.

With the standard mastopexy, the patient will have a scar around the areola, or brown area around the nipple, a vertical scar below the areola, and a scar in the crease where the breast meets the chest wall. In most women, most of the scars are well camouflaged; all of them fade to a great extent in time.

Immediately following surgery, there is decreased sensation in the nipple. Eventually the sensation improves but may not completely return.

Mastopexy is not covered by health insurance.

Reduction Mammoplasty

Women made uncomfortable by extremely large breasts may have been yearning for the aid of a plastic surgeon since puberty and only acquire the courage to ask for it after menopause.

Sonia W., fifty-eight, was a slender woman with very large breasts. Although she looked well in clothes and was admired for her figure by both men and women, she hated the size of her breasts and felt as if she were carrying two laundry bags: "They were so pendulous and heavy that every summer at the beach I thought I would die." She finally considered the possibility of having a reduction mammoplasty.

Her friends and relatives thought she was absolutely crazy. "Such a drastic procedure!" exclaimed a cousin. "She's already got a terrific figure," commented a disapproving friend. In spite of many admonishments, and her own trepidation, Sonia went ahead and had her breasts made smaller. A year later, when asked if she regretted the operation, she replied, "I don't know why I waited so long!"

Women with large breasts may want reduction mammoplasty because of pain in the back, neck, and shoulders; rashes of the skin under the breasts; or simply to look and feel more attractive with and without clothes.

Reduction mammoplasty is usually performed under general anesthesia, and the patient is admitted to the hospital for twenty-four to seventy-two hours. The common method of reduction mammoplasty results in scars similar to those occurring after mastopexy. The difference is that in reduction mammoplasty breast tissue is removed, leaving the breasts smaller as well as firmer. Occasionally the breasts may not be entirely symmetrical in terms of size, shape, or nipple location. There may also be a loss of sensation in the areola.

Reduction mammoplasty may be covered by health insurance; check with your insurance company.

Breast Augmentation

Some women want to increase the size of their breasts. A plastic surgeon enlarges breasts by surgically placing a sac filled with silicone gel under either the breast tissue or the pectoralis muscle of the chest wall. Implants do not impede early and accurate detection of breast cancer, either by physical examination or by mammography, because the implants are *under* the breast tissue or muscle and never on top of breast tissue.

Augmentation mammoplasty may be performed as an outpatient procedure. It is not covered by health insurance.

Abdominal-Lift

Abdominoplasty, or the tummy tuck, removes excess skin and fat and tightens the abdominal wall. The surgeon makes an incision just above the pubic hair, pulls the abdominal skin tight, and removes loose skin. Some stretch marks can be removed in the process, but that is not the aim of the surgery.

Abdominoplasty is performed under either general or spinal anesthesia, and the patient is hospitalized for twenty-four to seventy-two hours following surgery. Abdominoplasty involves pain and discomfort, a relatively long recovery period, and the possibility of complications. There is a scar across the lower abdomen and occasional numbness or tingling sensations in parts of the abdomen.

This procedure is not covered by health insurance.

Buttock-Lift and Thigh-Lift

If the skin is lax, a conventional buttock-lift and/or thigh-lift (the surgical removal of fat and trimming of extra skin) may be the only way to achieve an improved contour.

Suction Lipectomy

The newest procedure in fat removal is a technique that suctions out the fat cells. The ideal candidates are women with firm skin who have saddlebags on the thighs, drooping buttocks, sausage-roll abdomens, or generous flanks. The procedure is done under general or spinal anesthesia, takes about two hours, and can be quite painful for a few days afterward. Full recovery can take a few months, but the results are dramatic. If a woman has solid, firm skin, she is likely to have a good result and only a minuscule scar.

Should a woman gain weight at some time in the future, the weight is gained in all areas of the body, not in just the former problem area. The new proportions achieved by the contour surgery will not be lost.

General Cautions

Any woman contemplating plastic surgery should explore carefully the reasons she wishes such surgery, the realistic expectations of the procedure, and whether there might be simpler, safer alternatives to try first. Any surgery entails the potential for complications from bleeding, infection, and anesthesia. Plastic surgery is not a trivial matter, so carefully weigh the risks and benefits before making any decisions, and do the following:

1. Seek a qualified plastic surgeon, preferably one with experience in cosmetic surgery, who is frank, compassionate, and accessible. Do not hesitate to check the surgeon's references or seek a second opinion.

2. Become familiar with the details of the procedure, the options available within a given category of plastic surgery, and the possible risks and benefits.

3. Find out what the surgery will cost and whether any of the cost is covered by your health insurance.

4. If you feel doubtful after your investigations, postpone the plastic surgery. It can always be done at a later date; it cannot be undone.

ACHES AND PAINS IN YOUR BONES, JOINTS, AND MUSCLES

Even if we have dedicated ourselves to staying fit as we age—to improving our cardiovascular systems, muscle tone, and flexibility—we still will have occasional aches and pains. They are a part of life—"the thousand natural shocks that flesh is heir to." While we often think of pain as evidence of failure and imperfection in our bodies, or as a sign of severe illness, we should, instead, regard pain as an important warning signal. It is a language used by skin, limbs, and organs to signal their need for protection or a period of rest to preserve life and prevent disability.

Most often, aches and pains are gone before we begin to worry about them. It is only when they persist for days or weeks that we begin to feel very vulnerable and fragile.

Charlotte M., an active sixty-two-year-old used to playing tennis and carrying heavy bundles, was startled by a sharp pain below her right shoulder and in the small of her back as she reached for a can in the supermarket.

She tried to think what she might have done during the day to bring on this pain. Moving the heavy potted plant from the bedroom to the hallway? Hitting the ball too hard in the morning's tennis game?

The next day, the pain was not only present but more intense. She took two aspirin and used an electric pad for about twenty minutes, gaining some relief. For two days, she continued her home remedy, but the pain stubbornly persisted.

The third day, a friend came over to chat, and Charlotte described her worries. She was concerned that she should see her doctor and get an X ray. Perhaps something had broken, or maybe that tight knot she felt in her back was an early sign of a terrible disease, even cancer. Her friend was very reassuring. She had had a similar pain that lasted nearly two weeks and then disappeared completely. Charlotte relaxed, continued with her aspirin, and took hot showers, and in less than a week, the pain was just a memory.

Cassandra T., a robust grandmother age fifty-seven, continued planting small tomato plants in the garden despite a vague ache in the lower part of her back. The next day, the pain rendered her almost helpless. She could not get out of a chair without a severe, stabbing pain in the lower back. In fact, looking in the mirror, she saw that she was not even able to straighten her spine completely and looked somewhat like the Leaning Tower of Pisa. She remembered that six years ago, after moving furniture, she had had a similar problem, which had lasted for weeks.

Her daughter, a nurse in the local hospital, told her that bed rest on a hard mattress, aspirin, and warm baths would help. For several days, Cassandra watched the house get messier and her baby tomato plants languish. She worried about chronic back pain, slipped discs, back braces, and back surgery. But after a week, the pain was completely gone. A few days later, her house was straightened and the garden flourishing again.

Yolanda G., seventy-one, was a thin, graceful lady who prided herself on her dancing legs. One morning she slipped on a throw rug and banged her shin on a wooden edge of the couch. She watched a swelling develop; but despite some pain, she had no difficulty bearing weight on the leg. She remembered that either an ice pack or a hot pack was supposed to reduce the swelling but could not decide which. She was also worried about a fracture, but the thought of an expensive taxi ride to the local hospital, a long wait in the emergency room, and her share of the bill made her conclude that a period of rest and cool compresses would be a better approach. Over the next few weeks, the swelling changed from purple to green to yellow, and the bruise finally disappeared.

Older women are frequently confronted with physical symptoms and problems for which they must suddenly plan some course of action. Some women respond with intuition and common sense guided by their past experience. In the examples above, the first woman, Charlotte, tried to recall what might have caused her pain. Cassandra, the second woman, remembered a similar painful episode six years before. All three women examined their problems: Charlotte tried to think what she did before the pain started; Cassandra looked at her spine in the mirror; Yolanda checked the swelling on her leg and made the leg bear weight. Two of the women even sought advice from friends or children, much as physicians consult other doctors.

Each woman feared that her problem might be more serious than it was. Cassandra worried about the possibility of chronic back pain or a slipped disc. Yolanda was concerned about a fracture and tried simple home remedies in addition to one of the most healing treatments—a tincture of time. In all instances, these women used medical diagnostic techniques with correct, thoughtful approaches and treatments.

While we cannot and should not be our own doctors, the stories of these three women point out that we alone are the best caretakers of our bodies, the best sensors of what is wrong, and the first to benefit from the resolution of our problems. Each day we are obliged to use our best judgment about caring for ourselves. A woman who takes the time to understand her problems and learn as much as possible about what ails her is more likely to succeed in the art of aging in the best of health.

Certain qualities of pains suggest that a professional examination is worthwhile. By far the majority of aches and pains are not really serious but, rather, part of the normal wear and tear on our bodies. A doctor, however, may be able to alleviate short-term or chronic suffering by suggesting a specific remedy or therapy. Even more important, a doctor may be able to discover an underlying condition that needs to be recognized and treated.

When to See a Doctor
Contact your doctor if you have any of the following pains.

1. Persistent pains that will not go away despite one or more weeks of home remedies. For example, the severe and disabling shoulder pain that will not permit you to brush your hair could be bursitis, which often will disapper almost miraculously after a cortisone injection in the painful shoulder.

2. Pains that cause significant disability. Pains that prevent walking or seriously interfere with your usual activities should be

reviewed by a doctor in the hope of preventing long-term disability and regaining as normal an existence as possible.

3. Pains associated with redness and swelling in joints. These pains may require an X ray, blood tests, or laboratory examination of aspirated joint fluid (that is, fluid that a physician has removed from a joint with a syringe) to discover whether the fluid contains evidence of an infection, contains crystals associated with gout or pseudogout, or is typical of rheumatoid arthritis. All these problems have specific remedies.

4. Pains accompanied by chills, sweats, or fever that are more than the typical beginning of a virus. These symptoms may suggest an underlying disease.

5. Pains accompanied by weakness of muscles or numbness in parts of limbs. These symptoms may indicate that there is pressure on nerves, as in disc disease. It is important to recognize and treat such problems early, since nerves that have been crushed usually do not regenerate, and permanent disability is a possible result.

6. Pains that are unusually severe.

Although you might have one or more of the six classes of pain, in most instances, your problem is likely to be just a particularly nasty ache or pain rather than a sign of disease. With proper medications, therapy, and time, it will usually disappear. Many women let their minds race to the worst possibilities—paralysis, cancer, and the like—despite the relative infrequence of those conditions. Sharing these fears with your doctor and with friends will help put the problem in proper perspective.

Remember, the body generally heals itself in time.

What Kind of Doctor to See

Women wonder whether a particular problem should be checked by a general practitioner, an internist, or a specialist. Many believe that if a generalist is good, a specialist is better. Most often, this assumption is not true.

In most instances, your family doctor or internist is an excellent person to go to first for help with aches and pains. Since most health problems are fairly common, your regular physician can help you. When your problem is particularly complex or rare, or if the diagnosis is uncertain, your doctor will refer you to a specialist—an orthopedist (bone doctor), a rheumatologist (arthritis doctor), or a neurologist (nerve doctor).

Rheumatisms and Other Diseases

Some of us are visited by recurring pains in older age that aren't triggered by injury. We know a storm is coming more surely than does the local television meteorologist because our "rheumatism" or "arthritis" has acted up.

There are over twenty distinct forms of rheumatism specifically defined in medical textbooks. They tend to fall into three major classes, depending on the source of the inflammation: (1) wear and tear disorders; (2) infections or mineral deposits in joints; and (3) disorders of unknown source and of the body defense, or immune, system.

By far, the most common joint pains belong to the first class of disorders, which include degenerative arthritis, bursitis, and vertebral disc disease. Less common joint diseases such as gout and pseudogout belong to the second class, in which uric acid or calcium crystal deposits in joints cause inflammation. The inflammatory problems of unknown cause, the most common of which is rheumatoid arthritis, belong to the third class.

One condition that seriously affects one out of every four older women (and is especially severe in women with ancestors from northern Europe, the British Isles, Japan, or China) is not classified as arthritis or rheumatism at all. This condition is a progressive thinning of bone called osteoporosis and is more serious in women than in men, since women accumulate less bone tissue than men in youth and lose it more quickly after menopause. Osteoporosis itself causes no discomfort. It is an important condition because it makes some older women very susceptible to bone fractures, even in the course of the simplest everyday activity.

OSTEOARTHRITIS

Osteoarthritis, or degenerative arthritis, is the gradual wearing down of joints that accompanies the aging process. Although its other common name, degenerative joint disease (DJD), suggests illness, it is, in most cases, simply a condition of increasing cartilage and bone destruction resulting from years of routine wear and tear on a joint. Unlike common aches and pains, which come and go, the signs and symptoms of osteoarthritis are chronic and always with you.

All the bruises your joints suffer over a lifetime gradually damage the cartilage in your joints. The damage finally manifests itself in older age as regular pain in a knee or hip.

The Normal Joint

Cartilage is a flexible, thin layer of rubbery, resilient tissue that covers joint surfaces and acts as a cushion between bones. It forms a large part of the structure of the nose and ears. It is the white cap you've seen covering the ends of a chicken's leg bones. Normally, cartilage is very smooth. When it is injured or degenerates, the surface becomes irregular and thinner, as small parts break off or are worn off, leaving bones to crunch painfully against each other with movement.

Synovial membrane lines the joints and secretes a small amount of lubricating fluid so that surfaces can move smoothly over each other.

The Degenerated Joint

A severely degenerated joint is distinguished by several features (see figure 7):

• increased synovial fluid in the joint that pours out in response to inflammation. This extra fluid results in swelling of joints and sometimes needs to be removed with a needle.

• eroded joint cartilage that initially is roughened, then pitted, and finally worn away, leaving hard bone to rub against bone. This erosion results in painful, creaky, crunchy joints that do not have a full range of mobility.

• deformity through destruction of cartilage, stress, and damage to ligaments.

• deformity through erratic new bone formation. Bones continually reshape themselves, depending on the stresses on the joints. In response to these stresses, the bone grows abnormally, creating spurs that can cause pain and markedly thickened bones.

Risk Factors for Osteoarthritis

The following are documented risk factors for osteoarthritis:

1. Female sex. Studies in England have shown that while 87 percent of women and 83 percent of men over the age of sixty-four have X-ray evidence of osteoarthritis, 22 percent of all women have dramatically more accelerated breakdown of cartilage, erratic bone growth, and disability from osteoarthritis than men.

2. Family background. One unusual form of osteoarthritis that attacks the joints at the ends of the fingers usually runs in families. This results in bumpy, thickened deformities, called Heberden's nodes, that at first are soft and painful but eventually

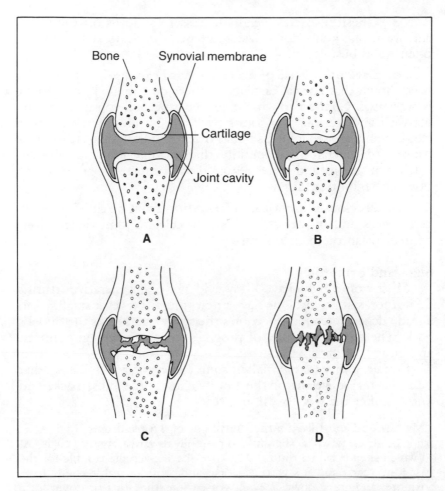

Figure 7. Joint Degeneration   Joint degeneration may eventually cause crippling. In a normal knee (**A**), bones slide easily in the joint cavity, which is lined with synovial membrane. Cartilage cushions the bone ends, and a strong membrane, the synovium, surrounds the entire joint. In degenerative joint disease, the cartilage roughens, and the joint cavity narrows (**B**). If the cartilage deteriorates further, spurs may develop at the margins of the joint (**C**). Finally, the cartilage may wear away entirely, leaving only bone against bone—and a crippling disability (**D**).

become painless. Women with large Heberden's nodes can no longer wear rings, and their hands appear misshapen. The cause of these nodes is unknown.

3. Obesity. Excess weight increases the loads on the joints and wears the joints down faster. Hence the heavy older woman often walks bowlegged.

4. Lack of exercise or excessive hard exercise. Experiments have shown that normal cartilage surfaces deteriorate if movement is prevented. Contrary to what might be expected, you are not sparing wear and tear on your joints by doing nothing. On the other hand, highly abused joints, such as those found in many athletes or dancers, degenerate more rapidly than normal joints. A normal balance of activity and rest is required to maintain the good condition of the joint cartilage.

5. Previous injury or malformation from birth. These circumstances add further stresses and accelerate joint destruction, particularly in the back and hips.

Signs and Symptoms

Most women who have X-ray evidence of degenerative arthritis do not feel symptoms. One day, a new injury, however small, to an already degenerated joint becomes the straw that breaks the camel's back. The tale is then one of progressive pain, swelling, stiffness, and limitation of activity.

Certain joints are especially prone to degeneration. Those that bear the major weight of the body—namely the hips, back, and knees—suffer the worst wear and tear.

"My husband and I live on the third floor of a triple-decker," said Gertrude F., seventy-two, as she shuffled painfully toward a large armchair, into which she sat with a thud. "My knees have given me trouble for the past four years, and it's getting worse and worse. I can't climb stairs anymore, and going down is even worse. Sometimes if I sit down for a good while, my knees are frozen when I stand up, and it takes me a few minutes to be able to bend them. You know, I haven't been out of the house in eight months, since my knee buckled under me when I was going downstairs. Thank God, my husband was right in front of me and broke my fall. I could have broken bones right and left. Well, now I take my trusty aspirin all day, I use my cane, and my Sam helps me with everything. He's a jewel. My doctor thinks I should have an artificial knee, but I'm scared. But how lovely it would be to see spring again."

Typically, women with hips affected by degenerative arthritis have difficulty getting in and out of the bathtub and in and out of low chairs or couches. They walk with a painful limp and have trouble climbing up and down stairs. The pain they feel can be referred pain—the knee hurts, but it is the hip joint that is losing cartilage.

Knee problems also cause painful, slow gait and difficulty with stairs. Because of the pain, people try to move less. The muscles weaken, producing a less stable joint, which is then more stressed and degenerates faster. This vicious cycle has to be stopped through treatment.

Knees, and even hips, can make creaky sounds on movement. The knees are often enlarged, hard, and knobby and sometimes swollen. The joints cause much discomfort, but they are rarely hot and tender. Osteoarthritis does not cause the fever and excessive fatigue characteristic of other rheumatologic disease, such as rheumatoid arthritis.

In rare cases, a woman can develop a painful bulge behind the knee, called a Baker's cyst, which may need to be drained or removed.

Treatment
Degenerative arthritis is an uncomfortable rusting of the skeletal machinery but need not be a serious crippling disease. Treatment includes the following:

Rest and Exercise
Frequent rest allows the healing process to occur. You can rest by simply lying on a couch in midmorning and midafternoon. Or you can rest a limb through the proper use of a cane, splint, or brace. If you are unable to get as much rest as you need because you are caring for others, try to get extra help at home (see chapter 17).

The way we "oil" our joints is through a regular balance of rest and exercise. Exercise strengthens muscles around a joint, making the joint more stable and improving the ability of the joint to move. Sometimes special corrective exercises are needed to undo bad patterns of movement that put undue stress on a certain joint. Usually a physical therapist prescribes these exercises and trains you to do them; the therapist may also train you to use special equipment that can alleviate symptoms and improve your joint function. You may have to go to the hospital physical therapy department or to a therapist's office; some therapists will see patients at home.

Ice and Heat
Ice and heat are useful old-fashioned remedies for inflamed joints. You should apply an ice pack to the affected area when your injury or swelling is new, or within the first twelve hours. The ice contracts your arteries, limits the blood flow to the injured area, and prevents further swelling.

Heat is useful for older, more chronic problems or for injuries after the first twelve hours, since heat draws blood into the area. The blood combats inflammation, limbers muscles, and promotes healing. Hot-water bottles, warm compresses, hydrocollators (cloth-covered pads for keeping moist heat next to the skin), warm showers and baths, and saunas and whirlpool baths are all good ways of applying heat. It is felt that moist heat penetrates tissues better than dry heat.

Drugs

The medical mainstay in the treatment of osteoarthritis is acetylsalicylic acid, or aspirin. This inexpensive and trustworthy medicine has been used in tablet form for nearly a hundred years, and as an extract of willow bark for hundreds of years before that. Used in low doses, aspirin acts as an analgesic, or painkiller. Aspirin also relieves inflammation, but, to do so, it must be taken regularly in higher doses, for example, two aspirin every four to six hours. A constant level of aspirin in the bloodstream counteracts inflammatory reactions.

Some people cannot take aspirin but may be able to tolerate buffered or enteric-coated aspirin. Taken regularly, the drug can irritate the stomach lining. For some women, small doses of aspirin (even if taken with food, such as a piece of bread or a glass of milk, which usually reduces its irritating effect) can produce heartburn. Women who have active ulcers or who have had bleeding ulcers in the past should not take aspirin. Women on blood thinners (Coumadin, or warfarin) must not take aspirin or other salicylates. Women who are allergic to aspirin must also avoid it.

When levels of aspirin are too high, people notice ringing in their ears, headaches, and dizziness. These are signals that the dose should be reduced.

Other drugs used for treatment include the following:

- *Nonsteroidal anti-inflammatory drugs.* Drugs such as ibuprofen (Motrin), naproxen (Naprosyn), indomethacin (Indocin), tolmetin sodium (Tolectin), piroxicam (Feldene), sulindac (Clinoril), fenoprofen calcium (Nalfon), and others have been marketed for pain relief and treatment of inflamed joints. They are usually much more expensive than aspirin (twenty dollars to forty dollars per 100 pills, compared with one dollar per 100 aspirin) yet do not appear to offer significant advantages other than a reduced dosage schedule. If salicylates do not work for you, however, try these medications. You may find relief with one pill and not with another. Like aspirin, these medications can cause irritation of the stomach and bleeding ulcers and should not be used if you are on blood thinners. Elderly women should use these nonsteroidal drugs cautiously, since they can impair kidney function and cause mental clouding. Your doctor should monitor your use of these drugs.

- *Nonacetylated salicylates.* Such salsalate drugs (Disalcid, Arthropan Liquid) are related to aspirin but do not cause stomach upset or bleeding problems. They are useful anti-inflammatory drugs for women who should not take aspirin and nonsteroidal drugs—that is, women who are taking blood thinners, women who have active ulcers, or women with a history of bleeding ulcers. These drugs are quite expensive.

- *Acetaminophen (Tylenol).* Acetaminophen is a drug that provides pain relief but has no ability to counteract inflammation.

Surgery

In a small percentage of osteoarthritis cases, the degeneration of hip, knee, or shoulder joints can be so severe that the patients feel

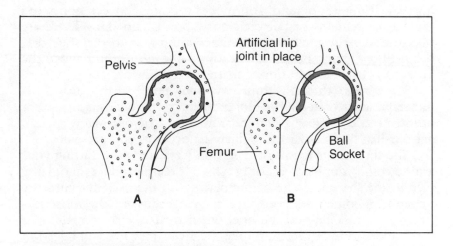

Figure 8. Artificial Hip   Repair of a hip joint badly damaged by arthritis (**A**) with an artificial hip (**B**) usually restores the ability to walk without pain. A new ball-and-socket joint is created by inserting a hip prosthesis in the joint cavity.

constant pain despite maximum treatment. These people often cannot move without pain in their joints, which severely curtails their activity. Recent technology has produced artificial joints, usually made of polyethylene or plastic (and metal), that can replace degenerated joints and thus allow freer movement and minimal or no pain (see figure 8).

The surgical procedure for replacing a hip joint or a knee joint is a major operation that is performed under general anesthesia. A woman considering a joint replacement must otherwise be in fairly good health (that is, have few cardiac and respiratory problems) to undergo a few hours of general anesthesia, about a week of bed rest, and one to three months of training in the use of the new joint.

This surgery has been successful in many women, most of whom are in their seventies or eighties by the time they require a new joint. It can offer freedom of movement and freedom from pain. As one seventy-eight-year-old said, "I've got a new lease on life. After years of being practically crippled, I am bouncing around on artificial knees."

BURSITIS

A bursa is a small sac or cushion lined with synovium and containing a small amount of fluid. It provides padding between bones and muscles or tendons or between bony points and skin. There are bursae under the muscle that connects the arm to the shoulder, behind the "funny bone" at the tip of the elbow, and above the kneecap. There are 140 bursae in the human body.

Sometimes, through injury or long-term wear, calcium, a mineral that circulates in the bloodstream, forms deposits around or near the sac, causing a painful inflammation. Anyone of any age can get bursitis, but it is far more likely to occur as you get older.

The shoulder is the most commonly affected area. Lifting your arm to comb your hair, eat, or brush your teeth produces agonizing pain in the shoulder. The pain radiates into the neck and into the upper arm, sometimes even into the fingertips. In the more fortunate, the disability can be brief when treated with rest, use of a sling, and aspirin or acetaminophen. Or you may need an injection of cortisone into the sac to lessen your pain dramatically.

Some people suffer a mild, long-lasting pain in the shoulder. A rare consequence of this chronic pain is muscle spasm, which produces a "frozen" shoulder. This condition means that the normal smooth arc you make when lifting your arm high above your side is severely restricted. A simple exercise that can help release the spasm is to stand at an arm's length from the wall and walk your fingertips up the wall.

An X ray of the bursitic shoulder often shows calcium deposits near the bone. If disability persists for months despite other treatments, this calcium must be removed surgically if you are to experience relief.

GOUT

A Frenchman once described the pains of rheumatism and gout as follows: "Place your joint in a vice; turn the screw until you can bear it no longer. That gives you an idea of rheumatism. Now, give the instrument one more turn, and you have gout." Since the time of Hippocrates, it has been known that gout is rare in women before menopause, though after the age of sixty, about one-third of those affected with gout are women.

Gout is a disease in which uric acid, which normally circulates in the bloodstream in small quantities, increases in quantity and deposits itself as crystals in joints. The crystals cause irritation in the joints, which produces intense pain, redness, and swelling. Gout usually affects the big toe (see figure 9) but may involve the ankle, hand, wrist, elbow, and knee joints.

Laura W., sixty-nine, an obese woman, awoke during the night with excruciating pain in her right big toe. The toe was swollen and red and felt warm to the touch. She could not remember banging it or injuring it in any way. Being a stoic, she took two aspirin and returned to bed. For nearly a week, Laura suffered with the pain in her big toe. The pain and redness lessened, and she was reluctant to bother her doctor. Finally, ten days later, she made an appointment because her toe was still swollen. The doctor was not able to make a definite diagnosis. He told her that she should have come in right away, when the problem had just started, since he would then have been able to diagnose the condition accurately. He presumed that she had gout and put her on medication. Fortunately for Laura, the toe improved, and four years later she had not had another attack.

A very hot, red, painful joint is potentially serious and should be checked by a physician immediately, since an infection or an inflammation can damage joints. In any case, an early examination can allow more accurate diagnosis. If there is fluid in the joint, the physician will remove some with a needle and examine it under a microscope. The definitive diagnosis of gout is made by finding uric acid crystals in the fluid.

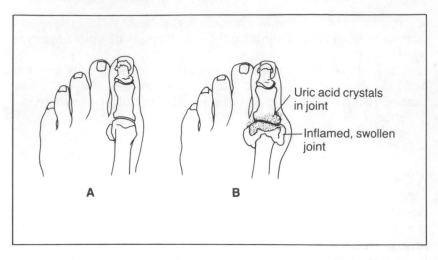

Figure 9. Gout   Gouty arthritis results when a normal big toe (**A**) is irritated by uric acid crystals, which cause soreness and swelling (**B**).

There are two phases of treatment. The first calms the inflammation with the use of drugs, such as colchicine, phenylbutazone (Butazolidin), or indomethacin (Indocin). The second lowers uric acid levels in the blood to prevent the deposit of crystals in joints. Drugs are often used to accomplish this as well. Allopurinol (Zyloprim) or probenecid (Benemid) are usually well tolerated in the older woman, though allopurinol can, in rare cases, produce serious rashes. This drug is also quite expensive.

Diet can help prevent attacks of gout. Women with gout should avoid alcohol, fasting, and diets that are high in protein and fat.

Women taking diuretics may have increased levels of uric acid in the blood. If necessary, the dosage may have to be decreased.

PSEUDOGOUT

Like gout, pseudogout is caused by crystal deposits in joints. In pseudogout, however, the crystals are a compound of calcium, not uric acid, and the joints involved tend to be larger joints, such as knees and hips, rather than smaller joints.

The disease is treated with colchicine, phenylbutazone, salicylates, and nonsteroidal anti-inflammatory drugs and by removing fluid from the affected joint. Pseudogout often runs in families and is more common in persons with diabetes, osteoarthritis, or sudden critical illness. The disease afflicts about 7 percent of men and women over sixty.

RHEUMATOID ARTHRITIS

Rheumatoid arthritis, unlike osteoarthritis, is a systemic, or total, body disease causing fatigue and fever as well as inflammation in many joints and fibrous tissues. The disease seems to reflect a disturbance of the immune system.

About 3 percent of the United States population is affected at one time or another with rheumatoid arthritis. In adults, the disease most commonly starts in middle age and affects three times as many women as men. Rheumatoid arthritis that starts after age sixty tends to be less severe than in younger people and may fade away within ten to twenty years.

An unfortunate 10 percent to 15 percent of people affected with rheumatoid arthritis have such severe joint inflammation that crippling deformity results. In desperation, such patients will sometimes seek miracle cures from all kinds of unusual treatments, such as undergoing bee stings or taking snake venom.

Cause

The cause of rheumatoid arthritis is unknown. Researchers have tried to identify viruses as the culprit but have not yet found a clear viral origin. The disease is thought to be, in part, a derangement of the body's defense system. The theory suggests that circulating defense bodies, or antibodies, combine with a virus or other particle and deposit on, or attack, our own body parts as though these parts were foreign elements, causing the pain and inflammation that are characteristic of rheumatoid arthritis.

Signs and Symptoms

Early symptoms of rheumatoid arthritis are fatigue, loss of appetite, and occasional fevers. Later, joint and muscle aches begin, and joints are very stiff in the morning. Some joints become red, hot, and inflamed for weeks. Inflammation tends to affect multiple joints and gradually migrates over weeks from one place to another. Commonly, symmetrical joints are affected, such as both hips, both knees, or the fingers on both hands, and permanent deformity of joints can result.

Sheila B., sixty-four, ordinarily athletic, and vigorous, realized that she had been tired for weeks and was slowly losing weight. Because she had occasional fevers, she thought she had a flu. Her hands were stiff and achy in the morning, and one day she noticed that both knees were warm to the touch, red, and swollen.

Her doctor took several blood tests and an X ray of her hands. The results showed a mild anemia and a positive test for rheumatoid factor, which suggested rheumatoid arthritis. Over the following years, several joints in her hands became deformed despite high daily doses of aspirin for pain relief. She functioned well in her routine activities, though it took her almost an hour to get rid of her stiffness in the morning.

The following ten years were difficult for Sheila. She had frequent painful swellings in multiple joints, muscle aches, and weakness. She developed little painful lumps called rheumatoid nodules under her skin. Over the years, she tried different therapies, such as cortisone, gold shots, and antimalarial drugs, each of which worked for some time. As a last resort, she had even taken a trip to Florida to try snake venom, but that treatment had not helped. An occupational therapist gave her forks, spoons, and knives that were specially adapted to her deformed hands so she could eat normally.

Finally, at the end of fifteen years, the inflammation left her joints, and no new nodules developed. The doctor told her that the disease had "burned itself out." She died nine years later at eighty-eight, having been able to care for herself until the end of her life.

Diagnosis of Rheumatoid Arthritis

Women who feel pains in their joints and experience ten minutes or more of joint stiffness in the morning, fatigue, and loss of weight should have a medical examination to look for rheumatoid arthritis.

Several laboratory tests help diagnose the condition. Rheumatoid factor—a combination of gamma globulins, part of the body defense system, and other uncertain compounds—is found through a test in the blood of 75 percent of people with rheumatoid arthritis. Women with high quantities of rheumatoid factor tend to have worse symptoms of the disease than those with low amounts. Anemia, measured by a blood test, is also common in patients with rheumatoid arthritis. The sedimentation rate (a measure of the rate of settling of red blood cells, which can increase in certain disease states) is also quite high.

X rays of rheumatoid joints often show typical features of the disease that help with the diagnosis.

Treatment

Rheumatoid arthritis is a disease that is nonfatal but cannot be cured at this time. Doctors can greatly help patients suffering from the disease by reducing their pain and disability and fostering their optimism. Treatment generally centers on rest and exercise, application of heat, medications, and surgery.

Rest and Exercise

During times of fatigue, fever, and active joint inflammation, rest is the appropriate therapy. Brief periods of bed rest during the day, a good night's sleep, and help with household chores will allow you time to heal the inflammation—and help you stay cheerful. Joints should be rested in positions that limit muscle stress on them. For example, a firm mattress or a bed board will support rather than strain your back. A straight-backed chair can rest your back and knees. Sleeping with small pillows under your head at night reduces the amount of bending of the neck. Occasionally, a particular joint can best be rested through use of a splint, sling, or cane. Your doctor will advise you in these matters.

Exercises done after the active inflammation subsides restore the full, normal range of movement and gradually build muscle power around a joint. Exercises reduce deformity and help maintain maximum function. For example, you can preserve and strengthen your hand function by holding and squeezing a soft ball.

Heat

Hot baths, heat lamps, and paraffin baths for hands and wrists can relax muscles and increase circulation to inflamed joints. These remedies can be utilized at home or in a physical therapy department of a hospital or clinic. Therapists will teach you exercises that help maintain normal range of motion for joints. They will also provide household devices that help you remain self-reliant.

Medications

Medications for rheumatoid arthritis serve two purposes: relieving pain and reducing inflammation.

As with osteoarthritis, acetylsalicylic acid (aspirin) helps the most. Large doses, such as eight to twelve aspirin per day (and sometimes as many as twenty), are usually needed to maintain enough aspirin in the blood to work effectively. If you develop a ringing in the ears, report this symptom to your physician. It can mean that the dose of aspirin is too high. When an adequate trial of aspirin has failed, one of the nonsteroidal anti-inflammatory drugs might be successful. In a small number of people, side effects include heartburn, ulcers, and bleeding from the stomach and intestine; kidney damage may occur.

Antimalarial drugs such as chloroquine and hydroxychloroquine sulfate can sometimes lessen the effects of rheumatoid arthritis. These drugs are given over a number of months—as the disease, one hopes, becomes less active.

Gold injections, given weekly over a few months, have helped about 40 percent to 60 percent of patients treated, for a period of time. Sometimes the injections cause skin rashes or blood problems, which may require discontinuing the drug.

Penicillamine (Cuprimine), taken by mouth, is another drug that can delay the progression of the arthritis. It can also suppress formation of blood cells, however, so women taking this drug need weekly blood counts.

Low doses of cortisone pills (prednisone) often help give pep and a sense of well-being as well as improve appetite and reduce fever and joint pains. Unfortunately, cortisone also causes side effects. In women, cortisone accelerates the thinning of bones that occurs with age, which can lead to fractures. Stomach ulcers and intestinal ulcers can develop with cortisone, as well as elevated blood sugar and high blood pressure. Rarely, the blood supply to the end of a long bone of an arm or leg can be cut off suddenly, leading to joint degeneration. For these reasons, cortisone is started as a last resort or, in small doses, as an adjunct to other treatment. Long-term cortisone therapy must be tapered off slowly over a period of months. Sometimes, your doctor may inject cortisone directly into a particularly nagging knee or shoulder.

Some rheumatoid arthritis patients have been treated successfully with drugs that inhibit the body's defense system. These drugs must be closely monitored, since they also suppress the formation of blood cells and expose the patient to a greater risk of infection.

Surgery

Surgery can transform deformed rheumatoid hands into more normal-looking, functional hands. Often tight tendons are loosened or transferred from one part of the hand to another. Preventive hand surgery often can ward off the worst effects of rheumatoid arthritis, as when the swelling of the synovium ruptures tendons of the hand. A surgeon can prevent such extensive damage and crippling by removing the synovium and replacing some of the joints in the hand. Or the surgeon can fuse the finger joints in a position of function so that one can still pick up objects. Wrist surgery can relieve pressure on nerves that has led to numbness and weakness of the fingers.

Knee, hip, and shoulder joints often are replaced with artificial joints, producing dramatic pain relief and improved function. As one sixty-eight-year-old said, several months after both her knees were replaced, "I did the fox-trot for the first time in ten years!"

Emotional Support

A sympathetic, accessible physician is vital to provide the maximum relief possible and to help the patient deal with this chronic, painful disease. Counseling is often helpful in the early phases of the illness, as the woman mourns the loss of her healthy body and tries to accept deformity, inability to do many familiar tasks, and the exchange of the role of nurturer for the role of dependent. A counselor also can help family members understand the patient's needs.

Women with rheumatoid arthritis can adapt to their illness and maintain an active and positive attitude toward life. It does take gumption, an ability to adapt to change, and patience and understanding on the part of those around you.

Judy L., fifty-eight, had always been the one to hold the family together. She organized and cooked for all the birthdays and holidays; she helped her husband, children, and grandchildren with their clothes shopping; she drove her family to their various appointments and activities. Now, suddenly a victim of severe rheumatoid arthritis, Judy could not even drive a car or stir her coffee in the morning. She felt useless and a burden and became so depressed that she did not want to get out of bed in the morning.

The social worker in the hospital rheumatology clinic began to see Judy once a week for counseling and organized a few family conferences. She also invited Judy to join several people with rheumatoid arthritis—all of whom were coping with their changed roles, images, and medical problems—for group therapy. Gradually Judy started feeling better. She learned that she could both accept help and retain her family's respect. She admired the courage of the other men and women in her rheumatoid group; their example gave her courage to deal with her own trials.

POLYMYALGIA RHEUMATICA

A rare disorder of the body's defense system, polymyalgia rheumatica is found mostly in people over sixty and most commonly in women. Pain, stiffness, and weakness of muscles of the shoulders, upper arms, hips, and legs are common. There is often headache in the temple area, on one or both sides.

The disease must be recognized and treated promptly. When it affects the blood vessels of the eye, sudden blindness can result.

This eye involvement can be identified early by blood tests and a biopsy of the temporal artery. Some women have telltale headaches in the temple area, but others who are affected have no head or eye symptoms. About 2.5 percent have clinical eye involvement; about 20 percent may have artery changes.

POLYMYOSITIS AND DERMATOMYOSITIS

Both polymyositis and dermatomyositis are diseases of older people that cause weakness and, sometimes, pain and tenderness of the muscles of the arms, shoulders, hips, and legs. The skin may be swollen and somewhat red; many women have joint pains, swelling, and fluid in joints as well. The diagnosis is made from visual observation, blood tests, and muscle biopsy.

Sometimes cancer of the breast, ovary, uterus, lung, or small bowel can be associated with polymyositis or dermatomyositis; hence anyone with either disease should be checked for cancer. These diseases often abate with removal of the cancerous tumor. Cortisone or immunosuppressive drugs may help the symptoms.

OSTEOPOROSIS

Bone is living tissue. Like other tissue in the body, it constantly replaces itself. Small cells in the bone break down old bone, while other cells form new bone from protein, vitamins, and calcium. During the course of a year, between 10 percent and 30 percent of your skeleton is replaced. As you advance beyond thirty-five years of age, the balance between destruction and formation of bone is upset. New tissue is not formed as quickly as old tissue is lost, and the total bone mass of your skeleton decreases.

When bone loss occurs at a slow, normal rate, we recognize its signs as normal aging—the gradual loss of the height of the spine, the mild hunch of the upper back. Sometimes, however, the bone loss is so severe that the bones become porous, and the skeleton becomes an unstable structure. Both falls and fractures of the spine and long bones become common, and X rays of the skeleton show thin bones. This severe bone loss is called osteoporosis (see figure 10).

Risk Factors

Several factors contribute to the development of osteoporosis.

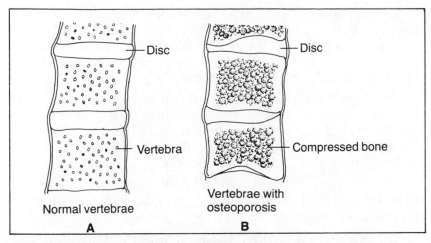

Figure 10. Osteoporosis   Osteoporosis can cripple the spine. Normal vertebrae and discs firmly support the body's weight (**A**). Vertebrae weakened by osteoporosis may break down (**B**), causing pain and deformity.

1. Amount of bone in early adult life. Not everyone has the same amount of bone tissue at maturity. Girls have 20 percent less bone mass per pound of body weight than boys; well-nourished, physically active children develop more bone mass than malnourished, diseased, or less active children. Black people have more bone mass than white or Oriental people. The less bone mass to start with, the greater will be the effects of thinning bones. Women, particularly Caucasian and Oriental women, and malnourished, inactive female children are, therefore, at greatest risk of osteoporosis.

2. Family background. Osteoporosis tends to run in families. If your grandmother or mother was stooped and broke her hip or wrist, you are likely to have osteoporosis in your background.

3. Postmenopausal bone loss. The hormone estrogen slows down the action of the cells that destroy bone. After menopause, the ovaries produce virtually no estrogen, and although the adrenal glands do make some, it is not enough to stop the destructive work of the cells. In the first ten years after menopause, women lose bone mass six times more rapidly than men of the same age, and more slowly after that.

Younger women who have had hysterectomies that include removal of both ovaries experience the same bone loss as postmenopausal women. If you are having a premenopausal hysterectomy, ask your surgeon if one or both ovaries can be kept. If not, ask why not, and get a second opinion.

4. Immobilization. When you move very little, your skeleton loses bone tissue more rapidly than usual. Women who become very sedentary in older years (from bed rest; confinement to wheelchairs, casts, or splints; or paralysis from nerve damage or stroke) increase their chances of bone loss.

5. Diseases. Diabetes, rheumatoid arthritis, alcoholism, thyroid disease, and Cushing's disease are all associated with more rapid bone loss than normal.

6. Nutritional factors. Calcium, which is needed in bone formation, is often poorly absorbed in older people or in those with lactose intolerance (see chapter 11). Excess protein or fat in the diet has been shown to cause calcium loss, as have both diet and regular soft drinks, coffee, alcohol, and nicotine.

Signs and Symptoms

The most common sign of osteoporosis is loss of height through compression fractures of some of the vertebrae; a vertebra whose bone has become thin can suddenly collapse as a woman reaches for a jar on a shelf or lifts a moderately heavy object. A severe pain erupts in the back and is intensified by any movement of the spine. The pain can last for weeks before it disappears completely. Some women are forced to take to bed, which weakens their bones even more. As more vertebrae collapse, the spine folds over, like a wilted flower stalk. The result is disfigurement (dowager's hump), pain, and some debility. In severe cases, more than six inches in height can be lost from vertebral fractures.

Older women with osteoporosis are much more vulnerable than men to fractures: vertebral fractures occur eight times more in women than in men; wrist fractures, two times more; and hip fractures, over three times more. As hip bones thin out, a fracture can result from a mere twisting motion. The resulting fall is blamed as the cause of the fracture, when in reality the fracture preceded the fall.

Diagnosis

On X rays, the bones of a woman with osteoporosis appear less dense than normal and sometimes even appear hollow. But by the time X rays can detect this decrease in bone density, more than 35 percent of the mineral content of the bone has been lost.

Therefore, it is very difficult to diagnose osteoporosis at an early stage. Sophisticated tests, while not totally accurate, do provide good estimates of bone density. These are usually done two or three years apart to check on the rate of bone thinning. Bone biopsy is accurate but quite painful, and may have complications.

Treatment of Fractures from Osteoporosis

Vertebral fractures are treated with pain relievers (codeine, aspirin, and others) for a period of weeks. During this time, it is important to do gentle exercises, even if they are slightly painful, since lying still leads to further bone loss.

Wrist fractures usually do not require surgery; hip fractures almost always require surgery. Sometimes traction is applied over a period of weeks if a woman is unable to undergo hip surgery because of a severe heart condition or other debilitating disease.

Prevention of Osteoporosis

Many clinical studies have shown that osteoporosis is a preventable disease if preventive measures are taken as early in adulthood (ideally before the age of thirty-five) as possible. Women over fifty should consider themselves at risk and should take preventive measures immediately. Women who already have signs of osteoporosis can significantly slow the progress of the disease by taking the same measures, suggested below. Unfortunately, you cannot replace bone tissue that has been lost.

1. **Diet.** You must have a calcium-rich diet, of 1,200 to 1,500 milligrams of calcium daily. This amount is equivalent to four to five cups of skim milk or four to five cups of yogurt per day. Oysters, sardines, canned salmon, collards, turnip greens, rhubarb, tofu, brown sugar, and molasses are all high in calcium. (See chapter 11 for a listing of the calcium content of various foods, and plan your daily menus accordingly.) Women who have had kidney stones are often placed on a low-calcium diet; they should ask their doctors how much calcium to ingest per day.

Avoid diets too rich in protein and fat. Twelve percent of your daily diet should be protein and 30 percent to 35 percent fat. Avoid coffee, alcohol, soft drinks, and cigarettes. Be sure that you have citrus fruit or other sources of vitamin C each day.

2. **Calcium supplements.** Many different types of calcium powders and tablets are available in drugstores and health food

stores. (Calcium lactate should not be used by women who have lactose intolerance.) You need to be aware of the amount of calcium each contains. Most tablets contain about 13 percent calcium. Calcium gluconate contains about 9 percent calcium. Calcium carbonate has the highest amount of calcium available in tablet form, about 40 percent. If you take this form of calcium, you won't need as many tablets as you would otherwise. Examples are Os-Cal, Calcet, Caltrate, and Tums. (About five Tums a day will supply your total calcium needs.)

3. Fluoride tablets. Fluoride—used in combination with calcium, vitamin D, and estrogen—can retard osteoporosis by replacing calcium in bone. Sodium fluoride stimulates bone formation and forms a tighter structure than calcium-based bone. However, fluoride treatments are still experimental, since fluoride is toxic in high doses, and its value in lowering fracture rates is still questionable. Consequently, it is reserved for women with severe osteoporosis who fail to improve on calcium, vitamin D, and estrogen.

4. Exercise. You must exercise every day to preserve bone mass. The best exercises are walking, gentle jogging, or dancing—upright, antigravity exercises that involve weight-bearing movement and muscles pulling on bone. Swimming, while promoting general fitness, does not retard osteoporosis, since your bones bear less weight in water than out of it. Exercise also helps you strengthen the muscles surrounding your spine and stomach—which helps you stand tall, relieves strain on your spine, and even adds inches to your height.

5. Estrogen replacement therapy. The decision to take estrogen by pill must be weighed carefully by you and your doctor. Estrogen can help you absorb calcium more efficiently and inhibit bone destruction; however, prolonged use increases the risk of uterine cancer. This risk can be diminished if you take an estrogen/progesterone combination instead. If you have severe osteoporosis that does not improve with calcium supplements, you may be a candidate for long-term (ten- to twenty-year) estrogen treatment, which can be safe under proper medical supervision (see chapter 9).

6. Sunshine. Sunshine helps your skin manufacture a potent form of vitamin D, which is important in helping your body absorb and use calcium. Spend time out of doors, walking or even sitting. If you cannot get out of the house, sit in front of an open window.

If you are even more restricted and cannot get sunlight, eat vitamin D–rich foods such as vitamin-enriched milk, take fish oils, or take vitamin D$_2$ in doses of 400 international units.

Whether you are fifty, seventy, or ninety, straight-backed or somewhat bent, it is never too late to support your bones' ability to support you.

LOW BACK PROBLEMS

The body is an awesome example of architecture. It is like a movable skyscraper whose supporting steel, the spine, must withstand vast, uneven stresses and motions without falling. Two parts of the spine that have the greatest freedom of movement, the neck and lower back, are also the most vulnerable to problems. Backache has afflicted people ever since early humans stood up on two feet to walk.

The spine is made up of thirty-three bones, the vertebrae, that are linked together and supported on the sides by strong fibers called ligaments. The vertebrae are separated and cushioned by sacs called discs. The spine's stability depends on the strength and integrity of the ligaments, as well as on the support of the back muscles, stomach muscles, and buttock muscles. The spine must be well protected by ligaments and discs not only to maintain the body's posture but also to protect the thick bundle of nerves, the spinal cord, that passes up and down through a canal in the spinal column and along which travel the electrical signals that command movement and feeling.

Symptoms of a Low Back Problem

Four major symptoms signify a back problem: pain, stiffness, restriction of movement, and deformity. An individual can have any or all of them. Each of the symptoms must be analyzed to identify clues that lead to the diagnosis.

Pain can be of several types. Local pain, which occurs right in the area of injury or inflammation, produces steady or intermittent aching. To protect the injury, muscles in the immediate area go into spasm and thus limit further movement. This type of pain usually occurs with sprains, fractures, or other trauma.

Pain from nerve roots can result from the irritation of nerves where they emerge from the spinal cord. This pain is often sharp and severe; its intensity can be increased by a sudden movement, such as a cough or sneeze. The pain generally shoots like an electric shock from a spot in the back to a buttock or down a leg, depending on the nerve involved. Numbness, tingling, and weakness are also common. Sciatica is irritation of the roots of nerves to the leg and foot. Disc problems, osteoarthritis, and skeletal defects are the more common sources of nerve root pain. It is always advisable to have a thorough medical examination and appropriate treatment as soon as possible after the flare-up of such pain, since chronic pressure on nerves can lead to permanent disability such as weakness, numbness, or, in extreme cases, the loss of use of a limb.

Pains from muscle spasms are felt as dull pain along the spine. A spasm produces stiffness in the back and limits easy movement; it sometimes can be seen as a tight bulge along one side of the affected spine. Sometimes spasms are the source of the back problem, occurring as a result of depression or anxiety. Spasms may also be a protective reaction to injury.

Pain felt in the back can, in fact, be referred pain—pain originating in abdominal or pelvic organs. It can be a deep aching, and its location is hard to pinpoint. Deformity of the spine, spasms, or limitation of movement almost never result from this type of pain.

Causes of Low Back Pain

Low back pain can result from a variety of causes.

1. Strains and sprains are the most common sources of backache. These bruises and tears of back muscles and ligaments are caused by lifting heavy objects or by sudden, unexpected motions. Strains and sprains will usually go away completely after two to four weeks of rest and care.

2. Collapse or compression fractures of one or more vertebrae, due to thinning of the vertebral bones from osteoporosis, cause severe back pain. The pain goes away when a solid scar of bone tissue finally forms, usually within weeks.

3. Obesity, especially when it involves a very heavy abdomen, puts undue stress on the spine, pulling it forward and weakening its ligaments. The muscles around the spine must then work very hard to maintain erect posture and often become fatigued and stressed. Women who have had many near- or full-term pregnancies often lose the muscle tone of the abdominal wall, which bulges forward and stresses the back.

4. Degenerated vertebrae, the result of osteoarthritis, often develop sharp bone spurs that cause pain in the back and pressure on nerve roots.

5. Depression and anxiety may be associated with increased tension and painful spasm of back muscles. In some cases, back pain originates solely from psychological stress.

6. Trauma to the spine from falls can result in fractures, muscle injury, or ligament tears that cause inflammation and pain.

7. Minor birth defects in the spine such as spondylosis, scoliosis, and spondylolisthesis may result in abnormal posture and lower back pain. Excessive curvature of the low back (lordosis) also can lead to backache in later life.

8. Aging or injured ligaments surrounding a disc may weaken to the point that a sudden cough or movement pushes part of the disc through the weak ligament. This puncture causes severe pain, a crooked posture, and difficulty in moving. Sometimes the disc presses on nerve roots.

9. Diseases of the pancreas, gallbladder, kidneys, lower intestine, uterus, or ovaries can lead to pain in the back, though the back is not at all involved.

10. Diseases that destroy parts of the spine are very rare causes of back pain. These diseases include infections (such as tuberculosis or staphylococcus) and tumors (either benign or cancerous) that have arisen in bone or have spread from other organs, such as the breast or lung.

Diagnosis of a Back Problem

To diagnose the cause of low back pain, your physician first will observe your posture as you sit, stand, and walk. Then he or she will have you perform a series of exercises to test the flexibility of your spine and to see which movements produce pain. You may be asked to bend forward, and backward, twist to the right and left, and lift each leg with the knee bent and then extended. The doctor may tap each bony prominence of the spine, from the neck to the tailbone, to see if any are out of line or tender. Finally, the doctor will check your muscles for spasms and examine your abdomen, pelvis, and rectum for evidence of internal problems.

X rays of the back will be taken in various positions to identify structural problems that may be the primary cause of the pain. Your physician may order a CAT scan. In rare cases, when protruded discs are suspected, you may need a myelogram. In a myelogram, dye is put into the spinal column by a neurologist, who watches its movement through the spine on X rays. A ruptured disc that encroaches on the nerve root is visible in the myelogram.

Finally, certain blood tests may reveal signs of infection or rheumatologic disease.

Treatment

Treatment of low back problems requires care, cure, and prevention of recurrence—in that order.

Muscle strains are the most common source of backache and usually go away within two to four weeks. The first day, put an ice bag on the painful area to limit swelling. Over the next few days, use hot packs to soften the spasmed muscles and bring blood to the injured area. Rest in bed while lying on one side, flexing hips and knees, and giving the spine the least amount of stress to allow healing. A bed board placed between the spring and the mattress will give the back extra support.

Acetylsalicylic acid (aspirin) offers relief from both pain and inflammation. Take it if you can tolerate it. Other painkillers, such as codeine, and muscle relaxants, such as diazepam (Valium), can help and may be prescribed by your doctor.

Gentle exercises can be started early. If your back pain is severe, you can support the back with a wide belt or brace bought at a surgical supply store on recommendation from your doctor.

Ligament tears are treated in much the same way but may require six to twelve weeks of treatment.

Ruptured discs demand strict bed rest and painkillers, often for a few weeks. Then you can resume activity bit by bit, taking frequent rest during the day. In the rare event that the pain does not subside, you may have to have the disc removed by surgery or have chymopapain injected into your spine to dissolve the troubling disc.

Chiropractic

The discipline of chiropractic holds that illness results from a misalignment of the spine. Postural defects put undue strain on the spine and lead to disability. The chiropractor will take X rays of your spine to make a diagnosis and then treat you in two phases. The first phase of therapy uses manipulations and exercises that reduce muscle spasm and produce better alignment of the spine. The second phase involves the regular practice of special exercises to improve posture and tone muscles, which increases the stability of the spine.

For many back problems, chiropractic, in the right hands, offers a rational approach. Check with your doctor to be certain that manipulation of your back will not be harmful. Ask your doctor for the names of some reputable chiropractors; be sure to let your chiropractor know that he or she is working as a member of a team with you and your doctor. Some doctors are reluctant even to consider the possibility that chiropractors have something to offer. In this case, if you still choose to go to one, you will have to get a referral from friends or by contacting the American Chiropractic Association office in your state or the national office at 1916 Wilson Boulevard, Arlington, Virginia 22201 (202-276-8800).

Acupuncture
A well-recognized art of Eastern healing, acupuncture has been accepted in the United States for about ten years. Acupuncture involves the insertion of very fine needles into special points in the body, along channels of energy called meridians. The needles stimulate these areas found near muscle groups, major blood vessels, and nerve groupings. Stimulating the points releases hormones (endorphins) that are the body's natural painkillers and that can relieve pain or muscle spasm. Usually several treatments are required.

Acupuncture may be a valuable treatment method for specific types of pain. A good way to get reliable acupuncture therapy is to ask your physician for a referral. Always inform your physician when you are seeing an acupuncturist.

Certification of acupuncturists varies from state to state. To assure yourself that you are seeing a certified acupuncturist, call the Board of Registration in Medicine in your state, or write or call the American Association of Acupuncture and Oriental Medicine, 50 Maple Place, Manhasset, New York 11030.

Prevention of Back Pain
Prevention is the key to long-term success in avoiding backache. The following suggestions should prove helpful.

1. Lose weight if you are overweight (see chapter 11).

2. Strengthen your abdominal and back muscles (see pages 72–75).

3. Maintain good posture. Look in the mirror to be sure your spine is straight and your lower back is not excessively curved. Stand with your stomach muscles tight, chest upward and outward and buttocks tucked in. This posture limits the hollow in the lower part of the back.

4. Avoid high heels or backless shoes. Learn to wear flexible, soft, flat shoes with thick crepe soles. Go barefoot as much as you can.

5. Do not spend long hours standing.

6. Sleep on a firm mattress, lying either on your side or back, with knees bent slightly, propped by a pillow if necessary. Do not sleep on your stomach.

7. When you lift heavy objects, do not just bend over. Squat down with your knees together and hold the heavy object close to your body as you lift.

EXERCISES FOR LOW BACK PAIN

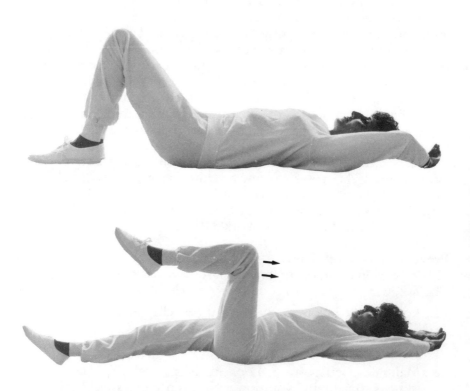

Lying on your back with your arms above your head and your knees bent, move one knee as close as possible to your chest and straighten the other leg. Alternate your legs.

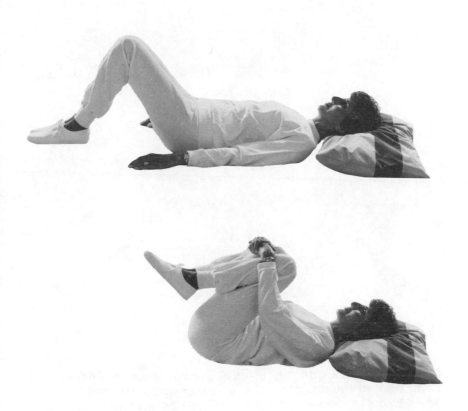

Lying on your back with a small pillow under your head, your knees bent, and your arms at your sides, bring your knees up to your chest, and with hands clasped over the knees, bring them toward the chest as tightly as possible. Hold for a count of thirty; return to the position of rest.

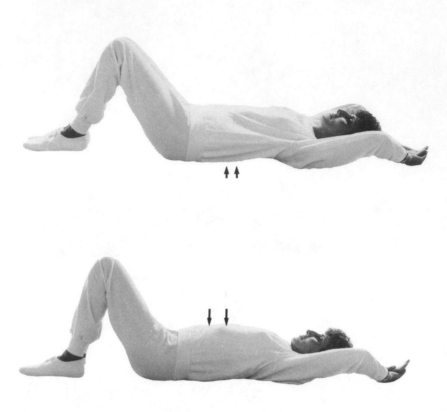

Lying on the floor with your arms above your head and your knees bent, tighten the muscles of your lower abdomen and buttocks so as to press the lower back tightly against the floor. Hold for a count of thirty; then relax. Repeat.

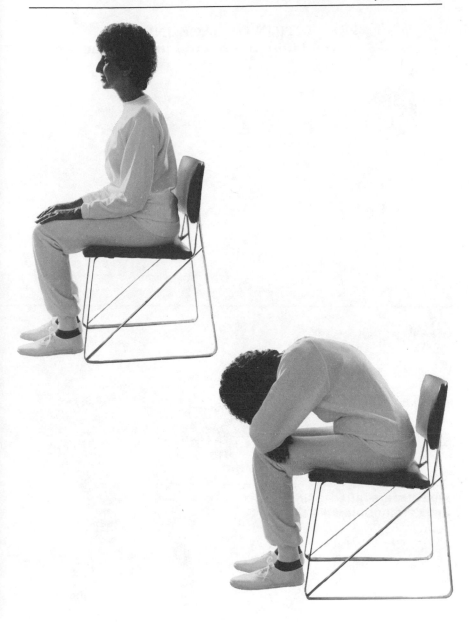

Sitting on a hard chair with your arms loosely resting on your thighs, let your body drop forward, with your head down. Pull your body back to the sitting position, keeping your abdominal muscles tight. Relax; then repeat the exercise.

PREVENTION OF BACK INJURY
Correct and Incorrect Ways to Lift and Stand

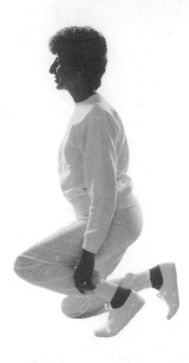

Objects are lifted using the knees rather than the back.

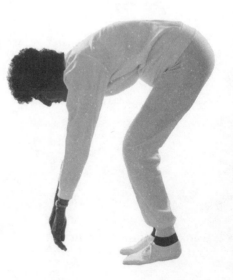

Objects are lifted straining the back.

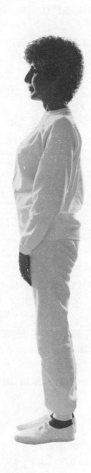 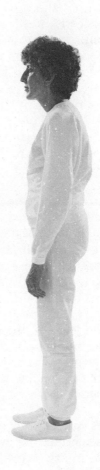

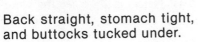

Back straight, stomach tight, and buttocks tucked under.

Excessive curvature of the back, weak stomach muscles, relaxed buttocks.

YOUR FEET

By the time we reach menopause, we have been standing on our own two feet for quite a few years. Sometimes we have refused to sit down and get off them; often we have stuffed them into stylish but narrow-toed shoes; occasionally we have danced on them until dawn. Mostly, we have offered them little support.

Then, one day in our older years, our feet rebel. An ache, a pain, a sore, a cut, an infection, or even numbness may be present (see chapter 5). Walking, which was once automatic, becomes deliberate, each step acutely felt as pain shoots up the leg. Belatedly, we abandon elegant shoes in favor of comfortable ones.

One-third of older people have significant foot disorders. Many of these disorders can be improved with simple measures; others require specialized care from an internist, podiatrist (chiropodist), or orthopedist.

Structure of the Foot

The feet bear a heavy burden from above (on the average, 140 pounds) and cushion our entire body from the shock of constant stepping on hard surfaces. The skin pads under the heel, the ball of the foot, and the toes act the way shock absorbers do in a car, giving a relatively smooth ride despite the many bumps underfoot.

The shock-absorbing capacity of the foot results from several elements acting together: the elastic properties of the skin and underlying tissues; the vascular system, which protects tissues from heat and mechanical energy that build up when tissues are rapidly compressed (for example, when you jump); and the arched bony structure of the foot, which allows it to absorb stresses rather than resist them.

Changes in the Foot with Aging

In a lifetime the average person walks the equivalent of four times around the world. Thus, by the time you are fifty, your feet have as good as circled the earth at least twice and are feeling their age and wear. As the feet age, the elastic elements of the skin and supporting tissues thin, as they do in other parts of the body, and the arch weakens and lowers. Spurs, or bony irregularities, form on some of the foot's twenty-six bones, causing tissue damage. Often poor circulation, evidenced in bulging veins that cause swelling of the skin and in poor arterial flow, diminishes the ability of foot tissues to respond to inflammation or injury. Finally, deformities can occur from a life spent in ill-fitting shoes.

The result of all these changes is that the older foot is less resistant to stress and injury.

Causes of Foot Pain

A common cause of painful feet in adults is acute or chronic foot strain. Excess pressure on the tissues of the foot, or even mild pressure on deformed parts of the foot, can lead to inflammation and pain.

Natalie R., sixty-eight and heavyset, was persuaded to take a course on historic buildings in her hometown. A friend had been trying to get her out to do things ever since Natalie's divorce. The course was to involve five days of walking tours of the buildings.

The group of walkers toured one or two large buildings each day, climbing up and down stairs and staying on their feet for hour after hour. After three days, Natalie's feet were sore, but she massaged them when she came home and took a warm bath. At the end of the five days, she not only had very sore feet but tender calf muscles too. Only after two weeks were her feet back to normal.

Pearl O., a fifty-year-old executive, was fed up with her weight and with her fatigue on climbing stairs. She was determined to start jogging. Pearl bought an expensive pair of running shoes and started jogging around a small pond near her home.

Pain or no pain, rain or shine, Pearl went out and jogged, starting with a half mile and working up to two miles a day in a month. Her feet were often sore; but then, she knew that joggers always had minor injuries, and she decided she was no exception.

A year later, twenty pounds lighter and decidedly in better physical condition, Pearl still had foot pain. Her doctor took an X ray and found degenerative changes of some bones. He sent her to a podiatrist, who diagnosed arthroses, or overgrown bone resulting in deformity. It was obvious that she had suffered chronic injury to the ball of her foot during jogging. The jogging had stretched out her ligaments and caused inflammation of her joints and the overgrowth of the tissue—the body's attempt to protect itself from injury.

Fortunately, with rest and properly padded shoes, her chronic foot problems subsided over several months. She even managed to keep her slim figure and fitness by swimming, doing floor exercises, and sometimes using the Y's rowing machine.

Calluses

A callus is a thickening of the skin in any area of the body (most often on the foot) that is exposed to pressure or friction. Calluses can form on the ball of the foot, when arches are weak; over hammertoes; and over bunions. Usually, the problem is preventable by wearing properly fitted shoes. For women who walk improperly and put abnormal stress on parts of their feet, corrective shoes may be the only way to avoid forming calluses.

A callus is treated with the application of a 40 percent salicylic acid plaster, which is covered by a felt pad to avoid further pressure on the callus.

Corns

Corns are soft thickenings between toes (usually between the fourth and fifth toes) or hard thickenings over bony prominences. They are cone-shaped—with the tip of the cone pressing into the foot tissues, making the corn very painful and tender to the touch. Corns can be removed chemically with the application of salicylic acid plasters or surgically by a competent podiatrist. You should never try to shave off your own corns, since dangerous infections can result. The best way to deal with corns is to prevent their occurrence by wearing properly fitted shoes and by reducing pressure on any protuberances by using corn pads on your feet or foam rubber pads in your shoes.

Ingrown Toenails

When the tissues near a toenail that has been cut in a curve (usually the nail on the big toe) press against the edge of the toenail, an ingrown toenail results. If the area becomes infected and produces a swollen, painful toe with pus in the tissues, treatment requires lancing the abscess, draining the pus, soaking the foot, and taking antibiotics for a week.

You can prevent ingrown toenails by cutting your toenails straight across, instead of cutting them curved down at the edges.

Plantar Warts

Plantar warts grow on the sole of the foot as clearly outlined thickenings. They are caused by a virus.

The key to treatment is to remove the wart with as little scarring as possible, since the scars left on the foot can sometimes be more painful than the original warts. Salicylic acid plasters can be applied to the warts and changed several times a day. Over a few weeks, the warts should disappear. The warts also can be pared back and either frozen or burned off. Hypnosis has been a successful treatment for plantar warts for some people, though the reason for its success is not fully understood. Many people, unfortunately, never succeed in parting company with these warts. For those with multiple warts, hypnosis may be a solution to try first, before undergoing the more painful alternative procedures.

Athlete's Foot

Athlete's foot is not necessarily a condition of athletes and is quite common in older women in the summertime. The condition is an infection caused by a fungus that grows between the toes when they are hot and moist. The infection causes itchy, scaly lesions, and sometimes painful fissures. The feet may appear dry and cracked; there is danger of additional infection entering at a bleeding crack.

It is important to keep your feet dry and clean. If you perspire readily, apply cornstarch, or cornstarch powder, which acts as a drying agent. Once the fungus has set in, it can be treated with antifungal powders, sprays, or creams, such as Desenex (undecylenic acid), Micatin (miconazole), and Tinactin (tolnaftate).

Bunions and Other Deformities of the Toes

If you have squeezed your feet into narrow-toed, high-heeled (over one inch) shoes for years, you may eventually suffer deformities of your toes. (Flat feet can also lead to these problems.) Your big toe can permanently slant inward, crushing the other toes or even overriding the second toe; you can develop bunions—bony, frequently painful knobs that protrude from the inner sides of the balls of the feet.

The treatment of bunions depends on the particular case. Some women have large bunions but no pain. Others have smaller bunions but may have pain, redness, and swelling of the protruding part of the foot, particularly after an active day.

Before you consider surgery to remove bunions, you should make every attempt to treat the problem by more conservative methods. These methods include wearing corrective shoes that support your arches; wearing shoes molded to your foot, which must be prescribed by a podiatrist, to prevent any pressure on your bunions; and improving muscle strength and circulation through exercises.

Hammertoes

A toe (usually the second) that becomes fixed in a flexed, or bent, position is called a hammertoe. Calluses form on both the tip and the bent part of the toe from its constant rubbing against the shoe. Often, women develop hammertoes by wearing shoes or elastic stockings that are too short or too tight, which causes the toes to curl under and upward.

Treatment requires wearing specially molded and padded shoes that ease the pressure on the hammertoe. When the deformity causes pain and/or disability, surgery is recommended. The toes are fused in a straight position, or tendons are transplanted to give the toes flexibility.

Heel Spurs

Pain under the heel is most often caused by inflammation of the tissues of the heel and by bony protrusions into the tissues. The condition is more common in people who stand or walk for long periods at a time.

These bony growths, sometimes called heel spurs, are diagnosed by the occurrence of pain in the front part of the heel and X-ray evidence of bone spurs.

Raising the heel about a quarter of an inch decreases the pressure on the heel bone and eases the condition. The soles of the shoes can be fitted with foam cushion pads with the part over the spur hollowed out. Occasionally, injections of cortisone and lidocaine (Novocain), a local anesthetic, will decrease inflammation and pain. A person rarely has to resort to surgical removal of spurs to get relief.

Morton's Neuralgia

Morton's neuralgia is a condition found most often in middle-aged women. A small tumor growing on one of the nerves to the toes, usually the third or fourth toe, produces pain that radiates toward the toes. At first, the pain is produced only when the woman bears weight, but, ultimately, pain persists even when she rests.

Often the tumor can be felt as a firm, small lump over the third or fourth toe. Some women get relief from aspirin or from cortisone injections to the area. Usually surgery is needed to remove the tumor.

The Ultimate Care of the Feet

Follow these suggestions to keep your feet in good shape and free from painful disorders:

1. Buy shoes that will fit you all day. At the end of the day, most women have some swelling in their feet, which can make a pair of shoes that fit properly in the morning agony by night. It is wisest to shop for your shoes toward the end of the day. Always try on both shoes, since your two feet are probably not the same size or width. Do not buy shoes that hurt when you try them on in the hope that you will break them in. Stay away from synthetic materials, which do not allow your feet to breathe and can contribute to infections. The tip of your shoe should be about a finger's width away from the tip of the big toe when you stand, giving you plenty of room to move your toes and preventing the pressing that can lead to hammertoes.

Running shoes make excellent, comfortable walking shoes.

2. Avoid high-heeled shoes whenever possible. High heels put great pressure on the balls of the feet. This pressure causes callus formation, weakening of the arch, and hammertoes.

3. Keep your feet clean and dry. Use cornstarch powder if you perspire a lot. Keep your toenails properly clipped. This is critically important for diabetics or for women with poor circulation (see chapter 5).

4. Massage your feet regularly. Your foot muscles are strained at the end of a day of standing and walking. A gentle massage relaxes them and relieves tension on your ligaments. A foot massage can also be a great source of sensual pleasure.

5. Keep the skin of your feet well lubricated with a light cream if your feet tend to be dry. Avoid putting cream between your toes, however.

SUGGESTED READINGS

Alexander, Dale. *Arthritis and Common Sense*. New York: Simon & Schuster, 1981.

Fredericks, Carlton, Ph.D. *Arthritis: Don't Learn to Live with It*. New York: Perigee Books, Putnam Publishing Group, 1985.

Fromer, Margot Joan, R.N. *Osteoporosis*. New York: Simon & Schuster, Pocket Books, 1986.

LaLanne, Elaine, with Benyo, Richard. *Fitness After 50: Elaine LaLanne's Complete Fitness Program*. Lexington, Mass.: Stephen Greene Press, 1986.

Lettvin, Maggie. *Maggie's Back Book: Healing the Hurt in Your Lower Back*. Boston: Houghton Mifflin, 1977.

Malkin, Mort. *Walking—the Pleasure Exercise: A 60-Day Walking Program for Fitness and Health*. Emmaus, Penn.: Rodale Press, 1986.

Notelovitz, Morris, M.D., and Ware, Marsha. *Stand Tall! The Informed Woman's Guide to Preventing Osteoporosis*. Gainesville, Fla.: Triad Publishing, 1982.

Rooney, Theodore W., D.O., and Rooney, Patty Ryan. *The Arthritis Handbook.* Dubuque: William C. Brown, 1985.

Schneider, Myles J., D.P.M., and Sussman, Mark D., D.P.M. *The Family Foot-Care Book: How to Doctor Your Feet Without a Doctor.* Washington, D.C.: Acropolis Books, 1986.

White, Augustus A., III, M.D. *Your Aching Back: A Doctor's Guide to Relief.* New York: Bantam Books, 1984.

Three

Your Eyes, Ears, Nose, Mouth, Teeth, and Voice

M ANY of the organs located in the head help us maintain contact with the environment. We can usually tolerate their temporary failure. We've all experienced a bad cold that is deafening or laryngitis that renders us speechless. When the failure threatens to be permanent, it is hard to maintain our equilibrium.

YOUR CHANGING EYES

In middle age, focusing your eyes can be more challenging than focusing your mind. You notice that you are having even more trouble reading the fine print than usual and need to hold it a bit farther away. This change is a normal consequence of aging, called presbyopia. The eyeball's crystalline lens (see figure 11), which adapts its shape to focus your sight, stiffens with age. As a result, objects must be held farther away to be focused on the retina, where the light-sensitive vision cells lie. If you already wear corrective lenses, you brave this latest indignity and purchase bifocals. Modern bifocals are made so that the division between the lens halves for far and near vision is not noticeable. If you have hitherto been blessed with perfect vision, you must now remember to carry along your reading glasses.

Apart from this common but benign change in the older woman's vision, there are three critical eye conditions all older

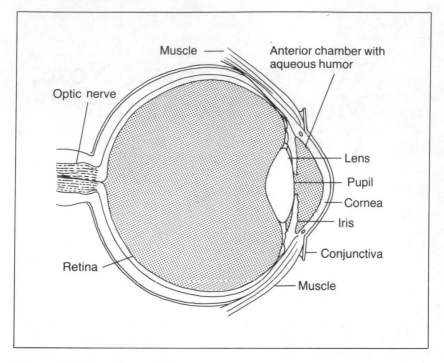

Figure 11. The Normal Eye

women should know about: glaucoma, cataracts, and macular degeneration.

Glaucoma

Untreated glaucoma (see figure 12) is one of the leading causes of blindness in older women. About 2 percent of all women over fifty have this condition in a mild form. Women with a family history of glaucoma and women with diabetes have increased risk of developing glaucoma. The loss of side vision, a symptom of the disease, can come on so slowly over a number of years that it may not be noticed.

Glaucoma is caused by the buildup of pressure in the chambers of one or both eyes. The front part of the eye (anterior chamber) is bathed in a thin liquid (aqueous humor), which is constantly made and circulated in the chamber and drains out into the veins. In the most common form of glaucoma (open-angle glaucoma), the pressure builds up gradually, compressing blood vessels that nourish the retina and permanently reducing vision.

Some of the early warning signals that suggest the possibility of glaucoma are these:

1. Reduced peripheral (side) vision. You may have more difficulty seeing people, cars, or objects approaching you from the side. (You can easily test your peripheral vision by looking straight ahead, bringing your arms up straight from the sides of your body, and wiggling your fingers. You should be able to see both hands moving simultaneously without moving your eyes to either side.)

2. Halos of light. You may see these distinct halos around streetlights and other outdoor lights even on very clear nights.

The other type of glaucoma (closed-angle glaucoma) is much rarer but much more dangerous. Most cases come on abruptly, causing severe pain in the eye, blurred vision, and a pink cast to the white of the eye. This group of symptoms is considered a medical emergency and should be evaluated immediately by an ophthalmologist, a medical doctor who specializes in diseases of the eye.

In closed-angle glaucoma, the canal draining the aqueous fluid suddenly shuts, causing a rapid and dangerous buildup of pressure. Permanent damage and even blindness can occur in a matter of twenty-four hours if the pressure is not relieved.

Many commonly prescribed drugs—such as Pro-Banthine, Librax, and Transderm-Scōp—can aggravate or precipitate closed-

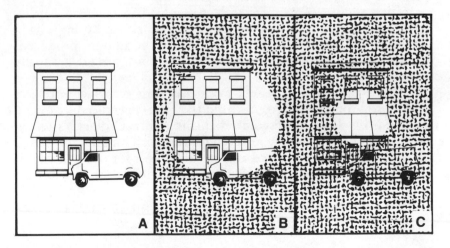

Figure 12. Glaucoma   Glaucoma need not affect normal vision (**A**) if it is treated. In untreated glaucoma, peripheral vision is lost (**B**) until finally only a small area directly ahead may be seen (**C**).

angle glaucoma. If you know that your eye pressure is high, mention this fact to any doctor starting you on a new medication. If you have never had your eye pressure checked, do so to learn whether or not yours is normal.

Diagnosis of Glaucoma

To check for glaucoma, a specialist must measure the pressure within your eyeball. Your optometrist (nonmedical eye doctor), ophthalmologist, or family doctor can measure the pressure with either a regular tonometer (a small instrument placed on your eyeball after it has been anesthetized with a few drops of medication) or an air tonometer (a device that blows a small jet of air onto the surface of the eyeball and evaluates eyeball pressure by measuring how much the eyeball is compressed).

After fifty, you should have your eye pressures measured every two years. If you are diabetic, have a family history of glaucoma, or are known to have even mildly elevated eye pressure, the measure should be done annually.

Treatment of Glaucoma

If your examination reveals elevated eye pressures but no evidence of any visual damage, you may not require treatment for some years. You should see your ophthalmologist about every four to six months for an eye checkup so that medicines can be prescribed to reduce the pressure in your eye at the earliest signs of injury.

The majority of women with glaucoma can be treated easily with eye drops that lower eyeball pressure either by improving drainage of aqueous fluid or by diminishing the amount produced. Drops and sometimes pills are given two to four times a day, usually indefinitely.

Many patients now benefit from laser surgery, which increases the drainage of the fluid from within the eye. This procedure can be done with little or no discomfort in the ophthalmologist's office. Nonlaser surgery is usually reserved for the small number of women who have an attack of closed-angle glaucoma or for those in whom laser treatments or pills and eye drops have failed to prevent damage to the vision.

Glaucoma should not be neglected. The visual damage or blindness it can cause is preventable.

Cataracts

Cataract, or clouding of the lens of the eye, is an inevitable accompaniment of age. Through the years, chemical changes occur in the protein of the transparent lens that decrease the amount of light passing through to the retina, making objects less clear. Ophthalmologists have speculated that if all people lived beyond their nineties, almost everyone would require cataract surgery to be able to see.

While most people get cataracts in their sixties and seventies, some get them earlier. Usually, this tendency runs in families. Diabetics who have prolonged periods of very high blood sugar can get early "sugar cataracts." Scleroderma, a rare skin disease that occurs more commonly in women than in men, can also produce early cataracts. More women than men have cataracts in older age groups.

Certain drugs—such as chlorpromazine (Thorazine), a medicine for psychiatric disorders, and cortisone—can produce cataracts. If you are taking these drugs for months or years, be sure to have periodic eye examinations. Treatments to slow down, prevent, and eliminate cataracts are improving all the time.

Diagnosis of Cataracts

You might not be aware that you have cataracts. All you may experience is some discomfort or temporary blindness at night with bright lights, particularly the lights of oncoming cars. Some people do notice their vision gradually fading.

When your doctor looks into your eyes with an ophthalmoscope and says, "There seems to be a very early cataract in your left eye," he or she will have seen some of the collected impurities that appear as thin, dark lines or spots on the lens of the eye. The diagnosis is made visually without further laboratory testing.

If your doctor describes your cataract as "young" or "not ripe," he or she is referring to a cataract that produces no, or very little, interference with your vision. Cataracts can remain young for many years, even the rest of your life. Mature, or ripe, cataracts cause blurred, clouded, or veiled vision.

Cataracts can form in both eyes or in one eye at a time. If you have cataracts in both eyes, each cataract can ripen, or mature, at a different pace and at a different time.

Treatment of Cataracts

The only cataracts that can be halted and possibly reversed are diabetic or drug-related ones. In diabetics, early "sugar cataracts" may be prevented or improved by carefully controlling blood sugar. Treatment of drug-related cataracts requires that you discontinue the offending drug or drugs.

Most people with cataracts can get by from year to year with a simple change of eyeglasses. Some women may benefit from eye drops that dilate, or enlarge, the pupil, allowing more light to reach the retina.

Cataract removal is the most frequently performed major surgery in the United States. Complications are extremely rare, and most women have good results after surgery.

There is no one best time to remove cataracts, and cataracts need not be mature before they are removed. In general, cataracts should be removed when decreasing sight interferes with normal life. Once cataracts are removed, light can reach the retina without blockage; however, there is no longer a lens to focus the image your eye receives. To focus your eyes, you have three choices: cataract glasses, contact lenses (either those used daily or the extended-wear kind), or lenses permanently implanted in the eye.

The majority of ophthalmologists advise daily or extended-wear contact lenses for younger women having cataract surgery. Most eye doctors will not recommend permanently implanted lenses for women under forty because there is insufficient evidence about how well these lenses are tolerated over decades. The lenses have, however, proven excellent for older people.

Most women can easily learn to use their contact lenses properly and will have excellent vision. Women with hand-coordination problems may prefer glasses, even though they are quite thick and may distort peripheral vision.

For about a week after cataract surgery, you will probably need a helper at home. In the first two months after recovery, you should see your ophthalmologist three or four times: after that, you should have an examination once a year.

Macular Degeneration

One of the leading causes of severely reduced vision in older people, macular degeneration is not usually well treated by either medications or surgery. You may notice a slow, painless decrease in your central, or reading, vision in one or both eyes; side vision, fortunately, is preserved, so even when macular degeneration occurs in both eyes, it does not lead to total blindness. An ophthalmologist examining your eyes will notice typical abnormalities in parts of your retina. Occasionally, laser treatments can help prevent further loss of vision. Or, you can learn to make use of special magnifiers and reading aids.

Dry Eyes

Women are particularly prone to developing dry, itchy, or

burning eyes. Tear glands stop working as effectively in older age and produce fewer tears. This is an annoying but not dangerous condition that can be treated with artificial tears that you can purchase in a drugstore and use a few times a day.

Dryness of the eyes is the major problem in continuing to wear ordinary contact lenses into late middle age and beyond. Diligent cleaning and disinfecting of contact lenses, prompt replacement of damaged lenses, and the purchase of new lenses every year are usually the key to prolonging the comfortable use of your lenses. By maintaining the quality of your contact lenses and using lens lubricating solution in your eyes every two hours, you can prolong their comfortable use.

Plugged Tear Ducts

Occasionally the ducts that collect tears become blocked or inflamed. You will notice that your eyes are very watery, with a tear rolling out now and then. The inner corner of the bottom eyelid may appear red. You may relieve the inflammation by applying warm compresses, using antibiotic ointments, or having the ophthalmologist unplug your tear duct. The ophthalmologist inserts a probe into your tear duct to unplug it; the procedure can be done in the office and is not painful.

YOUR CHANGING EARS

Deafness is often perceived as a sign of age and a hearing aid a dreaded presentiment of old age. If you experience a gradual hearing loss, you may be tempted to put off getting your hearing checked because you dislike the thought of wearing a hearing aid. Paradoxically, untreated deafness makes a woman appear far older than a hearing aid ever does. Any woman unfortunate enough to have lost hearing in both ears during a bad cold knows how depressing and isolating even a temporarily silent world can be.

Hearing Loss

From the age of thirty, hearing declines. One day, you may be surprised to see someone pick up the phone when you didn't even hear it ring. This hearing loss is due to one of the early aging changes your ear is undergoing—the growing inability to hear higher frequencies. With further impairment, you may have difficulty understanding speech, especially consonants, since they have higher frequencies than vowels. You might misunderstand words with the sounds *p, th, k, sh,* and *ch,* especially when there is distracting background noise in the room.

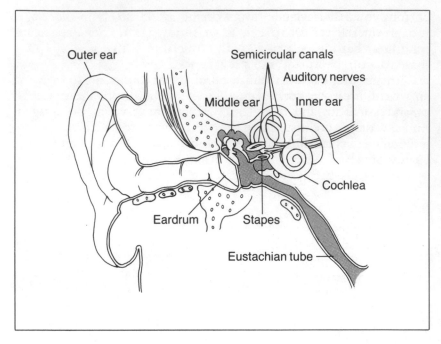

Figure 13. The Healthy Ear

When you are unable to hear a whisper three feet away, you have moderate hearing loss, and you probably don't hear some normal conversation.

You should never accept failing hearing without having a full medical checkup and a hearing evaluation. Hearing loss can often be treated, or it may be a valuable clue to underlying problems that need to be diagnosed.

Other factors that can cause hearing impairment include the following:

1. Noise pollution. The Environmental Protection Agency estimates that some forty million Americans are exposed to sound levels that cause permanent damage to the tiny hair cells of the inner ear, thereby threatening hearing.

2. Wax, cotton, or other material in the ear canal. Many people have excessive wax in their ears. Despite diligent cleaning efforts, and often because of them, wax can build up and impair hearing. In addition, if you wear cotton earplugs or clean your ears with cotton, you may leave behind small pieces of cotton that work their way down the canal to the eardrum (see figure 13) and interfere with your hearing.

A doctor or nurse can wash out the wax by squirting warm water into your ear with a syringe or Water Pik. If your earwax is very hard, it can be softened for a week or so with warm mineral oil or Debrox drops and then picked or washed out by a doctor or nurse. Cotton can usually be pulled out with an instrument or tweezers. It is inadvisable to put any hard objects or cotton deep in the ear canal.

3. Otosclerosis. Otosclerosis is a common cause of middle-ear deafness in older people. Excessive bone tissue forms around the cochlea, a structure in the inner ear. The use of a hearing aid is quite effective in these cases. A type of otosclerosis that starts in younger people results in paralysis of one of the small bones of hearing (the stapes) in the middle ear, which prevents sound waves from vibrating the stapes. You can have surgery to replace the stapes and improve your hearing.

4. Ménière's disease This disorder usually starts in the fifth decade of life, but it may affect younger women. It causes degeneration of sound-sensitive hair cells, progressive loss of hearing, ringing, pressure in the ear, and attacks of vertigo. Vertigo makes the room seem to spin around and can be provoked even by small changes in head position. You may be nauseated and occasionally vomit during attacks of vertigo. (Dizziness, on the other hand, is experienced as light-headedness, spinning inside one's head, or the feeling of intoxication.)

If you have an attack of Ménière's, you will feel better if you lie still in bed and take dimenhydrinate (Dramamine) or meclizine (Antivert) three times a day or wear a small disc of plastic containing scopolamine (Transderm-Scōp) behind your ear. The Transderm-Scōp can aggravate glaucoma, however.

In rare cases, the vertigo, nausea, and ringing can be so bad and resistant to medications that the doctor may recommend surgery for the affected ear.

5. Middle-ear infections. Middle-ear infection is generally, but not exclusively, a disease of childhood. Adults, like children, feel pain in the affected ear and may notice white or yellow liquid, which is pus, draining from the ear. You may have fever, swollen neck glands, or just mild hearing impairment on that side. By looking in your ear, a doctor or nurse quickly can confirm the presence of infection. Generally a ten-day course of antibiotics is prescribed.

A small number of women develop chronic ear infections and may need repeated courses of treatment, usually with cortisone ear drops, and occasional specialized cleanings by the ear-nose-and-throat doctor (otolaryngologist). Or they may need surgery if the infection has spread to neighboring bones or is due to a cholesteatoma, a benign tumor in the middle ear.

6. Diabetes or hardening of the arteries. These diseases can affect the circulation to the sensitive parts of the ear, producing nerve damage and deafness.

7. Nerve deafness. Many people deaf in one or both ears since childhood have some form of nerve deafness that is inherited or results from childhood infections. Nerve deafness can begin in middle age as well.

8. Medications. Many drugs—such as aspirin in high doses (eight to twelve pills a day), diuretics such as furosemide (Lasix) in large doses, or certain antibiotics such as gentamicin (Garamycin) used in the hospital—can cause hearing loss. If such deafness occurs, the drug doses can be lowered, or perhaps other medications can be tried instead.

Evaluation of Hearing Loss

If you suspect that your hearing is impaired, have a thorough medical examination that includes a review of your drug history to find out if you have contributing treatable conditions, such as some of those listed above. Ask for a referral to an ear-nose-and-throat specialist to have your hearing problem thoroughly evaluated—with audiology tests and X rays, if needed. (You should be checked at least every other year.) If your hearing is so bad that it interferes with conversations, work, or friendships, talk to the otolaryngologist about the best possible treatment before purchasing a hearing aid.

Hearing Aids and Other Helps

A hearing aid is a small electronic amplifier that increases the volume of sound in the ear of the wearer. It is mainly useful for amplifying face-to-face conversation and proves inadequate when sounds are farther away. The device does not distinguish between background noise and the sound you are trying to pick up. The devices used today can be so small and unobtrusive that they are unnoticeable with an appropriate hairdo.

A certified audiologist can best help you decide which hearing aid is most useful for you. Hearing aids cost between $300 and $800.

You might also do the following to make life simpler and more pleasant for yourself:

1. Buy or rent a telephone receiver with adjustable volume—all it takes is a call to the phone company. Wear a headset to hear the TV better. Consider light-flashing doorbells or alarm clocks and other modifications in your home.

2. Learn to be a good lip-reader. You can practice by yourself in the mirror or with a friend.

3. Learn to control the level of your voice and the quality of your articulation with a friend, audiologist, or speech therapist. If you are quite hard-of-hearing, your voice is likely to be too loud.

4. To cut down on noise pollution, consider investing in double-thickness windowpanes.

Tinnitus

"That buzzing in my ear is driving me crazy!" is a common complaint of at least 12 percent of women over fifty. The offending noises can be anything from high-pitched ringing to roaring, including whistling and buzzing. Most often the tinnitus is quite temporary and does not signify a hearing problem. Particular factors that can cause tinnitus are wax in the ears, inflammation of parts of the ear canals caused by common colds or influenza, and drugs such as aspirin or furosemide (Lasix).

Persistent tinnitus in a woman who otherwise hears normally can suggest more serious problems with the auditory nerves or other parts of the brain. Always report this symptom to your doctor and have him or her examine you for treatable causes. You may need a referral to an ear-nose-and-throat specialist for further testing. A pulsating tinnitus in one ear may suggest a malformation of a group of blood vessels in the brain and should also be reported to your doctor.

Assuming that no treatable cause is found, you must learn to live with the annoyance—always easier said than done. If you are healthy and have a positive outlook, you are much less likely to be bothered by tinnitus. When it is particularly distressing, you can listen to music, exercise, or take a mild tranquilizer prescribed by your doctor—such as oxazepam (Serax), chlordiazepoxide (Librium), or diazepam (Valium). If necessary, seek counseling to learn to cope with this disturbing physical problem.

YOUR NOSE AND SINUSES

One part of the body that exhibits little change in older age is the nose. There are, however, several nasal conditions that present problems to older persons with some frequency: nosebleeds; stuffy nose; and sinusitis, or inflammation of the sinuses.

Nosebleeds

Nosebleeds often surprise us. Most nosebleeds in mid-life and later years are transient and insignificant; however, they can occasionally signal an underlying problem.

Causes of Nosebleeds

A bloody nose can result from the following:

1. Injury to the delicate blood vessels lining the nose. This can result from picking the nose, vigorous blowing, common colds, or blows to the outside of the nose.
2. Excessive dryness of the air, particularly in winter. It helps to humidify the air either by placing pans of water on your radiators or near baseboard heaters or by using a two-gallon (or larger) humidifier that provides moisture through the night.
3. Rhinitis. This inflammation of the nasal passages is caused by dryness, pollens, dust, or other agents.
4. Clotting disorders of the blood. The platelets in your blood, which are essential for clotting, may be reduced by medications, viral illnesses, or cancer. If the number of these platelets is low, a nosebleed will be difficult to control. This condition is diagnosed by a blood test. If you are taking Coumadin, a blood thinner, a nosebleed can be an early sign that you may be taking too much medication. Again, a blood test will answer the question.

Treatment for a Nosebleed

To stop the bleeding, press the lower, wide part of the nose closed with a tissue; maintain continuous pressure for three to five minutes. Sit in a chair with your head tilted back. A cold washcloth or ice pack on the forehead may help.

If applying pressure doesn't work immediately, try it for another ten or fifteen minutes. Turn on some music to relax you. Do not release and then reapply pressure, as the blood will not have a chance to clot.

Occasionally, bleeding will continue despite your efforts. In this instance, it is best to see your doctor or go to the local emergency room. Your nose may need to be packed on the inside with cotton or Gelfoam for forty-eight to seventy-two hours. If you are sent home with a nasal pack, you should be prescribed antibiotics to assure that you will not get sinusitis.

Stuffy Nose

Your nose can become congested or swollen from allergy (to dusts, pollens, feathers, or cats, for example), sensitivity to dry air, viral or bacterial infection, sensitivity to alcohol, or just from hyperactive nasal tissue that swells with emotions.

Treatment depends on the cause of your symptoms. If you are allergic, skin tests can determine which factors produce your allergy. In all instances, try to eliminate the things you are sensitive to. If dust causes allergies, your home should be dust-free; if cats or dogs cause the problem, avoid contact with these animals; if feathers provoke reactions, avoid all feather pillows and down comforters and clothing; if dry air is the problem, humidification is the answer.

Nose drops or sprays that shrink your nasal membranes can help; when used too frequently, however, they can aggravate your symptoms. Most of these medications also can raise your blood pressure, speed up your heart rate, and even produce irregular heartbeats if you use them too much. It is safe to use them twice a day for three or four days.

Sprays containing cortisone, such as beclomethasone nasal spray, can halt your symptoms. Turbinaire sprays should not be used, since long-term use can slow down your own cortisone-producing adrenal glands, increase acid secretion in your stomach, and raise your blood sugar.

Milder nasal remedies such as Vicks VapoRub, Vicks Nasal Inhaler, oil of eucalyptus inhaled in a steaming pot of water, or even menthol candies may work less well but are much safer.

For more persistent cases, you can try medications—such as Contac, Sinutab, Dimetapp, Actifed, and Sudafed—that dry up the nasal secretions and shrink membranes. Since some of these medications can cause drowsiness, raise blood pressure, stimulate the heart, and aggravate glaucoma, you should take them under medical supervision if you have any problems in these areas.

Rhinitis caused by allergies can be helped by desensitization. Increasing doses of the factor responsible for the allergy are injected into your skin, causing you to produce antibodies that combine with the substance producing the allergy and make the substance nonallergenic. The whole process can be quite an undertaking, since treatments may be seasonal or may need to be continued throughout the year.

Sinusitis

Sinusitis is an inflammation inside the chambers of your face, surrounding your eyes and nose, that are ordinarily filled with air. When they are infected and filled with pus, they cause fever and pain in the forehead and nose, in the cheek, or in the upper and lower jaw and teeth, especially when you bend down.

Do not ignore sinusitis, particularly if you have fever and severe pain in the face or jaw. Your doctor will prescribe antibiotics, decongestants, and sometimes pain pills. Untreated sinusitis can lead to chronic, or long-term, problems with your sinuses. Worse still, the infection can extend to the brain, causing abscess or clotting of veins.

YOUR TEETH AND GUMS

Gum disease and tooth loss are not inevitabilities of old age. Although your gums naturally recede with age, there is absolutely no reason your teeth should not last a lifetime if you eat properly, brush correctly, floss regularly, use fluoride, and deal with dental and gum problems promptly.

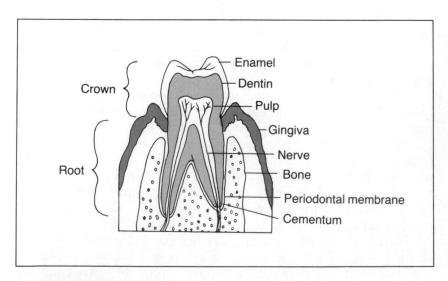

Figure 14. The Normal Tooth

How to Care for Your Teeth

To care for your teeth, you need to pay attention to your diet and to oral hygiene; in addition, you should use fluoride as a preventive measure against tooth decay.

Role of Diet

Your diet should contain adequate protein and vitamin C, to help your gums resist infection and replenish themselves, and calcium, to strengthen your teeth (see chapter 11).

Sweets cause tooth decay and need to be limited. Chocolate may not be as harmful as other candy; it has been shown to have some ability to slow decay. It is also better to eat a sweet as part of your meal rather than eat it as a snack. Sticky sweets such as caramels, gooey pastries, sugared dried fruit, and honey are particularly bad because they stick to your teeth and cannot be rinsed off easily. Try to brush your teeth after eating sweets or at least vigorously rinse your mouth with water.

Brushing

Brushing teeth doesn't whiten them but does remove some food particles and the destructive, acid-producing bacteria that collect on the gum line (see figure 14). These bacteria form a layer of plaque, which corrodes the enamel of the tooth. Bacteria can then enter the tooth and cause decay.

Your toothbrush should be in good condition and should have soft bristles. Since only the tips of the bristles do the actual cleaning, it is important not to squash the brush against the teeth. Place the bristles right at the gum line, and brush the outer and inner gum lines of all your teeth, using short, rotary motions. Replace your toothbrush at least every three months or sooner to be sure the bristles are straight and effective.

Use toothpaste sparingly. Although most toothpastes contain fluoride, which helps prevent tooth decay, many also contain abrasives that sandpaper the teeth to make them look clean. These abrasives can gradually wear off the protective enamel coat covering the teeth. Your dentist may, for this reason, prefer that you use a gel toothpaste.

Mouthwashes are not a substitute for brushing teeth. They may remove some food particles and freshen your breath, but they have no effect on the bacteria collected near the gums.

Flossing

You may wonder whether flossing is worth the minutes added to your daily routine. The answer is a definite yes. Flossing scrapes off plaque at and around the gum line and pries loose food particles stuck between teeth and out of reach of your toothbrush. Flossing leaves the gum margins clean, thus reducing the potential for developing irritated and inflamed gums.

Usually, unwaxed floss is better than waxed, since small particles of sticky wax can adhere to the teeth and serve as a feeding ground for bacteria.

Do not give up flossing simply because your gums feel tender and bleed easily. Ninety-eight percent of the time, the bleeding is a sign that your gums are swollen and inflamed from bacterial damage. Flossing and a visit to the dentist or dental hygienist for teeth cleaning are just what you need. Regular flossing between dental visits eventually will reduce gum tenderness.

Fluoride

Fluoride forms crystals that are much more resistant to bacteria or other destruction than normal tooth enamel. When absorbed daily, either in drinking water or from toothpaste or mouthwash, fluoride penetrates tooth enamel, strengthening its ability to resist decay. Fluoride also can slow the loss of calcium from bones in the body (see chapter 2).

The fluoridation controversy continues in the United States, years after scientific evidence clearly shows that communities with long-standing fluoridation demonstrate dramatic decreases in tooth decay and that fluoridation has no serious side effects. Despite these data, more than half of all Americans are not receiving fluoride in their drinking water.

You can take advantage of the benefits of fluoride even if your water is not fluoridated. Fluoride comes in tablet form both by itself or combined with vitamins and is available by prescription from your dentist or doctor.

The Dentist

Every person should see a competent dentist at least twice a year. Finding a good dentist is not difficult. You might ask people who take good care of their teeth for recommendations, call a dental school for the name of affiliated dentists (they are likely to be of high quality and aware of up-to-date technology and procedures), or call or write the Academy of General Dentistry, 211 East Chicago Avenue, Chicago, Illinois 60611 (312-440-4300), for referrals.

A good dentist will stress preventive care of your teeth, recommend regular teeth cleaning by a dental hygienist (one or more times per year, depending on your particular teeth), take periodic X rays of your teeth to locate hidden cavities (though most people need X rays only every few years or so, to limit radiation exposure), and check on the condition of your gums.

Bleeding Gums

A small number of women have bleeding gums from causes other than bacterial damage.

- Protracted head colds or similar illness can make gums feel sensitive and bleed more easily.
- Certain medications—such as phenytoin (Dilantin), given for seizures—can cause the gums to swell and bleed.
- Bleeding disorders—whether congenital, side effects of drugs such as aspirin or nonsteroidal anti-inflammatories, or rare toxic effects of drugs such as quinine or quinidine—can lead to bleeding gums.
- Rare cancers, such as leukemia or lymphomas, can cause bleeding gums.
- Diabetes can contribute to gum infection and bleeding gums.

Periodontal Disease

Periodontal disease, inflammation around the gums and in the bone supporting the gums, is the leading cause of tooth loss in people over thirty-five. Experts estimate that well over 50 percent of adults have this disease. The destruction of gums and bone can eventually cause loosening of the teeth to the point where many fall out or must be removed (see figure 15).

Periodontal disease (formerly known as pyorrhea) is caused by the interaction of certain bacteria in the mouth with your immune system. In fighting the bacteria, the immune system releases hormones, such as prostaglandins, that weaken the tissues that hold your teeth in place. Particularly vulnerable spots are the gum line; the gum between the teeth; spaces caused by a lost tooth, poor alignment of the teeth, or malocclusion (faulty closure of teeth); and the spaces in and around worn-down fillings and poorly fitting bridges or dentures.

Early periodontal disease causes bleeding gums and bad breath. Later, the teeth begin to move apart from one another, creating large spaces between teeth. Ultimately, the teeth wobble when hard food is eaten, causing bleeding and pain, and eventually they fall out.

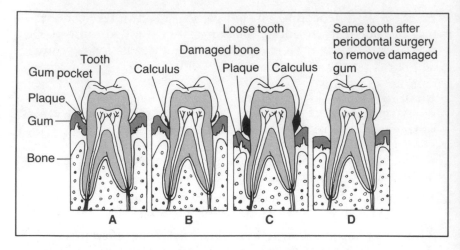

Figure 15. Periodontal Disease Periodontal disease begins when plaque builds up between the teeth and gums (**A**). Hard, chalky calculus may form with the plaque and pry gums and teeth farther apart (**B**). Irritation and infection may eventually destroy so much bone and gum that teeth loosen (**C**) and may even fall out. In periodontal surgery, diseased gum and bone are trimmed away to prevent further deterioration (**D**).

Prevention and Treatment

Prevention and early treatment of gum disease can save your teeth and your money. Caught early, gum disease can be controlled by following a regimen at home that includes the following:

- rigorous toothbrushing, starting with the bristles at the gum line, with small, rotary motions (ask your dentist or hygienist to demonstrate)
- daily flossing between the teeth and around the sides of the teeth
- eating a diet rich in fibrous foods that naturally clean the teeth (such as apples, lettuce, and most other raw vegetables) and in vitamin C, since deficiency of this vitamin is associated with poor gum condition
- limiting sweets, especially sticky sweets such as caramels, and good cleaning or rinsing after eating sweets

The other major road to control is to have your teeth cleaned twice a year by a dentist or dental hygienist.

Treatment of well-established gum disease requires surgery. The diseased gums are cut away, or opened. Bone may need to be reshaped, and bone and gum material may have to be grafted. Abnormal teeth may need to be capped. The procedures are time-consuming and expensive, but they are the only alternative to having your teeth removed and wearing dentures.

Researchers are investigating simpler and less costly methods of treatment. Some are testing antibiotics; others are studying the immune system to find ways of preventing the toxic damage to gums.

Dentures

About 20 percent of the people in the United States are toothless by age fifty, and most of these people wear dentures. Those who do not wear them should—to eat better, look better, speak better, and keep their jaws aligned properly.

Dentures must be fitted individually to your gums and jaw. The dentist takes X rays to look for bony deformities, bone cysts, or tooth roots that could cause future problems in the fit of the dentures. He or she makes wax impressions of your gum line so that the dentures can be fitted exactly to your mouth. Even small errors of fit can result in discomfort, irritation of the gums, pressure on the jaw, and erosion of the underlying bone.

The best time to get your dentures is several months after your teeth have been extracted, when your gums have had a chance to heal completely. Most women prefer to be fitted immediately after extraction and must put up with more frequent visits to the dentist for refittings as their gums heal and shrink.

If some of your teeth can be saved (especially those in the lower jaw), it is much better to have partial dentures than complete dentures. Partial dentures will feel more like normal teeth.

Your dentures should feel comfortable. Too many women struggle with dentures that feel too big, click during eating, or cause gagging. If your dentures bother you for as long as four months after you first get them, assume that they do not fit properly and return to your dentist. If you are still not comfortable after a refitting, get a second opinion, and even a third.

Keep these suggestions in mind when you first receive your dentures:

- Examine your gums daily before putting in the dentures. If you have a red, swollen area, give it a few days to heal before wearing your dentures again. If the redness does not go away, consult your dentist or doctor.

- Clean your dentures daily with a brush and a special dentifrice such as Polident. Keep them in warm water overnight. Rinse your mouth before you put the dentures in.
- At first, eat soft foods and chew slowly.
- Practice speaking at home, and learn ways of improving your speech.

You can reduce the expense of getting dentures by going to the clinic of a university-affiliated dental school. Fees are lower, and the work is good.

TASTE AND AGE

You may be surprised to learn that the organs of taste, the taste buds, are found not only on the tongue but on the palate, cheeks, the back of the throat, the upper part of the esophagus, and the lips. The tongue is most sensitive to sweet and salty tastes, the palate to sour and bitter; however, all parts of the oral cavity can sense all four tastes. The ability to smell affects your sense of taste.

As you age, you are unable to replace dying taste cells as rapidly as you lose them; consequently, your sense of taste diminishes. Some of this taste loss may also be due to a loss of sensitivity to odors.

The most common cause of loss of taste is viral infection.

Oral hygiene and smoking strongly affect taste. Poor mouth hygiene decreases taste by covering taste buds with decayed food and bacteria.

Many drugs such as antibiotics (tetracycline, ampicillin), painkillers (codeine, hydromorphone), blood pressure medications (captopril diazoxide), and muscle relaxants (baclofen) can affect your sense of taste and smell. If you notice a significant decrease in your ability to taste when you are on any medication, report the symptom to your doctor. Perhaps he or she can prescribe a different medication.

Both periodontal disease and a condition called Sjögren's syndrome, in which salivary glands dry up, can produce a bad taste in your mouth.

DRY MOUTH

A very annoying and common problem in older women, dry mouth is generally caused by breathing through the mouth in dry air. In the wintertime, use a humidifier night and day, or set pans of water on radiators or near baseboards. In addition, keep a glass of water at your bedside at night. Concentrate on breathing through your nose rather than through your mouth.

Another common cause of dry mouth is not drinking enough fluid during the day or taking diuretics. Gum disease, too, can cause dry mouth and bad breath. Try to drink six to eight glasses of liquid per day, especially if you are diabetic or are taking diuretics or tranquilizers. You can suck on low-sugar candies or chew gum to increase salivation.

VOICE CHANGES IN AGING

Voice changes in older age are normal. The typical changes in the aging female voice are a lowering in pitch (as opposed to men, who can experience a heightening in pitch), a hoarser quality (in about 30 percent of women versus 60 percent of men), and less clarity in speech. Occasionally stroke, nerve degeneration, parkinsonism, or cancer can cause voice changes. Other stresses such as smoking, drinking, and excessive use of your voice can aggravate these changes but can often be treated. Therefore, do not accept voice changes without having a thorough examination by your doctor, and, in some cases, by an ear-nose-and-throat specialist. The following situations may lend themselves to treatment.

1. Low level of thyroid hormone, which is not uncommon in older women, is associated with a deep voice and slow speech. The voice quality will improve dramatically with replacement of thyroid hormone.

2. Vocal abuse—such as loud singing, screaming, cheering, or talking—can stretch and tire vocal ligaments and cause swelling of the vocal cords, or even calluses on the vocal cords. Nervous tension can also cause swelling of the vocal cords. You should be careful not to strain your voice and to rest it after you have used it intensely.

3. Cigarette smoking can irritate the vocal cords, leading to a throaty smoker's voice and, in some cases, to vocal polyps, which may need surgical removal.

4. Poor physical condition and a sedentary life seem to be associated with overall poor voice performance. Conversely, remaining physically and mentally active will keep your voice strong.

5. Inflammation of the vocal cords from smoking, pollution, or infection can cause voice changes. Your doctor can treat such inflammation by prescribing cortisone spray or antibiotics, as well as rest.

If your voice is weak, you may be able to strengthen it with some simple exercises. Check with your doctor to be certain that these exercises will not aggravate other conditions.

- Sit in a chair near a table. Place your hands on the edge of the table. Push the table edge for three seconds and release. Repeat ten times. This exercise tightens the muscles of the larynx, thus improving voice quality.
- Practice breathing with your diaphragm. Rather than raise your chest to breathe, use your stomach muscles to push air in and out (see chapter 14).

If hoarseness from benign causes persists, you might want to consider consulting a speech therapist or voice teacher, who will help you learn how to use your voice in a way that does not strain your vocal cords.

SUGGESTED READING

Shulman, Julius, M.D. *Cataracts: The Complete Guide from Diagnosis to Recovery for Patients and Families.* Washington, D.C.: AARP; Glenview, Ill.: Scott, Foresman & Co., 1985. (An AARP Book)

Four

Your Circulatory System

A good heart is better than all the heads in the world.

—Anonymous

W E grant to the heart jurisdiction over provinces that right-
fully belong to the brain. The heart's symbolic nature is so
firmly rooted in our minds that to accommodate the turns of our
thought we have forced the language to flower in metaphor. We
speak of people who are all heart and complain about those who
have none. We take joy in a light heart and lament a broken one.
Hearts will always break, but for today's women, the pain is as likely to be organic.

Women's hearts are not as healthy as they used to be. The
twentieth century is bearing witness to a dramatic revolution in
women's lives that affects their hearts. Increasingly, as women take
up breadwinning roles, the common lore that men, not women,
die of heart attacks is becoming obsolete. Women are adopting the
traditional stresses of male lives and, in the process, are making
heart disease a woman's disease as well.

THE HEART

The heart is a remarkably durable muscular organ (see figure 16)
that recycles about 7,200 quarts of blood each day, providing all
tissues and organs in the body with life-sustaining oxygen.

Your heart has two sides, each with a receiving chamber
(atrium) and a muscular pumping chamber (ventricle) that are
separated by valves that open and close at appropriate times. The

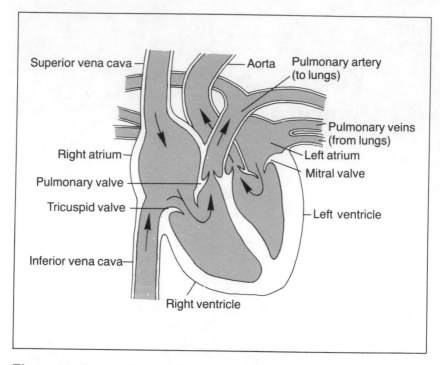

Figure 16. Circulation of Blood Through the Heart   Circulation of blood through the heart begins in the right atrium, where blood collects from two large veins, the inferior and superior vena cavae. The tricuspid valve admits the blood to the right ventricle, which pumps it through the pulmonary valve and pulmonary artery to the lungs. Blood returns from the lungs to the left atrium and flows through the mitral valve into the left ventricle. This powerful chamber propels the blood to the rest of the body via the aorta.

right side of your heart receives from your body's veins blood that has had much of its oxygen extracted in its travel through the tissues. The multitude of veins empty into progressively fewer and larger ones, until only two veins return blood into the right atrium: the superior vena cava, from the head and arms; and the inferior vena cava, from the legs, abdomen, and pelvis.

Blood collects in the right atrium, pushes open the valves, and flows into the right ventricle, which propels the blood into blood vessels that course through the lungs. In the lungs, your blood picks up oxygen and gives up carbon dioxide in preparation for the next cycle.

From the lungs, the pink, freshly oxygenated blood enters the heart's left atrium on its way to the left ventricle, the heart's largest muscular chamber. This powerful chamber collects about five tablespoonfuls of blood and, on an electrical signal from the specialized pacemaker nerves in the heart, squeezes this blood into a huge artery, the aorta, which branches into arteries all over your body, ending in the tiny capillaries in your tissues. The capillaries flow into rivulets that form veins. The veins return carbon dioxide, unused nutrients, and blood that needs fresh oxygen to the heart, completing the life-giving circuit.

Your heart must also feed itself by pumping blood containing oxygen and nutrients into its own muscle, through its own "coronary" arteries, to perform its monumental service to the body.

The coronary arteries are the first arteries to branch from the aorta as it leaves the left ventricle. Two coronary arteries go to the left side of the heart, and one goes to the right side of the heart, to provide its fuel. These arteries, so central and important, are also very vulnerable. Disease of the coronary arteries has been the leading cause of premature death in the Western world.

THE MEANING OF BLOOD PRESSURE

The circulation of your blood is propelled by the pumping action of your heart and maintained by the pressure in the walls of your arteries. Place your index and third fingers over the artery in your wrist, about one inch below the base of the thumb. When you feel a "pulse" striking your fingers, you are sensing the flow of blood pushed by the left ventricle's muscular contraction into the arteries, causing them to bulge. The time between pulses represents relaxation of the left ventricle as it fills with blood in preparation for the next contraction. This pumping and relaxing occurs 100,000 times a day, and nearly 3 billion times in the course of an average lifetime.

Unlike the veins, the arteries have considerably more muscle in their walls, giving them a strength that maintains pressure, or tension, even when the ventricle is in its relaxation phase. This muscle tone continues the pumping action of the heart and pushes blood forward. Blood pressure—which is, in fact, artery pressure—is expressed by two numbers, a higher one "over" a lower one. The higher pressure occurs when your heart's left ventricle contracts, propelling blood into the arteries. It is called systolic pressure and can be felt on your wrist as an outward push. When the ventricle relaxes, the muscle tone of the artery walls still maintains a pressure, though lower, and this is called the diastolic pressure.

When you look at a blood pressure apparatus as the doctor or health professional pumps it up, you will see a silver line of mercury rise up and slowly descend as the professional opens the instrument's valve. When your blood pressure reading is stated as "130 over 80," it means that during ventricular contraction, there is a force in the arteries that could push a column of mercury 130 millimeters high, against gravity. The number 80 means that during relaxation of the heart, the muscle tone of the arteries can push the mercury 80 millimeters high, against gravity. This lesser force continues to circulate the blood between pumps of the heart.

The greater the arterial muscle tone, the higher your blood pressure. For reasons that are not well understood, many people develop increased tone in their arteries as they age, which narrows the pipelines for blood, causing high blood pressure. Stress, fear, and other emotions also have a great impact on blood pressure, since the muscles of the arteries are affected by autonomic nerves and hormones, which in turn are sensitive to your emotions.

HIGH BLOOD PRESSURE

High blood pressure is one of the most common cardiovascular problems in the Western world and becomes even more common as we age. In all but a very few instances, its cause is unknown. Its consequences are, however, very well understood.

Blood pressure varies from second to second, depending on a myriad of circumstances. When you have high blood pressure, the muscular tension of your arteries is intense and constant. There is not precise agreement or sufficient knowledge about the long-term risk of occasionally elevated pressures, of mildly elevated pressures, or of high-normal pressures. The following table gives blood pressure ranges that are considered normal or hypertensive.

Range	Systolic Pressure	Diastolic Pressure
Normal blood pressure	80–140	50–90
Mild hypertension	141–165	91–104
Moderate hypertension	166–200	105–114
Severe hypertension	greater than 200	greater than 114

The accepted normal range increases with age and is still open to debate. A blood pressure of 140/90 may be normal in a seventy-year-old woman but not in a twenty-year-old. High pressure is defined, somewhat arbitrarily, as being above 140/90 for the late-middle-aged woman.

Risk Factors

Several conditions predispose an individual to high blood pressure. These include the following:

1. *A family background of hypertension.* If any of your blood relatives have hypertension, you are more likely to have it as well.

2. *Consumption of highly salted foods.* The sodium ion of salt swells the blood volume. When a larger volume has to squeeze through the arteries, blood pressure goes up. Recently, however, research studies have cast doubt upon the assumption that eating salt can raise blood pressure significantly.

3. *Cigarette smoking.* The nicotine released into your blood from smoking causes arteries to tighten and increases blood pressure.

4. *Obesity.* Being overweight increases your risk of developing high blood pressure, though most overweight women do not have hypertension.

5. *Stress, anxiety, and fear.* For most women, the increase in blood pressure that these feelings produce is transient and probably of no consequence. In some women, however, stress and emotions may contribute to damaging levels of blood pressure.

6. *Isometric exercise.* Lifting heavy objects such as grandchildren or shoveling snow—or contracting any muscles against resistance—can increase blood pressure.

Carol P., sixty, had lived in her rented apartment for thirty-two years. One day she received a sudden, dramatic increase in her rent that her Social Security check would not cover. Carol suspected that her landlady did not have the courage to tell her that relatives wanted the apartment and so was forcing her out by indirect means. Having no choice but to find another place to live, Carol began the search, and the chore of sorting the accumulations of over thirty years.

During a routine medical checkup two weeks later, Carol was surprised to discover that her usually normal blood pressure had shot up to 180/96. She returned for several appointments, and each time her blood pressure was still elevated. Finally, the doctor suggested treating her blood pressure, even though it clearly seemed related to the emotional circumstances surrounding her move.

Four months after Carol moved into her new apartment, and was beginning to feel that it was home, her blood pressure began to return to normal levels, even when she was off all medication.

Symptoms

Contrary to popular notion, you cannot feel high blood pressure. Even when you feel perfectly normal, you may have a very high blood pressure. When you feel a tight band of pressure around your head or throbbing in the temples, your blood pressure is often perfectly normal. Such symptoms are probably related to a tension headache rather than to tension in your arterial walls.

In extremely rare cases, women with dangerously high levels of blood pressure do feel symptoms. This rare syndrome is called malignant hypertension and can cause blurred vision or loss of vision, mental clouding, and even symptoms of stroke. This is a medical emergency, which needs immediate intravenous drug treatment to prevent serious complications.

Diagnosis

There is only one way to diagnose hypertension—by periodically checking your blood pressure. The pressure does not have to be checked by a doctor, though a doctor should make the diagnosis of hypertension.

In some communities, clinics offer blood pressure screening. For a few coins, blood pressure machines in drugstores and supermarkets will check you. And for about twenty-five dollars, you can purchase your own blood pressure cuff and, after taking a short time to learn to use it, accurately assess your blood pressure any time you wish.

If you do purchase a blood pressure cuff, do not become a "blood pressure fanatic," checking your pressure too often and worrying every time it is a bit elevated. Hypertension is not the infrequent elevated pressure that everyone has but a more sustained elevated pattern.

Treatment

Diet and exercise are simple, safe ways to control high blood pressure yourself, under the supervision of your physician. For many women, these are the only measures needed to treat the problem. Other women need to take additional measures.

1. Eat wisely. Try not to add salt to the foods you cook. More important, read food labels to see how much sodium the foods contain and try to avoid prepared foods that are especially high in salt, such as salad dressing, canned soup and vegetables, catsup, and salted peanuts, potato chips, or crackers. Also make an effort to stay away from luncheon meats and many cheeses—particularly provolone, feta, and process American. A number of salt substitutes that can make food more palatable, such as Co-salt, are available in pharmacies and grocery stores. You can use garlic, onion powder, pepper, and a host of other spices.

Baking soda contains a great deal of salt and should not be used for brushing teeth.

Some studies suggest that increasing roughage or fiber in the diet contributes to lowering blood pressure. You can add one or two tablespoonfuls of raw bran or other unprocessed grains to your meals. Bran cereals and muffins and granola snacks are also good sources of fiber.

If you are overweight, try to reduce on a reasonable diet that you can follow consistently. Generally, weight lost quickly returns quickly, so lose gradually and for good.

2. Exercise. Any exercise that stretches muscles and improves circulation can lower blood pressure. Such exercises include walking, swimming, jogging, bicycling, and dancing. Exercises that tighten muscles—such as weight lifting, pushing, shoveling, and digging—clamp down on arteries and can raise blood pressure.

Don't feel you need to exercise until pain and exhaustion set in. It is best to integrate exercise into your daily routine (see chapter 2).

3. Stop smoking. Breaking an old habit is no easy task, but you will be doing yourself immeasurable good if you can succeed (see chapter 6).

4. Try meditation or biofeedback techniques. Such forms of treatment can lower blood pressure for some people whose hypertension is caused by stress. *The Relaxation Response* by Dr. Herbert Benson (New York: William Morrow & Co., 1975) describes meditation techniques. Some major hospitals or alternative treatment centers (which are often listed in health food stores) can teach you to reduce your tension-increasing responses through the use of biofeedback techniques.

5. Take the drugs prescribed by your physician. Many women require blood pressure drugs in addition to the above measures. Drug therapy usually starts with the simplest, safest, and least expensive medications; other drugs are added as needed. All drugs carry some risk of side effects, no matter how minimal.

The first drug generally prescribed for hypertension is a mild diuretic in the thiazide family (hydrochlorothiazide, or Hydro-DIURIL; chlorothiazide, or Diuril) taken once or twice a day. This class of drug helps eliminate salt and water from your body, reducing your blood volume and thus lowering your blood pressure.

Most women experience no ill side effects from diuretics. A small number of women experience fatigue, weakness, or a loss of sexual desire; rarely, a woman will suffer an attack of gouty arthritis, affecting the big toe, ankle joints, or other small joints in the body. Some women with a preexisting diabetic tendency may have higher levels of sugar in their blood while taking thiazides.

Thiazide pills cause a loss of potassium, an important element in the blood and in the cells of the body. Most women can replace the lost potassium through a regular diet supplemented by fruit juices, bananas, apricots, dates, or unsalted olives. Other women have a greater potassium loss and need to take potassium tablets (such as Slow-K and Kaon) or a potassium drink daily.

You should have your blood potassium level checked a few months after starting diuretic pills and at least yearly thereafter.

If your blood pressure is still not low enough, the second drug generally prescribed is a medication that lowers blood pressure by opening arteries. Some medications act directly on the muscle walls of arteries; some interfere with the autonomic nerves that act to constrict the arteries; still others interfere with the body's production of epinephrine, which also constricts arterial walls. Common examples include methyldopa (Aldomet), hydralazine (Apresoline), propranolol (Inderal), metoprolol (Lopressor), clonidine (Catapres), guanethidine (Ismelin), and reserpine. Common side effects of drug treatment for high blood pressure include fatigue, weakness, loss of sexual desire, gout, nightmares, and hallucinations. You should not accept such side effects as inevitable, however.

Many drug treatments and combinations of treatments are available; some may work well for you, and some may not. The art of treatment is to tailor the choice or combination of these drugs to your individual needs. You need to be a partner with your doctor in this effort. Tell your doctor how each treatment makes you feel and how well you can tolerate any side effects, the costs, and the medication schedule. Do not shy away from discussing these issues with your physician; otherwise, you may decide to stop treating your blood pressure. That can only harm you in the long run.

COMPLICATIONS OF HIGH
BLOOD PRESSURE

Arterial pressure that is continuously elevated causes predictable damage to the arteries. The higher the blood pressure, the greater and more rapid the damage. But the damage occurs slowly over many decades, and there is plenty of time and opportunity for safe, effective, inexpensive treatment and prevention. Generally, the lower the pressure (even within accepted "normal" ranges), the less will be the wear and tear on your arteries.

With age, the arteries stiffen. The inner, smooth lining becomes uneven and jagged at certain places. These places along the walls of the arteries become the sites where cholesterol and other fatty material mixed with blood platelets accumulate (the condition of atherosclerosis). The effect is irregular narrowing of the arteries (arteriosclerosis), which creates the risk that a blood clot could form as blood cells are blocked and injured along their course.

With severe high blood pressure, such irregular arterial walls can weaken and, in some places, balloon out, forming aneurysms that can burst, rupturing the artery itself.

The arteries most affected by such wear and tear are those that bring blood to the heart, brain, kidneys, and limbs. This is why inadequately treated high blood pressure plays such an important part in the development of the following conditions.

1. *Coronary artery disease*. The accumulating fatty plaques reduce the much-needed blood and oxygen flow to the heart muscle and can lead to heart attack.

2. *Strokes*. Damaged arteries that nourish the brain develop blockages that prevent the flow of blood to it, causing injury or death to those parts of the brain affected. The result is paralysis of limbs, speech problems, or loss of brain function and intellect.

3. *Brain hemorrhage*. Weakened arteries or aneurysms in the brain can rupture when blood pressure is very high, spilling blood into the brain and causing injury and death of brain tissue.

4. *Kidney disease*. The vessels supplying the kidney with blood to be filtered and cleansed of toxic materials become thickened, injured, and blocked. The kidney is unable to cleanse impurities from the blood, and these impurities build up, causing mental cloudiness and fatigue.

5. *Limb disease*. Arteriosclerosis narrows the arterial blood supply to the legs, producing cramping, stiffness, ache, or tiredness in

your calves when you walk long distances or climb stairs or hills. A brief rest usually relieves the symptoms, allowing you to continue the activity until the next cramping and aching. As the arteries become further narrowed, less and less activity is needed to produce the ache in your legs. Also, sores, cuts, and bruises on your feet heal slowly because your circulation is poor.

Medication and/or surgery can help combat limb disease. Pentoxifylline (Trental) can help you feel fewer symptoms and increase your ability to exercise. If the problem is severe, you can have surgery to bypass the narrowed sections of arteries or to open the narrow parts. The surgery is complex, involves a long recuperation, and is usually only undertaken when symptoms are severe and good results can be expected.

HARDENING OF THE ARTERIES AND HEART DISEASE

Coronary artery disease occurs when the critical arteries feeding the heart muscle develop many tiny irregularities in the inner linings of their walls. Cholesterol, fats, and blood platelets stick to the walls,

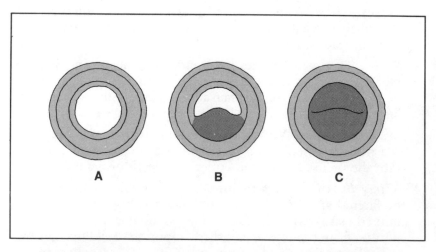

Figure 17. Atherosclerosis   In artherosclerosis, a normal artery (**A**) gradually becomes clogged with a hard film called plaque (**B**). Eventually the deposit and the blood clot forming around it may block the artery completely (**C**).

causing damage and decreasing the size of the arteries. This is the process of arteriosclerosis, or hardening of the arteries, which, over the course of decades, impedes blood flow and delivery of oxygen to the heart and converts arteries from open, smooth pipelines to narrow, partially or even completely blocked ones. Premenopausal women are less susceptible to heart disease because, somehow, female hormones exert a protective effect on the arteries.

Risk Factors for Coronary Artery Disease
Included among the risk factors for coronary artery disease are the following:

1. *Family history of heart disease.* The stronger the family background of heart disease (especially if family members experienced heart attacks under age fifty-five), the greater the risk.

2. *High blood pressure.* Elevated pressures accelerate damage to the coronary arteries.

3. *Diabetes mellitus.* This disease is associated with accelerated hardening of the arteries, especially the smaller arteries.

4. *Diet high in animal fat and low in fiber.* Such a diet may predispose certain people to heart disease. It contains a greater amount of low-density lipoproteins, which aggravate arteriosclerosis, relative to the amount of high-density lipoproteins, which protect against arteriosclerosis (see chapter 11).

5. *Smoking.* Cigarette smokers have a 60 percent greater chance of developing heart disease than nonsmokers.

6. *Lack of exercise.* If you get little or no physical exercise, you may increase the chances of coronary artery disease.

Angina
Angina is pain or pressure in the chest from an insufficient supply of oxygen to the heart muscle. It is a signal that there is disease of the coronary arteries that, at times, prevents your heart muscle from getting the oxygen it needs.

When you have coronary artery disease, the coronary arteries can usually supply enough blood and oxygen to allow you to go about routine activities. However, if you try to exercise strenuously, go out into wintry weather, try shoveling snow, or get very nervous and excited, you suddenly feel a tight pressure in the chest. In most cases, no damage is done to the heart muscle. If you stop your activity and let your heart rest, the pain usually goes away.

Certain conditions and activities reduce the amount of oxygen supplied to the heart muscle. These include the following:

1. *High blood pressure.* This condition forces the heart muscle to pump against a greater resistance.
2. *Anemia.* The heart must beat faster to circulate the diminished number of red blood cells more rapidly through the body.
3. *Fever.* The heart beats faster and requires more oxygen because all metabolic processes are sped up.
4. *Cold weather.* Cold detours blood from the skin into blood vessels of deeper, more vital organs, increasing the pressure in these vessels.
5. *Stress, anxiety, and fear.* These feelings speed up the heartbeat and tighten the arteries.
6. *Exercise.* Those exercises that make your muscles clamp down (isometrics) rather than stretch are especially risky.
7. *Smoking.* If you smoke a pack a day or more, about 10 percent of the oxygen carried in your red blood cells will be replaced by carbon monoxide, which does not nourish your tissues.
8. *High thyroid activity.* The thyroid hormone speeds up your metabolism and increases the work of your heart.

Symptoms of Angina

The typical angina attack is often described as a pressure, more than a pain, that occurs in the center of the chest under the breastbone. It feels as if a weight is standing or pressing on the chest wall. An individual may even feel the pressure—or a dull, aching sensation—in the upper abdomen, upper back, neck, jaw, shoulder, both arms, or left arm only.

Teresa O., sixty-two, always felt that she was as strong as a horse. She was not the type to wait for a man to carry her groceries or suitcases. One cold November day, she was carrying two parcels up the hill to her home. First she felt a bit queasy; then she noticed a tight, pressing sensation right in the center of her chest. Her breathing was rapid, and she felt sweaty. "Oh, Lord, am I having a heart attack?" she wondered. She put the bundles down and caught her breath. The pressure slowly retreated.

A passing gentleman noticed her pallor and offered to carry her bundles home. She called her doctor, who asked to see her in his office right away. He found her blood pressure elevated, and Teresa admitted that in the past few weeks, she had not been faithful about taking her blood pressure pills. The doctor took an ECG and found it to be completely normal, which he said only meant that she had not had a heart attack.

He asked Teresa to come to the hospital two weeks later for a stress test. She had to walk at ever faster paces on a treadmill. Pretty soon, she was huffing and puffing, and suddenly the pressure returned. She stopped, and the doctor gave her a nitroglycerin pill to put under her tongue. The pressure was relieved within a minute. He told her that her ECG had looked somewhat abnormal when she had felt the pain in her chest and diagnosed her pain as angina.

From that time on, Teresa learned to take things a bit easier. She had her groceries delivered. She stopped moving heavy furniture. Most important, she decided to give up smoking and take her blood pressure pills regularly.

Diagnosis of Angina

The key to diagnosing angina lies in the history of the pain. The doctor asks you to describe the pain or pressure you've experienced: its intensity, its duration, where it arose and where it radiated (the arms, upper abdomen, upper back, shoulders, neck, or jaw), what made it come on, and what made it go away.

The distinguishing features of angina are the consistency of the intensity of the pressure; the consistency of the duration of the discomfort, usually two to five minutes; the consistency of the location of the discomfort; and the consistency of the amount of exercise, cold, or anxiety causing the pain.

Many other organs can produce chest pain that feels very much like heart pain. What distinguishes heart pain from these other types of chest pain is its consistency and its association with activity that increases the oxygen demands of the heart muscle.

Your doctor will take an electrocardiogram, or ECG, which may show either a normal pattern or some slight changes in the heart's electrical waves that suggest strain on the heart. You may also have to take a stress ECG, which records your heart's electrical activity while you exercise—either on a treadmill or an exercise bicycle. Sometimes, dye is injected into an arm vein, and pictures are taken of your heart after exertion to reveal impaired areas in the heart muscle. Your doctor may still be unsure whether you have angina and, for diagnostic purposes, prescribe nitroglycerin, to be used at the time of pain. If the pill relieves your pain within minutes, the pain is likely, though not certainly, to be angina. In time, the diagnosis is usually clear.

Occasionally, if the diagnosis is unclear or if the doctor wants to evaluate the condition of your coronary arteries with the possibility of surgery in mind, he or she will request coronary angiography.

This technique involves passing a tiny tube through a major artery of a limb to your coronary arteries. Dye is injected, and X-ray pictures are taken. The procedure carries some risk of causing abnormal rhythms or a heart attack.

Treatment of Angina

You relieve angina by reducing the oxygen demand on your heart—by diminishing its work. If you suffer an attack, do the following:

- Stop whatever you are doing—exercising, working, or any other activity.
- Get out of the cold.
- Use meditation, mind control, or relaxation exercises to decrease anxiety or stress. Take several slow, deep breaths; close your eyes, and concentrate on relaxing your body (see chapter 14).
- If your doctor prescribes nitroglycerin, put a pill under your tongue when you have chest pain. It will open up blood vessels in your body within seconds, making it easier for your heart to pump, and thus reducing its oxygen needs. Nitroglycerin tablets must be protected from too much light and should be less than a year old to be effective. Usually, you feel a burning under the tongue as you take one and a pounding headache afterward. Some women may feel dizzy when they take the pill, so it is best to sit down first.

Attacks of angina can be reduced or eliminated by additional drug treatment. Three classes of medications are used separately or in combination: long-acting nitroglycerins, beta blockers, and calcium channel blockers. Because of the possible side effects and the importance of closely monitoring the drugs' effectiveness, women taking these medications should see their doctors at least every six months.

Long-acting nitroglycerins can be patched or pasted on the skin—as are Nitro-Dur, Nitro-Derm, Nitrodisc, or Nitro-Paste—or swallowed as tablets, as is Isordil. They reduce the work of the heart by relaxing the muscular walls of the arteries into which the heart must pump blood. The major side effects, headache and low blood pressure, can usually be handled by adjusting the dose.

Beta blockers such as propranolol (Inderal), metoprolol (Lopressor), atenolol (Tenormin), and nadolol (Corgard) decrease the heart rate and reduce the force with which the heart muscle pumps, thereby reducing its work. Some women experience fatigue, low blood pressure, slow heart rates, hallucinations, worsening asthma, and/or weakening of the heart muscle—symptoms that make these drugs unacceptable for them.

Calcium channel blockers such as nifedipine (Procardia), verapamil (Isoptin), and diltiazem (Cardizem) also ease the work of the heart by opening up the coronary arteries. These drugs may have less risk of weakening heart muscle and fewer side effects than many of the beta blockers.

Angina as a Warning Signal

If your chest pain comes on at rest, or with much less than the usual and predictable activity, if you feel much more intense or longer lasting pain, or if you have many episodes of angina within hours or within one day, call your physician immediately or go to the emergency room of the nearest hospital. Your symptoms may signal the possibility of an impending heart attack.

Often, you will merely need a period of observation and an adjustment of your medications.

Surgical Treatments for Angina

Debate still exists within the medical community about when more risky procedures or surgery should be undertaken. When angina cannot be prevented by treating all the factors that might worsen it (high blood pressure, anemia, high thyroid activity, stress, and others) and when, despite medications, you are unable to do the things you would normally like to do, it is time to consider further investigations.

Cardiac catheterization permits doctors to evaluate the condition of the muscle, valves, and chambers of your heart. It is a necessary procedure before any heart surgery is done. A tiny plastic tube is passed into your heart chambers through a major limb vein and artery, and the pressures in the chambers are measured.

Coronary bypass surgery reroutes blood around partially blocked coronary arteries through a new channel (usually a leg vein that the surgeon grafts to the coronary artery, attaching one end before the block and the other end just after the block).

The surgery can restore normal blood flow and is, in a very real sense, a second chance. Unfortunately, its risks can include heart damage, stroke, pneumonia, and, in rare cases, death.

The significant medical and surgical achievements of recent years have brought the agony of difficult choices. You and your doctor must make these decisions together, and you need to

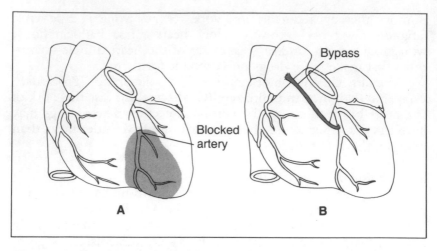

Figure 18. Coronary Bypass Surgery   Coronary bypass surgery is performed when plaque in a coronary artery blocks most of the blood supply to part of the heart (shaded part of **A**). A blood vessel taken from the leg is grafted above and below the blockage, allowing the blood to bypass it (**B**).

become informed and knowledgeable if you are to participate. Explore libraries and bookstores for books on heart disease, cardiac catheterization, and coronary bypass surgery that will help you make an informed choice.

Preventing Heart Disease
    The following precautions should be taken in an effort to prevent heart disease.

1. If you have high blood pressure, go on a low-salt diet, watch your weight, and take any medications your doctor prescribes.
2. If you are a diabetic, strive to achieve good blood-sugar control. Also, exercise on a regular basis (see chapter 5).
3. Try to remain active and "in shape." Walk every day instead of riding and develop hobbies that require moving so that you can reduce stress as well as get some exercise (see chapter 2).
4. Eat less red meat, less animal fats, and less cholesterol; eat more roughage (see chapter 11).
5. Stop smoking. If you cannot stop, at least avoid high-tar, high-

nicotine cigarettes, and limit yourself to no more than ten per day.

6. Reduce your weight, slowly and permanently, to within five pounds of ideal weight.

HEART ATTACK

A heart attack is caused by the sudden closing off of a coronary artery, usually by a blood clot, that results in injury or death to parts of the heart muscle.

Usually there is intense "crushing" pressure under the breastbone, often radiating into the neck or left arm, or both arms, and accompanied by shortness of breath, sweating, nausea, and a feeling of doom. Women who have had angina instantly recognize the pressure as more intense. If you have any of these symptoms, you need to take immediate action:

- Call an ambulance—you need hospital care.
- Put one or two tablets of nitroglycerin under your tongue and repeat this in five minutes if there is no relief.
- If you have shortness of breath, try to sit up or elevate your upper body, rather than lie down.
- Try to have someone stay with you. If this person knows CPR (cardiopulmonary resuscitation) techniques, he or she should be prepared to perform them if your pulse stops or if you stop breathing.

The ambulance personnel will check your blood pressure and pulse and put an oxygen mask over your mouth or oxygen prongs into your nose. In the emergency room, you will probably have many nurses and doctors working on you at once, taking an ECG, taking blood tests, putting in intravenous lines, giving you pills, and setting you up on a heart monitor. All this can be very frightening. The medical personnel are trying to work as quickly as possible to make a diagnosis and begin treatment. Then you will be transferred to the coronary care unit and monitored intensively for several days.

CONGESTIVE HEART FAILURE

Healthy heart muscle has a lot of strength and ability to stretch. Heart muscle that has been weakened from heart attacks or from long-standing high blood pressure loses its elasticity, becomes flabby, and is unable to pump blood effectively. The result is that blood backs up, and fluid leaks into the lungs. This condition is called heart failure, though the heart has not actually failed and is still pumping. Symptoms of congestive heart failure include these:

- Shortness of breath when lying flat. You may need to sleep propped up on two or more pillows for comfort.
- Wakefulness during the night. You may have to sit on the edge of the bed or near an open window to catch your breath.
- Shortness of breath when exerting yourself—climbing stairs, walking up a hill, making a bed, and so on.
- Swelling in the ankles. If you press your finger into the skin, it leaves a depression for a few minutes.
- Feeling "blah," without energy or desire to do any of your usual activities.
- Lack of appetite.
- Falling from weakness.
- Losing the will to live.

Treatment of Heart Failure
    The following is recommended for treatment of heart failure:
- Reduce your salt intake.
- Slow down. Your heart is stressed, and you should avoid excessive exertion or anxiety.
- Sleep with your head on two or more pillows. You will rest more comfortably.
- Put your legs up on a small stool when you sit during the day.
- Take medications. A drug often used to treat heart failure is digoxin, an extract from a plant (foxglove, or digitalis) that may be growing in your garden. It has been used effectively since the latter part of the eighteenth century. Digoxin increases the pumping force of the failing heart and slows your heart rate. Because too much digoxin can cause harmful disturbances in heart rhythm, you should never take more than what is prescribed, and you should be monitored closely by your doctor. If your pulse feels irregular, if you feel dizzy, or if your vision seems

"yellow," call your doctor, who can check your blood for an excessive level of digoxin and check your heart rhythm on an ECG.

Diuretics are usually prescribed to remove salt and water from your blood and body tissues. Some common diuretics are furosemide (Lasix), hydrochlorothiazide (HydroDIURIL), and chlorthalidone (Hygroton).

Vasodilators such as hydralazine (Apresoline), long-acting nitrites such as isosorbide dinitrate (Isordil), and nitroglycerin (Nitro-Dur) open up the blood vessels and make it easier for a weakened heart to pump blood through the body.

With proper care of a failing heart, a person can live comfortably for years and years.

STROKE

Stroke causes the death of brain cells by cutting off their blood supply. Although stroke is the third leading cause of death in older people in the United States, after heart disease and cancer, the death rate from stroke decreased by 46 percent between 1968 and 1981, perhaps because Americans are eating better, exercising more, smoking less, and treating high blood pressure earlier.

Until recently, doctors were unable to interfere in the progression and outcome of stroke. The paralyzed victims were watched and then sent for rehabilitation to learn to live with their disabilities. Fortunately, today we can recognize warning signs of stroke that can save lives and improve outcomes.

Blood supply to a part of the brain can be interrupted by three kinds of events: thrombosis, embolism, and hemorrhage.

Thrombosis is the most common cause of stroke and occurs when accumulating clots (thrombi), which form on the fatty deposits inside blood vessels, block the arteries. Embolism refers to a blood clot (embolus) that travels from a fairly large artery to a more distant, narrow artery, where it causes blockage. Hemorrhage is the rupture of a major cerebral blood vessel that causes bleeding into the brain. Brain hemorrhage accounts for less than 5 percent of all stroke in older women and results from inborn weakness of the walls of large arteries, or from arterial walls weakened by the ravages of years of high blood pressure.

Stroke afflicts men and women equally, and its incidence increases with age. Of the Americans who suffer different types of strokes, two-thirds survive, and about one-third of those who do make a nearly complete recovery.

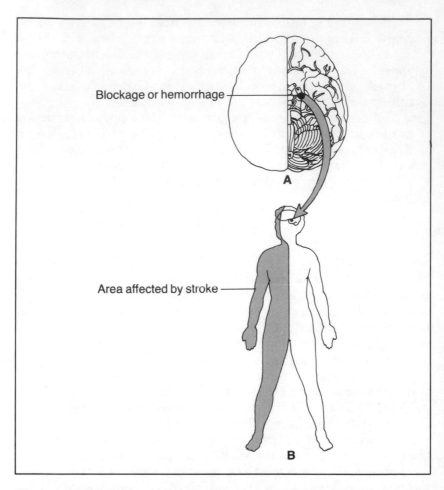

Figure 19. Stroke   A stroke occurs when part of the brain is damaged because its blood supply is interrupted (**A**). In some cases, an artery is blocked by a blood clot or another obstruction; in others, a blood vessel bursts and bleeds into surrounding brain tissue. Abilities governed by the affected brain area are temporarily or permanently impaired; often impairment occurs on only one side of the body—the side opposite the location of the stroke (**B**).

Approximate Rate of Strokes per Age Group in Women

Age	Number of Strokes per 1,000
55–64	3
65–74	8
75 and over	22

Risk Factors for Stroke

Stroke is associated with several risk factors.

1. *High blood pressure.* This condition is the most significant cause of stroke in women aged forty-five to seventy-four. Women who neglect even mild high blood pressure are apt to suffer more stroke than those with normal blood pressure. Treatment of the high blood pressure can prevent recurrences and diminish fatalities.

2. *Heart disease.* Women who have rheumatic heart disease and irregular heartbeats or who have had a heart attack run a high risk of developing clots that can travel to the brain.

3. *High blood cholesterol and high blood sugar, when associated with high blood pressure.*

4. *Obesity.* Being more than 30 percent above your ideal weight increases the tendency to hypertension and diabetes, conditions that augment the risk of having a stroke.

5. *Estrogen pills taken after menopause.* Studies have shown that estrogen-replacement therapy can elevate blood pressure in some women and increase the tendency to clotting in others. Both these factors predispose you to strokes.

6. *Smoking.* While smoking has been proven to increase stroke risk in men, it has not yet been so proven for women. Nevertheless, it is wise to consider smoking a potential risk factor for women as well.

7. *Severe migraine headaches.*

Symptoms of Stroke

Alla R., sixty-eight, got out of bed one morning and found that she was unsteady on her feet. She called her husband and noticed that her speech was very slurred, almost as if she were drunk. Her doctor recommended that she go to the emergency room right away, where her blood pressure was found to be 180/96. She was admitted to the hospital with a diagnosis of stroke.

For the next few days, Alla felt weakness on the left side of her body, particularly in her left leg. Her speech continued to be slurred. The doctors tried to control her blood pressure and her blood sugar, which was quite erratic, despite the Orinase tablets she was taking.

On the third day, a young woman from the physical therapy department came up and began to help her stand and walk again with the aid of a walker. A speech therapist gave Alla instruction in speaking. When Alla left the hospital a week later, she was speaking quite well and walking with the aid of a cane only.

Mary M., sixty, came into the hospital with a ten-year history of high blood pressure. For a few days, she had noticed blurred and sometimes absent vision in her left eye and, on the day she came in, some weakness of her right arm and leg. She was limping, and her hand shook when she tried to hold a cup of coffee. The same thing had occurred a month before, but it had completely disappeared within ten minutes, so she had put the whole episode out of her mind.

She was admitted to the hospital and treated with blood thinners. She then had some diagnostic studies, which showed that her left carotid artery was almost completely blocked. The doctor started some treatments and recommended a surgical procedure to remove the blockage.

The symptoms of stroke depend on which parts of the brain are affected. Certain areas control subtle functions such as the size of the pupil of the eye; other areas control more sweeping functions such as movement of the leg, sensation in the arm, or balance. Still other areas of the brain regulate breathing, blood pressure, or your state of alertness.

Sometimes stroke symptoms can progress slowly over many hours or days and then very slowly start to disappear—a common pattern with thrombosis. Or, the symptoms can appear all of a sudden, which is often the case in strokes caused by embolism. A severe brain hemorrhage can start with a sudden severe headache and confusion, with a resulting progressive decrease in consciousness.

These are some of the symptoms of stroke:

- double, blurred, or absent vision
- loss or decrease of sensation in parts of the body
- weakness of an arm, leg, or several limbs at once
- loss of balance
- thick speech or trouble controlling the tongue
- difficulty in finding words or garbled speech
- difficulty in understanding words
- drooling or trouble swallowing
- sudden loss of memory
- diminished alertness
- seizures (convulsions)
- severe pain in the head

- sudden loss of consciousness
- extremes of emotion without cause (laughing, crying, or acting out of control)

Three-fourths of people who have strokes have experienced some of these symptoms as early warning signals prior to the stroke. One-third of people who have these signals—transient ischemic attacks, or TIAs—go on to have a full stroke within a year's time. A woman with a TIA might suddenly have trouble reading, writing, speaking, or thinking. She might have one or more symptoms, such as trouble understanding what is said; garbled speech; double vision; or numbness or weakness in an arm, a leg, or in both.

The symptoms of a TIA begin very suddenly, reach a peak within five minutes, and start to fade within minutes to half an hour. On rare occasions, symptoms can last as long as twenty-four hours.

It is always important to alert your doctor if you have any one or a combination of the symptoms listed above. Your doctor may want to start you on treatment and observe you carefully for a while. If you cannot reach your doctor, go to the emergency room of your hospital.

Diagnosis of Stroke

The diagnosis of stroke requires a careful history and a physical and neurological examination. The doctor checks your level of alertness and memory, your ability to perform certain tasks, your ability to feel and differentiate a touch from a pinprick in many places on your body, your muscle strength, and your coordination and balance.

The doctor will look into your eyes with a special light to see the condition of your blood vessels and optic nerves and will listen to the carotid arteries in your neck for blockages of the flow of blood to your brain.

Next, the doctor will try to make sure that there are not other or additional explanations for your symptoms—a heart attack that may have caused a stroke, an infection that has extended to the brain, an immune disorder that also affects blood vessels in the brain, or a tumor. The full diagnosis requires further tests, including blood analyses, an electrocardiogram, and X rays.

These are several specialized neurological tests that help diagnose a stroke:

1. A spinal tap, which removes for analysis the fluid from the spine that bathes the brain and spinal cord.

2. Skull X rays, which help diagnose fractures of the skull that may have caused bleeding on the brain.

3. CAT scan (computerized axial tomography), a sophisticated examination in which a radioactive dye is used to illuminate the blood vessels to the brain and brain tissue itself, allowing recognition of damaged areas and diagnosis of even small interruptions in brain blood flow and, possibly, blood clots and brain tumors.

4. EEG (electroencephalogram), an examination that records brain waves to diagnose seizures, or abnormal electrical signals, from parts of the brain.

5. Oculoplethysmography, which records the blood pressure in the eyes, to determine whether the pressures are roughly equal. A dramatically lower pressure in one eye suggests blockage of one of the major arteries (carotid artery) to the brain.

6. Arterial angiography, which involves taking X rays of the brain as dye courses through its arteries. The procedure permits blockages or abnormal patterns of blood flow to be seen and diagnosed. In rare cases, the plastic tube through which dye is injected may dislodge small plaques that are present in arteries and cause a stroke.

7. Intravenous digital angiography, a new test, gives a computerized analysis of arterial pattern in the brain to see if there is any blockage. Whether the results are as good with this safer technique remains to be seen.

Treatment of Stroke

The treatment of stroke victims is still controversial in medical practice; however, research in this decade should clarify some of the debated issues.

Any patient undergoing a stroke is given oxygen through the nose or mouth. The doctors try to lower the blood pressure to normal ranges to prevent spread of the damage. In some instances, blood thinners, such as heparin, given intravenously, or Coumadin (warfarin), dipyridamole, or aspirin, given by mouth, are used to prevent enlargement of the blood clot causing the stroke and to prevent new clots from forming.

Neurosurgery can be helpful in transient ischemic attacks or in certain types of stroke. Doctors can reopen large clogged arteries by threading tiny balloons through them, by cleaning out plaques from the walls of the arteries, or by using lasers to unclog the arteries. They can even create an alternative route around blockages.

Some Swedish researchers have been able to reduce the degree of brain injury during a stroke by injecting dextran or other drugs into the veins of stroke victims to thicken their blood. These drugs draw fluid out of the brain, diminishing its swelling and allowing more blood to flow to the injured area. Some American researchers have used the spinal fluid as a vehicle to bring more oxygen and nutrients to injured brain tissue.

Rehabilitation of the Stroke Patient

Stroke conjures up terrible fears: of being handicapped and losing independence, of losing the love of a spouse or family, of having another stroke and ending up in a nursing home, or of dying. The disabilities produced by a stroke combined with these fears can result in profound discouragement and depression.

Nothing helps a stroke patient more than to start focusing on her strengths. Within a few days of a stroke, physical and occupational therapy begins. Paralyzed or weak limbs that cannot be exercised voluntarily are moved by a therapist to keep the joints limber and to maintain tone in the muscles. Patients are taught to use the strong arm or leg to exercise the weak one. Depending on the extent of the stroke, a patient may have to relearn all kinds of basic skills, including getting out of bed, sitting up and dressing, and bathing, grooming, feeding, and toileting herself properly and safely. The patient may need speech therapy to help her pronounce words better or find the proper words. The occupational therapist may give the patient special instruments that make life easier: a device for reaching high objects; forks, knives, and spoons with thick handles; plates with suction cups on the bottom; clothes with Velcro closures rather than buttons, and so on. As motivation and confidence return, the individual can train healthy muscles to take over the work of those that are stricken. The patient may need to simplify home routines and use memory aids such as notes, special pill dispensers, and appointment calendars. When the stroke patient returns home from the hospital, she may need help in the house (see chapter 17) and may benefit from the service of a visiting nurse, social worker, and/or therapist for a period of time.

The hardest adaptation for the patient is getting used to the image of herself disabled—using a cane or walker, wearing a leg brace, or sitting in a wheelchair. A depressed patient might benefit from psychotherapy or group therapy with other people who have had strokes. Antidepressant medication may also be used (see chapter 14).

Stroke clubs are a haven if you have had a stroke and currently are learning to adapt to your new circumstances. Organized by people who have recovered from strokes, the clubs help others cope with common difficulties such as how to get help in the home, how to cope with the tensions that a disability can put on relationships, and when and how to resume sexual activities. The American Heart Association in your area can tell you whether such a group is available locally.

Prevention of Stroke

Since the risk factors for stroke are very similar to those for heart attack, striving to reduce these risk factors helps you attack two killer diseases with one major effort. In addition, you may want to take two aspirin a day, unless you have reason not to take aspirin (are taking blood thinners, have allergies, or have a history of bleeding tendencies or bleeding ulcers). Check with your doctor to see that taking aspirin will not be harmful in your particular case.

VARICOSE VEINS

Rarely does a woman go through life without being plagued at some time or other by her veins. For reasons that are not well understood, women are more susceptible to varicose veins than are men. This susceptibility is aggravated by pregnancy, when the enlarging uterus partially obstructs the veins draining the legs and causes the veins to stretch out and drain less effectively.

Varicose veins are seen as unsightly distensions of the surface veins that have lost the normal tone in their walls and that bulge out against the skin's surface. You can see them as bluish bulging lines, often causing a discoloration or darkening and thickening of the overlying skin.

The surface varicose veins are not, themselves, the root of the problem, but rather a consequence. The real problem lies in the deep veins, which are usually swollen, weakened, and unable to effectively return blood up your legs.

Normal Blood Flow Through the Leg Veins

Veins drain blood from the legs to the heart. The largest veins in the legs, the deep veins, are embedded in the muscles of the legs. Just under the skin are the superficial veins, a series of smaller veins that drain blood from the skin and underlying tissues. Blood from these surface veins flows into the deep veins through perforating veins.

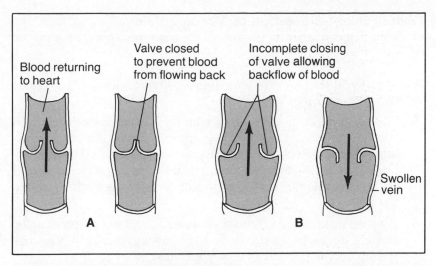

Figure 20. Varicose Veins   Varicose veins result from damage to valves in the veins. These valves normally prevent the backflow of blood (**A**). If they do not close completely, blood pools below the damaged valve, stretching and twisting the vein (**B**).

There is a steady flow of blood from the superficial veins, through the perforating veins, into the deep veins. The muscles of the legs, squeezing and exerting pressure on your deep veins as you go through your regular activities, push blood uphill against gravity (when you stand) into your pelvis. The veins have baggy valves at frequent intervals; these valves keep the blood from flowing backward (see figure 20).

Swollen Legs

When the deep veins lose their ability to return blood efficiently to the pelvis and ultimately the heart, the amount of blood in your legs builds up and prevents fluid that is in the leg tissues from returning to the leg veins. Your tissues then swell. The swelling, or edema, can become so great that the skin overlying it breaks down, forming blisters, and, finally, a sore that may take months to heal (a venous ulcer).

Characteristically, the swelling in your legs worsens as the day goes along and disappears by the time you awaken from a night's sleep. This change occurs because when you lie down, your blood no longer has to travel uphill to get to the heart; it can flow from your legs much more easily than when you stand.

Treatment and Prevention of Varicose Veins
Several measures can be taken to treat and prevent varicose veins.

1. When you rest, elevate your legs as often as possible to reduce the pressure of gravity.
2. Put pressure on the outside of your legs to help blood flow into your deep veins. You can buy support hose, or elastic stockings, in pharmacies or from surgical supply houses. Do not buy hose that end below the knee, since the strong elastic top will act as a tourniquet, slowing blood from flowing back up above the knee.
3. Exercise regularly. Exercise such as walking, or even pressing or tapping your feet on the floor while sitting, can help push the venous blood upward out of your legs.
4. Reduce if you are overweight, since a heavy abdomen or obese legs press down on the veins and block the flow of blood back to the heart.
5. Avoid standing in one place for long periods of time, since the force of gravity against the veins is the worst in the standing position. If you must stand much of the day, wear support hose and keep moving your feet and leg muscles.

For years, women have sought cosmetic relief from varicose veins by vein stripping or injections. Today doctors feel that there is rarely justification for the risk, discomfort, and expense that are associated with the surgery. All vein stripping does is remove the ugly superficial veins. It does nothing to solve the real problem, the incompetent deep veins, so within months, new varicosities return close to the places where the old ones were stripped away. You are left with the scars of surgery and new varicose veins.

PHLEBITIS

Phlebitis is an inflammation of a vein, which can either result from or produce a blood clot inside the vein. In superficial veins, this will appear as a hard, perhaps tender, warm bulge in the area of a vein. Although quite uncomfortable, superficial phlebitis is not a serious problem and will go away if you use warm compresses and elevate and rest your leg.
When the blood clot forms in the deep leg veins, particularly in

the thigh area, the problem can, in fact, be life-threatening. Usually blood returning from the leg is almost completely blocked, producing dramatic swelling, tenderness, redness, and warmth of the calf or thigh that do not disappear or improve with overnight sleep or elevation of the legs. These are important warning signals, requiring immediate medical attention from your physician or from doctors at a hospital emergency room.

A deep clot can be serious because part or all of the clot can dislodge from your leg vein and travel through your abdominal veins, into your heart, and then out to your lungs. Blood clots in the lungs (pulmonary emboli) block the flow of oxygen from large segments of lung tissue into your blood, leaving the blood oxygen-poor. Your heart, brain, and other body tissues become starved for oxygen and can malfunction, threatening your life.

Deep vein clots are diagnosed by your physician after careful examination and are confirmed by one or both of two tests: a venogram or an IPG. A venogram, which is an X ray of the veins of your leg taken after dye has been injected into a foot vein, will reveal any major vein blockages. A less complicated but also less accurate test is an IPG (impedance plethysmogram), which can estimate the pressure and the flow of blood in different parts of your leg by use of a machine placed on the outside of the leg.

If deep clots are diagnosed, you will be hospitalized in order to be given intravenous blood-thinning medication (heparin) for a few days. The doctor will prescribe oral blood-thinner medication—warfarin (Coumadin)—to be taken for three to six months to prevent new clots from forming.

ANEMIA

All cells of the body need oxygen to survive and do their work. They receive this oxygen from the red blood cells—which transport it on their major protein, hemoglobin. Hemoglobin is formed by the union of iron and a protein, globin. Other minerals and vitamins, principally B_{12} and folic acid, are also vital in the manufacture of blood.

The production of red blood cells is controlled by a hormone, erythropoietin, made in the kidney and released when oxygen levels in the blood are low. Blood cells are manufactured in the bone marrow, the spleen, the lymph nodes, the liver, and specialized cells scattered throughout the body. They circulate an average of 120 days before they are removed by the spleen and the liver. The amount of red blood cells present in the bloodstream depends on the balance between their production and their destruction.

When you have insufficient red blood cells to transport the oxygen, you are said to be anemic. Your body compensates by circulating your blood more quickly. Your heart pumps faster, and your lungs breathe more rapidly. The result is more stress upon your body.

Causes of Anemia
Anemia can be due to any of the following causes.

1. Loss of blood.
2. Production problems. These can include iron deficiency, vitamin B_{12} and folic acid deficiency, and severe protein deficiency.
3. Disorders of underproduction and overdestruction. Such disorders may include defects in hemoglobin (sickle-cell anemia and thalassemia), chronic disease (cancer, rheumatoid arthritis, and infection), liver or kidney disease, glandular disorders (low thyroid and low cortisone), invasion and takeover of bone marrow (leukemia, lymphoma, and metastasis), and hemolysis (G-6-P-D deficiency of red cells or drug-related destruction of red cells).

The most common causes of anemia in older women are iron deficiency, blood loss, and vitamin deficiency. In the United States, as many as 13 percent of adult women and 55 percent of pregnant women are deficient in iron.

Symptoms of Anemia

Juanita D., fifty-six, was used to active gardening, golfing, and swimming at her summer home. Before one vacation, the pressure and deadlines of her job were particularly stressful. She had bad headaches, which she treated with aspirin. Her old ulcer also kicked up, and Juanita gobbled antacids, hoping that these would treat the harmful effects of the stress and aspirin.

Now that she was on vacation, she found to her surprise that she was exhausted after twenty minutes of pulling up weeds. The next day, while golfing with friends, she huffed and puffed up small inclines and developed a bad headache. She went home early and tried to read but was distracted by black spots in front of her eyes, a headache, and a sense of faintness.

A close friend who stopped by that evening was upset by her pallor and took her to a local doctor. The doctor found Juanita severely anemic from a bleeding ulcer. She was immediately admitted to the hospital for blood transfusions and stronger ulcer treatment. The doctor felt that by taking aspirin for her headaches, Juanita had probably worsened her ulcer, causing it to bleed. He warned her never to take aspirin again.

The symptoms of anemia depend on its severity and on a person's physical reserves. Headaches, faintness, spots in front of the eyes, ringing in the ears, loss of appetite, nausea, drowsiness, and exhaustion are common symptoms. The anemic woman appears pale, has pale nailbeds and conjunctiva (the normally pink rims inside the eyelids), and is very sensitive to cold. Long-standing anemia can cause hair loss and thin skin that bruises easily.

If a woman is basically healthy with only slight anemia, she may just feel a bit of fatigue and shortness of breath when exerting herself. Women with mild heart disease as well as mild anemia may feel very tired, grow short of breath when walking, and feel some chest pain. Anemic women with heart disease may also develop heart failure in conjunction with even mild degrees of anemia.

Diagnosis and Treatment of Anemia

Anemia should not be self-diagnosed or self-treated. Most anemias have an underlying cause, and treating symptoms alone does not resolve the basic problem. (If Juanita, in the case above, had simply treated her symptoms with iron, she might have ended up with a perforated ulcer.)

If you suspect you are anemic, you need to have a thorough medical examination that explores all your symptoms and your drug history. Your blood, stool, and urine samples should be checked, and you should have rectal and pelvic examinations.

In some instances, you may need to be hospitalized for more complex investigations such as a bone marrow examination, X-ray studies of your intestines, or a liver-spleen scan.

Anemia Caused by Blood Loss or Low Iron Stores

When your anemia is caused by blood loss, the source of bleeding must first be found, the bleeding stopped, and transfusions given, if needed. Transfused blood cells survive only 30 to 60 days, as opposed to the usual 120 days, so they must be replaced quickly.

If your diet has been low in iron over months or years, your marrow produces smaller red blood cells containing less hemoglobin, and ultimately fewer red cells, causing anemia. You will need iron pills or injections to replace your body stores as well as vitamin C to help you absorb iron.

Anemia Caused by Vitamin Deficiency

You are more prone to pernicious anemia, a deficiency of vitamin B_{12}, as you age. This deficiency is caused by an abnormality in part of your stomach that prevents it from producing acid and from producing the hormone that allows the absorption of vitamin B_{12} from your food. To compensate, you will need monthly injections of vitamin B_{12}, since your intestines will not absorb enough of the vitamin taken by mouth.

Deficiency of the vitamin folic acid can also result in anemia. Your body stores enough folic acid to last only a few months, so you must regularly eat fresh vegetables in which folic acid is found or take folic acid tablets until your stores are built up again.

Anemia Caused by Destruction of Blood Cells

About 10 percent of black women and a smaller percent of Caucasian women of Mediterranean extraction have an inborn deficiency of a chemical called G-6-P-D (glucose-6-phosphate dehydrogenase). This deficiency makes the red cells especially prone to destruction when exposed to common drugs such as acetylsalicylic acid (aspirin) or sulfonamides (Bactrim, Gantrisin), phenacetin (in Anacin, Fiorinal), and probenecid (in Benemid). Fava beans contain a chemical that can also destroy the red cells in women with G-6-P-D deficiency.

The destructive anemia ends about a week after you have stopped ingesting the offending drug or food. You can have a simple blood test to determine whether you have G-6-P-D deficiency. If you do, carefully avoid the drugs and beans mentioned above.

Occasionally, drug allergies (such as to penicillin) or sensitivity to drugs like quinine, found in quinine water, quinidine (used to treat some heart conditions), phenacetin (used in A.P.C. tablets or Fiorinal for headache), and methyldopa (used in Aldomet for lowering blood pressure) can cause massive destruction of red blood cells. If you have known drug sensitivities, avoid the offending drugs.

Sickle-Cell Trait

Sickle-cell anemia is a blood disorder almost exclusively of blacks. Red blood cells exhibiting the sickle-cell trait have an abnormal hemoglobin molecule that causes the normally doughnut-shaped cells to assume bizarre sickle and crescent shapes under conditions of low oxygen. These odd-shaped cells get trapped in the small blood vessels, are destroyed early, and cause damage to the body organs. If you have sickle-cell trait (for which you can be tested), pay extra attention to your diet and get enough iron, folic acid, and vitamin B_{12}.

SUGGESTED READINGS

Alpert, Joseph S., M.D. *The Heart Attack Handbook: A Commonsense Guide to Treatment, Recovery, and Staying Well.* Boston: Little, Brown, 1984.

American Medical Association. *Straight-Talk No-Nonsense Guide to Heartcare.* New York: Random House, 1984.

Heimlich, Henry J., M.D., with Galton, Lawrence. *Dr. Heimlich's Home Guide to Emergency Medical Situations.* New York: Simon & Schuster, Fireside Books, 1984.

Warren, James V., M.D., and Subak-Sharpe, Genell J. *Surviving Your Heart Attack: The Duke University Complete Heart Treatment Program.* Garden City, N.Y.: Doubleday, 1984.

Yalof, Ina L. *Open Heart Surgery: A Guidebook for Patients & Families.* New York: Random House, 1983.

Five

Diabetes Mellitus

Y OUR body has to convert the food you eat into the energy that keeps you going. The chemical processing plant inside you can suffer the breakdown or loss of some of its machinery (such as numerous teeth or feet of intestine) and the shutdown of some of its laboratories (such as the gallbladder). It can even sustain significant damage in others (the liver), yet still keep functioning and supplying you with energy that causes the muscles to flex, the heart to pump, and the lungs to breathe. But if certain labs close or certain supplies are unavailable, the workings of the whole factory—and therefore your health—are in jeopardy. This is what happens when you develop diabetes.

Insulin from the pancreas enables cells all over your body to take the glucose in your blood and convert it into energy. Insulin also allows your body to store excess nutrients in the liver and in the muscles as glycogen, ready to be converted into glucose during times of need.

When fuel, in the form of food, enters the intestinal tract and is absorbed, your blood-glucose level rises, and signals are sent to your pancreas. Specialized cells in the pancreas (islet of Langerhans cells), which test your blood-glucose level continuously, release the necessary amount of the hormone insulin into the bloodstream.

In diabetics, insulin is either absent or poorly utilized. Consequently, glucose builds up in the blood, unable to get into the cells that so sorely need it for energy. The diabetic eats excessively, yet feels hunger and fatigue. Unfortunately, this eating cannot satisfy the cells, since the sugar still cannot enter them but instead spills over into the urine. When urine is full of sugar, water is drawn along, so the diabetic becomes dehydrated and is always thirsty.

TYPES OF DIABETES

Diabetes is a disease that afflicts 1 percent to 3 percent of the general population of affluent societies, but 5 percent to 10 percent of people over forty years of age. The proportion is higher among Jews. The disease takes two distinct forms: insulin-dependent diabetes mellitus (formerly called juvenile diabetes because it arises mostly in childhood and adolescence) and non-insulin-dependent diabetes (also called adult or late-onset diabetes mellitus).

Although insulin-dependent diabetes mellitus usually starts in childhood or adolescence, it occasionally appears in older years, especially in women. The disease seems to be caused by a gradual destruction of the islet cells in the pancreas and is triggered by a viral infection or other stresses.

The onset is abrupt, with excessive eating, drinking, urination, and loss of weight. You can have a level of sugar in your blood that is so high that it impairs brain function or causes coma. You need immediate treatment with insulin and are likely to need daily insulin injections. Even after treatment has started, it can be difficult to control your blood-sugar levels.

Non-insulin-dependent diabetes mellitus generally starts in older age, particularly in women who are overweight. It usually begins gradually, and you may have few or no symptoms for some time before becoming diabetic. If you have this kind of diabetes, you often can be treated without drugs if you carefully regulate your diet. Only 20 percent to 30 percent of these diabetics require insulin.

RISK FACTORS FOR DIABETES

A family history of diabetes puts you at greater risk for developing the disease. Your pregnancy history can also indicate a risk factor. Women who have had high blood sugar during pregnancies or who have had babies weighing over ten pounds at birth or who have had premature deliveries, toxemia, or miscarriages are at risk for developing diabetes. Also at greater risk are women who weigh more than 25 percent over their ideal body weight.

In addition, stress, infection, lack of exercise, and improper diet can convert a tendency to diabetes into the condition itself.

SYMPTOMS OF DIABETES

General symptoms of diabetes may include the following:

- excessive thirst
- weight loss despite increased appetite in some women, or weight gain in others
- excessive urination
- recurrent skin infections such as boils, furuncles, and carbuncles behind the neck, under the arms, in the creases between the abdomen and thighs, or around the fingernails
- persistent fungal infections of the nails on the hands or feet
- persistent fungal infections of the vagina, with severe itching and discharge
- infected gums
- frequent urinary tract infections
- low blood sugar, or hypoglycemia, which may produce weakness, tremors, headache, or a washed-out feeling about three to four hours after a meal
- occasional cloudy mental consciousness and, in rare cases, signs resembling a stroke (weak arms or legs) or coma
- heart trouble or hardening of the arteries prior to menopause

DIAGNOSIS OF DIABETES

Diabetes is diagnosed by measuring the level of blood glucose. A fasting blood glucose level of 140 milligrams or more measured after a night's sleep and before breakfast, or a glucose level of 200 milligrams or more two hours after a sugar load (called a two-hour postprandial blood-sugar level) identifies the presence of the disease.

Glucose levels in the range of 140 to 200 milligrams identify borderline diabetes, also called impaired glucose tolerance. About 10 percent to 15 percent of the U.S. adult population has borderline diabetes that can become overt under conditions of stress.

Clinitest tablets, or urine dipsticks, which test for sugar in the urine, or blood fingersticks are not an adequate way to diagnose diabetes. They can, however, be a useful tool for diabetics to check on their glucose control.

The glycosylated hemoglobin test (HbA-1c) is a relatively new blood test that indicates whether diabetes has been controlled on a long-term basis, or over several months.

TREATMENT OF DIABETES MELLITUS

The goal of treatment is to help your body mimic normal physiology—that is, to maintain as normal levels of blood sugar as possible.

Diet

Most people can fast one day and feast the next, and their pancreas automatically adjusts the amount of insulin they need. If you are diabetic, you cannot allow yourself that freedom. Instead, you must standardize the amount and type of food you eat because you cannot finely adjust the amount of oral or injected medication you take.

Your diet must be individualized to meet your specific insulin requirements, your weight goal, your exercise pattern, and your likes and dislikes. Nevertheless, there are several common principles of diet treatment.

- If you need to lose weight, try to do it slowly while following a balanced diet. Maintaining your ideal weight is important because the fat cells and muscle cells of obese people are less sensitive to insulin than those of leaner people.

- Eat small meals throughout the day rather than one or two big meals. A large meal will tax your pancreas's short supply of insulin much more than will several small meals with snacks in between.

- Avoid simple sugars (such as honey, sugar, and candy). They are very rapidly absorbed into the bloodstream and may overwhelm the insulin-producing capacity of the pancreas. When you require extra energy (during strenuous activity, when you are under stress, or when you have an infection), consume more calories at regular intervals and increase your medication as needed.

- Establish and maintain regular and dependable nutritional habits (see chapter 11). The American Diabetes Association's booklet

Exchange Lists for Meal Planning can help you vary your diet while maintaining the proper number of calories and balance of carbohydrates, proteins, and fats. You and your doctor can decide which meal plan is most appropriate to your energy needs—the 1,000-calorie diet, the 1,500-calorie diet, the 1,800-calorie diet, or the 2,400-calorie diet.

When purchasing food items, do not confuse the term *dietetic* with *diabetic* on food labels. Dietetic foods are simply somewhat lower in calories and in sugar content than regular foods of the same type, but they are seldom sugar-free and are expensive. Always read labels, and remember that the words *fructose, dextrins, disaccharides, sorbitol,* and *sucrose* all mean some form of sugar.

Exercise

Exercise helps the muscle cells of diabetics absorb more blood sugar and call for less insulin. Exercise helps obese diabetics lose weight by burning up calories, and it helps lean diabetics by letting them use the food they eat instead of their own muscle cells for fuel.

Plan to adjust your diet and medication to your level of exercise. You may need to eat a little more, take a little less insulin or medication, and have some honey or candy bars on hand in case of an insulin reaction. (See "Reactions to Insulin" on page 147.)

Pills (Oral Hypoglycemics)

The sulfonylureas used to treat diabetes act by urging the pancreas to produce more insulin. These drugs are useful in older diabetics, who often have some islet cells in the pancreas, as opposed to the juvenile diabetics, who have few or none.

Chart of Oral Sulfonylureas

Generic (Brand) Name	Average Dose	Duration of Action
Tolbutamide (Orinase)	500–1,000 mg twice a day	6–12 hours
Acetohexamide (Dymelor)	250–1,000 mg per day	12–24 hours
Tolazamide (Tolinase)	100–500 mg per day	16–24 hours
Chlorpropamide (Diabinase)	100–500 mg per day	24–36 hours
Glyburide (DiaBeta)	1.25–20 mg per day	4–24 hours

Precautions with Oral Hypoglycemics

Hypoglycemic reactions are not common in patients taking oral agents, but they can occur—especially at night with the longer-

acting pills, or when you eat very little. You can prevent the night-
time hypoglycemia, which can induce nightmares or early morning
headaches, by having a small snack at bedtime. Aspirin and alcohol
can increase the sugar-lowering effects of the sulfonylureas, so these
drugs should be taken only when necessary. If you have liver or
kidney disease, you may also develop hypoglycemic reactions and
should be monitored closely by your physician. Pills do not replace
proper diet and exercise; they offer help when diet and exercise
alone have failed to control blood sugar.

Insulin

The several types of commercially available insulins vary according to how long they act.

Chart of Insulins

Type of Insulin	Time Usually Given	Peak Action Time	End of Action Time
Short-acting			
Regular	before breakfast	2–3 hours later	6 hours
Semilente	before breakfast	3–6 hours later	12 hours
Intermediate-acting			
NPH	before breakfast	8–10 hours later	18 hours
Lente	before breakfast	8–10 hours later	18 hours
Long-acting			
Ultralente	before breakfast	12–20 hours later	36 hours
Protamine Zinc	before breakfast	12–20 hours later	36 hours

Insulin is usually prescribed after a trial of diet, exercise, and
hypoglycemic pills has failed to maintain a reasonable blood-sugar
level. The majority of diabetics who require insulin can be properly
treated with one injection per day. Usually NPH insulin is used, to
provide effective action over the waking hours. If your diabetes is
more difficult to control, you may need a combination of NPH and
regular insulin in the morning. Rarely will you need two injections a
day.

If you are starting on insulin for the first time, keep the following in mind:

- Make sure you get adequate instruction (from your doctor,
  nurse, or visiting nurse) in the use and monitoring of insulin. If

you need more information, contact your local chapter of the American Diabetes Association.

- Change the site of injection each day to prevent the formation of scar tissue, which might prevent absorption of the insulin into the bloodstream.

- If you develop redness, swelling, pain, or a lump at the site of an injection, use warm compresses. Should these local reactions to the injections persist, you may have to change the type of insulin you use.

Reactions to Insulin

An insulin reaction usually occurs when the amount of insulin injected is too high for the available glucose in the blood. The symptoms of a reaction include the following:

gnawing in the stomach	sweating
rapid heartbeat	nervousness or shaking
weakness and pallor	headache
uncontrollable yawning	
mental confusion or signs resembling a stroke or coma	

Fortunately, your body has its own way of dealing with an insulin reaction. Epinephrine from the adrenal glands pours into the bloodstream and causes the liver and muscles to release all the glucose they have stored, remedying the situation somewhat.

You can relieve an insulin reaction within minutes if you eat some sugar, candy, or a chocolate bar or drink some orange juice—all provide readily absorbable glucose. If your symptoms do not abate, call, or have someone call, your doctor immediately or go to the hospital.

If you take insulin, you should maintain these safeguards:

1. Carry a card or wear a Medi-Alert bracelet or necklace that identifies you as diabetic.

2. Keep with you at all times several lumps of sugar, soft candies, or honey packs to eat immediately if you suspect that you are having an insulin reaction.

3. Learn about the symptoms and treatment of insulin reactions and give close family and friends instructions on what to do if they suspect that you are having a reaction.

4. Check your blood glucose level with a fingerstick test if you are having symptoms of an insulin reaction.

COMPLICATIONS OF DIABETES

Numerous complications can result from uncontrolled or long-term diabetes.

Disorders of the Large Blood Vessels

The arteries of the body bear the brunt of diabetes. Disorders of the larger blood vessels result in increased heart attack, stroke, and blockage of the arterial circulation to the legs.

The high incidence of these disorders in diabetic women is probably due to their likelihood of having certain risk factors: increase in blood cholesterol and triglyceride levels; significant decrease in high-density lipoproteins, which tend to protect against heart disease; and a greater incidence of hypertension than in the general population.

Disorders of the Small Blood Vessels

Long-standing or poorly controlled diabetes can damage the retinas of the eyes, which can lead to impaired vision and, in severe cases, blindness. Factors influencing the development of eye disease are diabetes of long duration with very high blood sugars and diabetes coexisting with high blood pressure, a systolic pressure over 170 (see chapter 4). Diabetics also develop cataracts at a younger age than nondiabetics and experience a more rapid progression of the condition.

Treatment of retinopathy requires controlling blood pressure and blood sugar, following a low-fat diet, and having laser beam treatments.

Long-standing diabetes damages the small blood vessels of the kidneys, causing protein to leak into the urine. Older diabetics with hypertension are especially prone to this form of kidney disease, which can lead to kidney failure and the need for dialysis.

Problems with the Feet

The feet of diabetics are particularly vulnerable to problems. Poor circulation can retard or severely impair healing of even small cuts, bruises, or burns. In addition, blocked blood flow in the smaller blood vessels can cause decreased sensation in the nerves of the foot, resulting in the diabetic being unaware that there is a foot injury. Diabetics, therefore, must take extra special care of their feet. Consider these precautions:

1. Buy shoes that fit properly when they are new. Do not expect them to "stretch out."

2. Do not walk barefoot. Do not wear shoes without stockings. Do not wear sandals with thongs between the toes.

3. Wear properly fitted stockings, without mends in the foot area.

4. Inspect your shoes for nail points, small pebbles, or torn linings, which can cause unnoticed foot damage to the diabetic with impaired sensation.

5. Take special care of your toenails. The first signs of infection often start when long, curved, or irregular nails cut the surrounding skin; fungal infections (common in diabetics) lead to irregular thickening, breaking of nails, and growth of bacteria in the dry, dead skin.

6. Inspect your toes and the skin between the toes daily for cuts, scratches, and blisters. If you find any wounds that do not improve within a few days with first aid, see your doctor.

7. Wash your feet daily and dry them carefully, especially between the toes, to prevent fungal infections.

8. Use a lubricant on your feet to keep the skin soft and smooth, but do not lubricate between the toes.

9. Avoid extremes of temperature—freezing ocean water or very hot bath water, for example.

10. If your feet are cold at night, wear woolen socks. A hot-water bottle or a heating pad may cause burns.

11. Do not cut your own corns and calluses. Do not use chemical agents to remove corns or calluses.

12. If your vision is impaired, ask a family member or friend to inspect your feet regularly and help you with foot care as prescribed by your physician or podiatrist.

13. Make sure that your doctor and podiatrist know of each other and can consult about your infections, ulcers, nerve damage, or circulatory problems.

Prevention of Diabetic Complications
While experts disagree about how well conscientious control of diabetes can prevent or retard vascular disease, it makes good sense to do the following:

1. Try to maintain as normal a blood-sugar level as possible through diet; exercise; and, when needed, insulin or oral hypoglycemics.

2. Avoid obesity. Try to achieve ideal body weight (see below).

3. Eat less saturated fat (found in foods such as red meat, butter, egg yolks, chocolate, and vegetable shortening) and more polyunsaturated fat (found in corn oil, safflower oil, fish oil, and margarine). Avoid high-cholesterol foods.

4. Eat more complex carbohydrates (found in whole-grain breads, fruits, and vegetables) and fiber (found in bran and grains).

5. Make sure that your blood pressure is in the normal range. Lower your salt intake and take medications if prescribed.

6. Stop smoking.

7. Consider taking two aspirin a day, if you can tolerate it (see chapter 2 for cautions). Aspirin seems to reduce the incidence of cataracts in diabetics.

Age-Specific Height-Weight Table

Gerontology Research Center
Age-specific Weight Range for Men and Women

Height (ft and in)	50–59 yr	60–69 yr
4 10	107–135	115–142
4 11	111–139	119–147
5 0	114–143	123–152
5 1	118–148	127–157
5 2	122–153	131–163
5 3	126–158	135–168
5 4	130–163	140–173
5 5	134–168	144–179
5 6	138–174	148–184
5 7	143–179	153–190
5 8	147–184	158–196
5 9	151–190	162–201
5 10	156–195	167–207
5 11	160–201	172–213
6 0	165–207	177–219
6 1	169–213	182–225
6 2	174–219	187–232
6 3	179–225	192–238
6 4	184–231	197–244

Notes: Values in this table are for height without shoes and weight without clothes. Until more data are available, the weight range for people in their sixties should be used for people seventy and older.

SUGGESTED READINGS

American Diabetes Association. *Diabetes Forecast* (a bimonthly magazine). New York: American Diabetes Association (600 Fifth Ave., New York, NY 10020).

American Diabetes Association and American Dietetic Association. *Exchange Lists for Meal Planning*. New York: American Diabetes Association (600 Fifth Ave., New York, NY 10020), and Chicago: American Dietetic Association (430 N. Michigan Ave., Chicago, IL 60611), 1976.

Biermann, June, and Toohey, Barbara. *The Diabetic's Sports & Exercise Book: How to Play Your Way to Better Health*. New York: Harper & Row, 1977.

Duncan, Theodore G. *The Diabetes Fact Book*. New York: Scribner's, 1982.

Six

Your Respiratory System

AMERICAN women enjoyed the air of freedom that followed World War I. They made great strides socially as well as politically and began to frequent not only the voting booth but also the speakeasy. In gestures of defiance that were typical of the era, the flapper generation publicly drank and smoked, as the 1920s first roared and then crashed.

In the more than fifty years since, the flappers' daughters and their daughters have kept lighting up as they've crowded themselves into increasingly industrialized, automobile-clogged space. Only in the last fifteen years have we begun in earnest to clear our lungs and clean our air. Publicly, we are struggling to find safer ways to burn fuels and eliminate wastes; privately, we are struggling to kick the smoking habit and throw away our cigarettes.

THE LUNGS

Every time you breathe in, your balloonlike lungs expand and take in oxygen-rich air. Every time you breathe out, your lungs retract and let out air rich in carbon dioxide. The main function of your lung cells is to exchange carbon dioxide, the blood's waste product, for oxygen, without which your body's cells would die. To reach the lung sacs, or alveoli, your breath travels through your windpipe into a series of tubes, much like an upside-down tree, called the bronchial tree (see figure 21). Large branches (bronchi) divide into

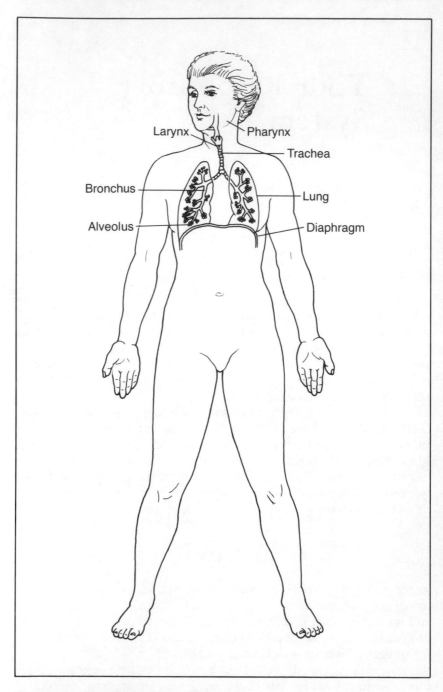

Figure 21. The Respiratory System

smaller and smaller branches and terminate in small air sacs that are each surrounded by tiny blood vessels. Oxygen from your breath moves across the membranes that separate the air sacs from the blood vessels into the blood. At the same time, carbon dioxide is released from your blood into the air sacs. When you exhale, the carbon dioxide returns to the atmosphere.

CHRONIC LUNG DISEASE

A disease that blocks the bronchi or destroys the tiny air sacs will interfere with your body's ability to receive life-sustaining oxygen and release carbon dioxide. The most common lung diseases, chronic obstructive pulmonary diseases, either obstruct the bronchial tubes (chronic bronchitis) or destroy the air sacs (emphysema). Smoking causes or seriously aggravates these conditions.

Chronic bronchitis is a disease caused by long-standing inflammation of the bronchial tree and is characterized by profuse secretions of mucus, or phlegm (see figure 22). Emphysema is a disease of the lungs in which air sacs gradually break down and the lungs grow less able to move fresh air in and out. Dead air becomes trapped inside the lungs and occupies the place of the destroyed lung cells.

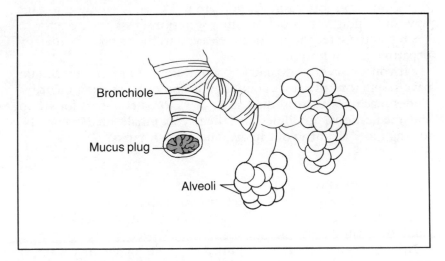

Bronchiole

Mucus plug

Alveoli

Figure 22. Bronchitis Bronchitis is caused by inflammation of the bronchial tree. The inflamed tissue secretes mucus, which blocks off many bronchioles. As a result, air cannot reach some alveoli.

With bronchitis and emphysema, as with other chronic conditions, the degree of disability varies. Most women are only bothered by the need to bring up phlegm or by shortness of breath when they climb the stairs. Some, however, need regular oxygen treatment and live a bed-to-chair-to-bed existence.

Treatment of Secretions

The normal color of bronchial secretions is white; any other color suggests infection. If you have chronic bronchitis, the phlegm interferes with the passage of air to your lung cells. You can cough up a cup or two of phlegm each day. Your breathing will improve if you can reduce the production of mucus or clear it out of your lungs.

To do so, avoid irritants, such as smoke, pollution, or infection. During heat waves, stay indoors, preferably in an air-conditioned room. Stop smoking and ask others not to smoke in your presence, since you will inhale their smoke.

Use expectorants, which are cough syrups that contain glyceryl guaiacolate, to help liquefy your phlegm and make it easier to cough up. You can buy expectorants in your local pharmacy without a prescription.

Learn lung treatments and exercises, such as coughing techniques and deep breathing, that help loosen your secretions so that they come up more easily. If you are weak, your family can learn ways of helping you cough up lung secretions. Ask your doctor to teach you these techniques or to refer you to the respiratory therapy department of a hospital.

If you are severely disabled by your lung condition, you should have respiratory therapy equipment at home. Such equipment includes machines that produce mist or vapor, nebulizers for steam and medications, machines that help you inhale medications by forcing more air into your lungs, and oxygen tanks.

Treatment of Infections

Early treatment of lung infections can prevent more serious infections and respiratory complications. If you notice a change in the color or quantity of your phlegm, run a fever, or have trouble breathing, notify your doctor immediately. He or she may want to start you on antibiotics—such as ampicillin, erythromycin, or tetracycline—as soon as possible.

Prevention of Chronic Obstructive Pulmonary Disease
Fortunately, you can do many things to prevent chronic lung disease.

1. *Stop smoking.* Smoking causes the greatest interference with your lung defenses.

2. *Avoid heavy drinking.* Alcohol impairs body defenses and increases your risk of infection.

3. *Get early treatment for infection.* Call your doctor if you notice a change in the color, quantity, or consistency of your mucus or if you have fever and/or increased cough.

4. *Drink enough fluids to loosen your phlegm and allow you to cough it up.*

5. *During winter, humidify the air in your home, at least in the room where you spend the most time.*

6. *Do not spend too much time in bed and, when you sit, try not to slouch.* Both reclining and slouching prevent you from breathing deeply, which can result in collapsed lung cells that can get infected easily.

7. *Avoid pollution as much as possible and any irritants to which you are allergic (pollens, animals, and so on).*

ASTHMA

The bronchial channels leading to the lung cells contain small muscles in their walls that can tighten in response to infection, stress, or irritants such as smoke or pollens. When they do, less fresh air reaches your air cells, and dead air is trapped in your lungs, leading to wheezing and shortness of breath.

Your doctor can prescribe any of a number of medications that will help open your bronchi. Some are pills or capsules, such as Aminophyllin, Theolair, Theo-Dur, Slo-Phyllin, Tedral, and Marax. Others are inhaled through tiny aerosol containers that deliver puffs of air mixed with medication, such as Ventolin, Isuprel, Alupent, and Bronkosol.

ANXIETY, STRESS, AND LUNG DISEASE

It is very frightening to have difficulty breathing, and the fright itself can cause the muscles of the bronchial tree to tighten, making breathing even harder. The harder breathing leads to more anxiety, establishing a vicious cycle. Some women with chronic lung conditions develop stress ulcers of the stomach and intestines.

One of the best remedies for anxiety is knowledge. If you understand your disease and know what can go wrong and how to cope, you are less likely to be overwhelmed (see chapter 14). Another remedy for anxiety is support—from your doctor, your family, your friends, your neighbors, other people with lung disease, or a visiting nurse. Your physician should be available to answer your questions and prescribe medical treatment as soon as you require it.

Depending on your needs and the severity of your illness, your doctor may prescribe a homemaker to assist you with shopping, cooking, and cleaning; a visiting nurse to check on your medical condition; or a respiratory therapist to assist you with the use of respiratory equipment.

PNEUMONIA

When you have a bad cold with a cough that gets progressively worse with increasing chest pain, you may wonder whether you have developed pneumonia. Nine times out of ten, you only have bronchitis. Pneumonia is not very common in otherwise healthy, active, older women.

Pneumonia is an infection of the lungs' air sacs caused by viruses or bacteria, or, in rare cases, other organisms such as mycoplasmas, fungi, or rickettsias. These organisms usually invade people whose body defenses are already weakened. Those most susceptible include the following:

- heavy smokers, since smoke paralyzes the tiny hair cells lining the bronchial tree that sweep bacteria and viruses out of the lungs

- heavy drinkers, since alcohol impedes body defenses against certain types of pneumonia-causing bacteria

- users of drugs such as barbiturates, which in large doses depress respiration, or cortisone, which suppresses the body's defense system

- bedridden people, since parts of the lung collapse when a person lies down

- women with diabetes, congestive heart failure, chronic lung disease, or cancer

- elderly and very frail women, who have little strength to breathe deeply or cough effectively and whose defenses are weak

Viral Pneumonia

In most forms, viral pneumonia is mild. However, when it is caused by the type A influenza virus, it has resulted in many worldwide epidemics and thousands of deaths.

If you have viral pneumonia, you may feel exhausted, cough up clear or yellowish phlegm, run a fever, and feel chest pain when you cough or breathe deeply. Your doctor may or may not hear specific sounds in your lungs, but a chest X ray will confirm the presence of inflamed lung tissue, usually in more than one place. If you have viral pneumonia, your doctor will advise you to follow these suggestions:

1. Stay home and rest. You do not have to stay in bed. Give your body some time to fight the infection and heal itself.

2. Drink plenty of fluids.

3. Take an expectorant cough syrup if you have lots of phlegm.

4. Avoid smoking.

An antiviral drug, Amantadine, may ward off a viral illness (including type A influenza) if taken within twenty-four to forty-eight hours of its onset. Taken later, it can shorten your illness. Older people experience frequent side effects of the drug, however, such as light-headedness and irritability, so Amantadine is not frequently prescribed. It should not substitute for vaccination.

Occasionally, a bacterial infection starts while your lungs are weakened by a viral pneumonia. You may suddenly get a worse cough, a darker-looking phlegm, or more fever or fail to improve after five to six days. Do not hesitate to see your doctor immediately for a reevaluation. Bacterial pneumonia must be treated quickly.

Bacterial Pneumonia

Bacterial pneumonia starts more quickly and worsens more rapidly than viral pneumonia. You may have persistent high fever and even delirium, chills, and chattering teeth. You cough frequently, and your phlegm may be white, green, or rust-colored and may contain tiny specks of blood. You may feel pains or a heaviness in your chest and have nausea, headache, a bloated stomach, and a complete lack of appetite. With a severe pneumonia, you may feel short of breath, appear pale, and have bluish fingernails—all suggesting oxygen deprivation.

Most bacterial pneumonias need hospital treatment so that necessary intravenous antibiotics and intense chest therapy can be given to clear the patient's lungs of secretions. All but the weakest and sickest women (usually those suffering from other serious underlying diseases) recover completely.

Vaccinations

There are two types of pneumonia vaccines: the influenza vaccine, given to prevent influenza that can result in viral pneumonia, and the pneumococcal vaccine, given to prevent pneumonia that is caused by the pneumococcal bacteria.

Influenza Vaccine

The influenza vaccine is about 60 percent to 70 percent effective. There are many strains of influenza, and different ones surface each year. No one can predict which new strain is about to come, so the vaccine is made against a variety of viruses from years before. The flu vaccine should be taken each year in October or November.

You should be vaccinated against the flu if you fit into one of these categories:

1. women over age sixty-five
2. residents of nursing homes, chronic-care hospitals, or other crowded facilities
3. women with heart or lung disease, chronic kidney failure, diabetes, severe anemia, or cancer, or who are taking medications that suppress body defenses (anticancer drugs and cortisone, for example)
4. medical personnel who have close contact with people likely to have influenza

In 1976, when the swine flu vaccine caused severe neurological side effects in a small number of people, a great cloud of mistrust enveloped all influenza vaccines. Very few complications have been associated with subsequent vaccines; however, it is wise to note that the following may occur as possible side effects of the influenza vaccine:

1. Redness, swelling, and/or pain in the area of the injection (usually the upper arm) may last one or two days.

2. Fever, muscle aches, or headaches may occur about six to twelve hours after vaccination and last one or two days. This reaction affects less than 5 percent of those inoculated.

3. Immediate allergic responses such as swelling and redness in the arm, generalized rashes, and, in rare cases, wheezing can develop if you are allergic to eggs or feathers (the vaccine is made in egg albumin).

The neurological complication of paralysis (Guillain-Barré syndrome) has not been a problem with the influenza vaccine since 1976.

Pneumococcal Vaccine

The pneumococcal vaccine is about 80 percent to 90 percent effective against the pneumococcal bacteria, which are often the culprits in the pneumonias of nonsmokers. The pneumococcal vaccine is given only once to adults and is good for ten or more years. There are few complications. The vaccine can be administered at the same time as the influenza vaccine.

LUNG CANCER

The respiratory illness that engenders the greatest fear is lung cancer—now as common in women as in men and the leading cause of death from cancer in both sexes.

Lung cancer, if detected early, can sometimes be operated on and cured. But the options for treatment of lung cancer that has spread are quite limited; they are, essentially, radiation treatment and chemotherapy.

Whether lung cancer is detected early or late, the chances of surviving for five years are only about 10 percent to 20 percent and depend more on the particular type and location of the cancer than anything else. Unlike other cancers, lung cancer cannot be detected early through routine checkups, including chest X rays. Chances of curing the disease are no greater today than twenty years ago.

Your best hope is not to get lung cancer. The best way of not getting lung cancer is not to start, or at least to stop, smoking.

Cigarette Smoking

Cigarettes are probably responsible for 80 percent of all lung cancers. It is not fully understood why some people can smoke and escape lung cancer while others cannot. In general, the number of cigarettes you smoke and the length of time you smoke increase your risk. Cigarette dose and time can be expressed in terms of "pack-years":

> 1 pack a day for 1 year = 1 pack-year
> 1/2 pack a day for 2 years = 1 pack-year
> 2 packs a day for 5 years = 10 pack-years

Generally, smokers who have accumulated more than twenty pack-years have statistically significant increases in lung cancer rates. There is evidence, however, that the risk of getting lung cancer decreases in proportion to the number of years since the smoker stopped smoking.

Quitting the Habit

It is very difficult for some people to quit smoking, since it fosters psychological and physiological addiction. Smoking can be your habitual way of handling stress and anxiety—not to mention boredom. Efforts to stop are more likely to succeed when your discomfort from smoking or your fears about its consequences become intolerable. Your physiological addiction can resemble that of a drug addict. Quitting can make you feel quite ill, temporarily. Your psychological addiction can be more tenacious, plaguing you for months and even years after you've "quit."

The rewards of quitting are greater than just lowering your risk of lung cancer. You will smell better, feel better, and breathe easier. You will also lower your risk for heart disease.

If you want to quit smoking, there are several methods you can try.

1. The "Cold Turkey Method" works for the most motivated. You may have greater success if you pick a target date for quitting.

2. Support groups that require a fee, such as "Smokenders," provide you with company while you struggle and an economic incentive to succeed.

3. Hypnosis works for some. There are hypnosis clinics in many major hospitals in larger cities, as well as independent hypnosis clinics.

4. Acupuncture may help certain women stop smoking. Used for this purpose, acupuncture entails placing small needles in specific spots in your ear and leaving them in place for weeks. The acupuncture may relieve some of the stress associated with quitting.

5. Nicotine-containing gum (such as Nicorette) helps you quit by diminishing your physiological craving or addiction, leaving you free to struggle with your psychological and social addiction to cigarettes. Whenever you crave a cigarette, you chew the nicotine gum. After about a month, your physiological addiction is over, and you can abandon the gum. Some women find, however, that they cannot tolerate the gum's bitter taste.

> Warning: The Surgeon-General Has Determined That Smoking Is Dangerous to Your Health.

Seven

Your Gastrointestinal System

THINK of the gastrointestinal system as a complex processing plant that manufactures building materials and energy by chemically converting raw materials (food) into usable products (sugars, amino acids, and lipids) and waste products (feces and urine). (See figure 23.) The main corridor of this plant, the alimentary canal, turns and coils almost mazelike for thirty feet through the human torso, from the mouth to the anus. At points along the canal or near to it, we find wrecking equipment (mouth, teeth, and tongue), transport devices (esophagus), processing depots (stomach, intestine), and miraculously intricate chemical laboratories (gallbladder, liver, and pancreas).

THE DIGESTIVE PROCESS

Once food is delivered to the plant, the mouth and teeth tear and grind it. The esophagus, or food pipe, delivers the ground material to the stomach, a large muscular organ that further mashes and mixes it with acid and enzymes to break the food down into its basic parts—proteins, carbohydrates, fats, vitamins, and minerals. The stomach pushes the ground mixture into the small intestine, where most of the absorption into the bloodstream takes place and from which the blood carries nutrients to the liver for processing or storage. The pancreas sends enzymes and the gallbladder bile into the small intestine to improve the absorption of proteins and fats,

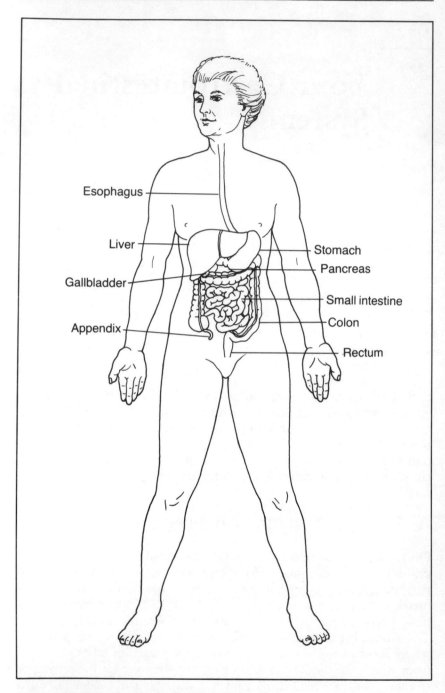

Figure 23. The Gastrointestinal System

respectively. Vitamins, minerals, and water also seep into the bloodstream from the small intestine all along its length. Bacteria residing in the large intestine, or colon, process the undigested residue of food and turn it into waste.

DIGESTIVE PROBLEMS

By and large, the gastrointestinal system works extraordinarily well. But its machinery is affected by the stresses and strains of our lives, the vagaries of our diets, and the predisposition of our genes. The gastrointestinal system reacts by producing indigestion, constipation, loose bowel movements, painful spasms, and ulcers. Weaknesses in the corridor walls can develop and cause hiatus hernia; bulging pockets called diverticula can cause bowel irregularities and occasionally inflammation and rupture. The gallbladder occasionally develops stones and may become infected. And the entire system is vulnerable to cancer.

Hiatus Hernia

Hiatus hernia, a common but usually minor problem in older women, occurs when a part of the stomach lining bulges up into the bottom portion of the esophagus, or food pipe. This bulging, which exposes the unprotected esophagus to stomach acid, can occur after eating large meals and when lying down or bending down.

Symptoms, Diagnosis, and Treatment

Some of the symptoms of hiatus hernia are heartburn, belching, and even vomiting, but the condition need not be accompanied by symptoms. Those symptoms that do arise can be controlled.

Diagnosis of hiatus hernia requires an X ray of the esophagus, called a barium swallow. The purpose of treatment is to prevent a backup of the acid-filled stomach contents into the esophagus and may include one or more of four remedies:

1. eating more frequent but smaller meals, since larger meals can back up into the esophagus

2. refraining from lying down for at least two to three hours after eating

3. elevating your upper body when in bed to keep the esophagus well above the stomach

4. taking antacids every few hours

Heavy women should lose weight and avoid girdles, which can aggravate the backup of stomach contents.

Complications

Occasionally, serious problems develop as a result of hiatus hernia. The following symptoms should be reported to your doctor right away.

1. Severe pain, which seems to mimic the pain of a heart attack but which, in fact, is more likely to be evidence of an ulcer. This pain, caused by stomach acid backing into the esophagus, can be felt in the chest area and sometimes in one or both arms. If you can connect the pain to posture (does it hurt more when you lie down?), eating (is it worse after a meal?), or antacid medications (do they help you feel better?), you can assure yourself that the pain is more likely to be coming from your esophagus than from your heart.

2. Difficulty in swallowing food. Your sense that food is sticking in your chest as you swallow can be the result of long-term ulceration that causes scarring and stricture of the esophagus. This condition is diagnosed by X ray. Treatment involves stretching the tightened area with long rubber tubes called bougies.

3. Bleeding (resulting in anemia). Sudden brisk bleeding will produce vomiting, a black or tarry-looking stool, and dizziness on standing after sitting or lying down. Slow bleeding may produce no symptoms or just mild fatigue, pallor, and pale nailbeds and conjunctiva (the insides of the lower eyelids).

Peptic Ulcers

Peptic ulcers are festering wounds that develop in the areas bathed by the stomach juices, most commonly in the stomach, duodenum, and esophagus. If these highly acidic stomach juices are produced in large quantities or if the surrounding tissues have lost some of their protective coating because of inflammation, the juices can corrode normal tissues.

Stress, alcohol, and nicotine increase acid secretion; alcohol, aspirin, and nonsteroidal anti-inflammatory drugs can damage the protective stomach coating.

Women now develop peptic ulcers as often as men, possibly because women smoke more, drink more, and work under pressure more than in the past.

Symptoms, Diagnosis, and Treatment

The symptoms of peptic ulcers are burning or grinding pain in the upper abdominal area and frequent burping, belching, and flatulence. In a classic case, the pain wakes you up at 2:00 A.M. and can be relieved by food, antacids, or milk. The very elderly woman with a peptic ulcer may experience none of these symptoms and may suffer only from vague abdominal cramps and lose weight.

Diagnosis is made by observing your response to treatment or by seeing the ulcer on a barium X ray called an upper G.I. Small ulcers may not show up on an X ray but may be visualized directly through a long, flexible tube called a fiber-optic endoscope inserted through the mouth. Diagnosis of stomach ulcers, as opposed to duodenal ulcers, usually requires visualization with the scope and then a biopsy to be certain that the ulcer is not cancer.

Ulcers that are treated conscientiously can heal completely in two to six weeks with the use of one of the following treatments:

1. Take two tablespoonfuls of antacids or two tablets every hour while awake for the first two or three days; then every two hours for two days; and, finally, four times per day, an hour after meals and before bedtime. Read the ingredients on the antacid container. Since antacids containing magnesium produce loose bowels, and antacids containing aluminum produce constipation, alternating these two kinds of antacids is the best treatment—or use one that contains both magnesium and aluminum. Antacids can be bought without a prescription.

2. Take 400 to 600 milligrams of cimetidine (Tagamet) four times a day or 150 milligrams of ranitidine (Zantac) twice a day for about six weeks. These drugs effectively reduce acid secretion but may cause confusion in elderly women. They should be used with caution and in reduced doses in women with kidney impairment. These drugs must be prescribed by your doctor.

Successful treatment also requires that you do the following:

1. Eat frequent small meals daily instead of two or three large meals.
2. Maintain a regular diet; you need avoid only those foods that cause you irritation or indigestion.
3. Avoid alcohol, coffee, tea, and nicotine—all of which increase acid production.

4. Avoid any form of aspirin or nonsteroidal anti-inflammatory drug, which can erode your stomach lining. Instead, use drugs such as acetaminophen (Tylenol), salsalate (Disalcid), or arthropan (Trilisate).

5. Try to relax. If you feel tense and nervous, practice meditation or relaxation techniques or ask your doctor to prescribe a mild antianxiety pill for a short period of time (see chapter 14).

Complications

If you have a peptic ulcer, you need to be checked regularly by your doctor. Ulcers can cause slow bleeding, which can result in anemia. The bleeding is diagnosed by noting microscopic blood on a stool sample stained with special dye and by doing a blood count. Ulcers can also cause rapid bleeding when the acid erodes a larger blood vessel and produces vomiting of large amounts of material that looks like coffee grounds or red blood. Rapid bleeding can make you excrete dark, tarry stools. The low blood pressure caused by an eroded blood vessel produces dizziness, weakness, and even collapse. Emergency surgery may be needed to stop the bleeding.

Severe ulcers can sometimes erode the wall of the intestine, causing perforation and peritonitis as intestinal contents and acid spill into the abdominal cavity. Symptoms are severe abdominal pain and fever. Occasionally ulcers cause so much scarring that intestinal obstruction occurs. The abdomen becomes rapidly distended and tender, and the person vomits intestinal contents. Emergency surgery is needed for both complications.

You should call your doctor if any of these conditions occur:

1. You have severe and recurrent abdominal pain that does not go away despite several days of diligent antacid use.

2. You have bloody vomitus or tarry stools.

3. You have weakness, dizziness, or pallor accompanying ulcer pain.

4. You have severe abdominal pain with persistent abdominal distension or with fever and vomiting.

Gallstones

Medical schools teach that the person most likely to develop gallstones is "forty, female, fertile, and fat." While women do not "own" gallbladder disease, they are more susceptible to it than men. About 20 percent to 25 percent of women over fifty-five have gallstones.

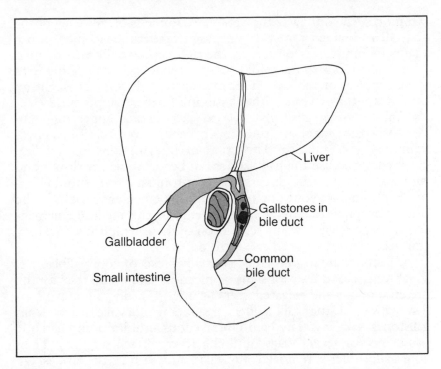

Figure 24. Gallstones   Gallstones form in the gallbladder or in the bile duct, which drains the bile into the intestine. The stones often produce no symptoms, but those that lodge in the common bile duct may cause sharp pain, fever, or abscess and may rupture—a rare medical emergency.

The gallbladder is a small sac beneath the liver that stores bile salts made from water, cholesterol, fats, and other salts. These bile salts assist in the digestion of fats and are emptied into the small intestine through a small duct called the bile duct. A person can live very well without a gallbladder because the liver will take over its function.

Stones are most common in women who have had many children, who are obese, who have diabetes, who eat lots of sweets, or who have a very strong family history of gallbladder disease. Stones can develop in the gallbladder when cholesterol levels in the blood get high and the cholesterol crystallizes (see figure 24). Sometimes bacteria travel from the intestine to the gallbladder, and chemicals crystallize around them, forming stones or gravel.

Symptoms, Diagnosis, and Treatment
Gallstones may be "silent" in many women. If they produce no

symptoms, the only way they might be noted is on an X ray of the abdomen obtained for other purposes. Sometimes women notice vague abdominal discomfort in the right upper abdomen or mild pain that extends to the middle of the upper back after eating fried foods, apples, or cabbage. This intermittent discomfort might go on for months or years without causing further symptoms.

Gallstones can also give rise to excruciating upper right abdominal pain, pain in the upper back, fever, chills, nausea, vomiting, and jaundice. This complex of symptoms is a medical emergency because the gallbladder can become filled with pus and rupture, causing life-threatening peritonitis. You should immediately contact your doctor or go to the emergency room of the nearest hospital. Elderly women undergoing this medical emergency may experience a far milder version of these symptoms, but they still need immediate medical attention.

Gallstones are diagnosed by X-ray dye tests of your gallbladder, sonar tests, blood tests for signs of infection, and blood tests for the presence of bile and elevated liver enzymes. Usually, if you have inflammation of the gallbladder or blockage of bile ducts from gallstones, you are treated with intravenous antibiotics and narcotic painkillers for several days until the severe attack subsides. Then your gallbladder is removed surgically, and with it, the stones.

Gallstones causing symptoms should be removed surgically, preferably before you are sixty. Sooner or later, these stones will cause problems, and surgery poses fewer risks when you are younger.

The Big Debate—Surgery for "Silent" Gallstones?

There is disagreement about the advisability of surgery for "silent" gallstones. While most women reasonably wish to avoid surgery, there are risks to watching and waiting. Close to half the women with "silent" stones will have significant trouble within five to twenty years, and almost all these women will end up losing their gallbladders. Perhaps 10 percent to 20 percent of these gallbladder patients who develop problems will have serious complications of the disease or surgery. These complications can include abscess or gangrene of the gallbladder; perforation of the gallbladder, causing peritonitis; inflammation of the pancreas; and pus in the lining of a lung.

Since the odds of developing problems within twenty years are nearly 50–50, the elective surgery makes sense, particularly if you are under sixty or if you are older but in good physical shape and have no other major medical problems.

Nonsurgical Approaches

Some treatments for gallstones that are being studied and used may offer a better and safer alternative to surgery. Chenodiol tablets (Chenix) and other related chemicals taken orally for six months to two years can dissolve some gallstones. They seem to work best in thinner women, who tend to have many small gallstones, as opposed to heavier women, who tend to have one or two larger stones. The gallstones can, however, recur.

More recently, some doctors have removed gallstones through a long tube that is passed through the mouth and small intestine to the bile duct to the gallbladder. This procedure is called endoscopic papillotomy and seems to be especially useful for elderly women and other persons for whom surgery would be very risky. Other doctors are experimenting with dissolving gallstones by injecting a drug into a tiny tube passing right through the liver and into the gallbladder. In both procedures, the gallbladder remains in place, and the gallstones can form again.

The newest technique for removing gallstones (and kidney stones too) is not yet widely studied as of 1986. This technique breaks up stones with laser or sonar beams. There are still complications with these procedures, but they are promising for the future.

Prevention

Obesity predisposes women to forming gallstones. This is especially true for obese women who go on and off diets and experience rapid weight gains and losses. Avoiding gallbladder disease is an additional good reason overweight women should try to lose weight gradually and permanently. Pregnancy, birth control pills, and estrogen taken for menopausal symptoms have also been associated with greater risk of developing gallstones.

Many researchers have explored the possible link between gallstone formation and diet. Some evidence suggests that diets low in natural fiber and high in refined carbohydrates contribute to stone formation. Conversely, it may be true that diets rich in fiber and low in refined carbohydrates may help prevent gallstones and gallbladder disease. Since such diets also offer some protection against heart disease, diabetes, and colon disease, you can only help yourself by following them.

Constipation

Constipation describes two conditions: infrequent bowel movements and hard, difficult-to-pass stools. Usually symptoms range from mild abdominal discomfort to a feeling of bloatedness to straining hard for bowel movements. Often a person who is constipated just doesn't feel right.

When thousands of American women were asked to describe their normal bowel movement pattern, the responses described patterns that ranged from three times a day to twice a week, with two-thirds of the women claiming one bowel movement per day.

Even though there is such variation in normal bowel habits, more than 50 percent of older women use laxatives regularly. Many of these women do not even consider themselves constipated but wish to maintain "regularity."

Prevention

Various factors foster constipation:

1. too little time on the toilet
2. diet low in fiber
3. too little fluid intake
4. too little activity
5. stress, anxiety, or depression
6. dependence on laxatives
7. weak abdominal and pelvic muscles
8. use of iron supplements and certain medications

The factors causing constipation are generally under your control. You need to allow time in your day, preferably early in the day, for an uninterrupted session on the toilet. Regular bowel habits cannot be restored overnight. Don't strain when nothing happens after ten or fifteen minutes of sitting on the toilet. Try later in the day. Try adding more natural fiber to your diet in the form of fresh green, leafy or deep yellow vegetables or fruit, coarse-grain breads and cereals, or even raw bran, available in most health food stores. The fiber increases the speed at which stools pass through the bowel and adds to the bulk of the stool.

If you're fighting constipation, drink at least eight to ten glasses of fluid each day; drink more on very hot days, when you lose more fluid through perspiration. Fresh fruit and fruit juices, especially prune juice, can produce a laxative effect.

Try walking more and driving less. An inactive body produces inactive bowels. Exercise and activity do not have to be strenuous to have a positive effect on the bowels. A little exercise each day is better than occasional vigorous exertion. For women disabled with arthritis, even walking around the house can be helpful. You can buy tapes or records of exercise programs or watch exercise programs on local TV stations. Do the exercises that you are comfortable with (see chapter 2). An excellent source of exercises from low-intensity to high-intensity levels is *Fitness for Life: Exercises for People Over 50* by Theodore Berland (Washington, D.C.: AARP; Glenview, Ill.: Scott, Foresman & Co., 1986).

You can learn to lessen stress, anxiety, and depression (see chapter 14). Exercise relieves stress and improves the motility of your intestines.

Abdominal and pelvic muscles are often weak in women, especially in those who have had multiple or late pregnancies. You can evacuate better if you strengthen these muscles (see chapter 2 and chapter 8). Exercise books will outline many appropriate exercises for them.

Using laxatives too often encourages laziness in bowels—they come to depend on laxatives. If you are used to laxatives, try tapering off slowly, while increasing your level of physical activity and your intake of fiber and fluid. Another reason laxatives should not be used regularly is that they interfere with the body's absorption of vitamins, minerals, and important medications.

Many medications slow down the bowels—in particular, pain pills, such as codeine, oxycodone hydrochloride (Percocet), meperidine hydrochloride (Demerol), and pentazocine hydrochloride (Talwin). Try to use as little pain medication as possible. If necessary, you may need stool softeners or bulk laxatives while you are on these pills. Iron supplements also cause constipation and dark stools. Taking vitamin C with the iron will help alleviate the constipation.

Treatment with Laxatives and Enemas

Four main types of laxatives are used to treat constipation: bulk, lubricant, salt, and irritant.

- Bulk laxatives add bulk to the stool. An example is Metamucil.

- Lubricants, such as DSS (dioctyl sodium sulfosuccinate, or Colace), encourage water to enter the stool, thereby increasing its bulk and softness. Mineral oil coats the intestine with oil, making the passage of stool easier. However, it can prevent the absorption of fat-soluble vitamins and can produce severe pneumonias if it is accidentally aspirated into the lungs during vomiting. Glycerin suppositories provide a safer way of lubricating stools.

- Salt laxatives such as magnesium sulfate, carbonate, or hydroxide (milk of magnesia) hold on to water, making the stool softer and bulkier.

- Irritant drugs work by stimulating the intestinal nerves, thus increasing bowel activity. Cascara, castor oil, Senokot, and bisacodyl (Dulcolax) are four common examples. Dulcolax is also available in suppository form.

Enemas act by stretching the rectum, lubricating the stool, or irritating the colon lining. You can use an enema safely, provided you do not do so more than once a month and provided that you do not use large quantities (more than a quart) of water or irritating soapsuds. Fleet enemas (packaged enemas with premeasured ingredients) are gentle and easy to use.

Hemorrhoids

Hemorrhoids, or piles, cause pain and embarrassment to about 60 percent of older American women. Millions of dollars are spent each year in search of relief.

Hemorrhoids are simply varicose veins of the rectum—baggy, overstretched veins that result from excessive pressure within the abdomen. External hemorrhoids are the little tags of skin around the anus that are painful to touch when stretched with blood. Internal hemorrhoids develop inside the anus, though they can protrude outside of it, and are less painful because they are covered by a relatively insensitive mucous membrane. Many women first develop piles during the third trimester of pregnancy, when the fetus and uterine sac compress the rectal veins. Most of the time, fortunately, hemorrhoids cause little or no discomfort.

The low fiber content of the North American diet, resulting in constipation and straining at bowel movements, as well as the sitting posture we assume on the toilet contribute to the development of hemorrhoids. Other, more serious conditions such as cirrhosis of the liver, congestive heart failure, and lung disease accompanied by lots of coughing also predispose you to hemorrhoids.

You usually first discover your hemorrhoids when you see spots of bright red blood on the toilet paper after a painless bowel movement. Your rectum may itch, and you may feel small skin tags that had not been there before. Occasionally you may have several days of painful bowel movements; feel an almond-sized, very tender lump protruding from your anus; and, after a bowel movement, notice a lot of bright red blood in the toilet bowl.

Diagnosis

Most women are able to diagnose their own hemorrhoids. But the danger in doing so is that they may ignore a serious condition such as colitis, polyps, or cancer that announces itself with the same symptoms. Therefore, diagnosis of hemorrhoids should be left to your physician, who will examine your rectum, look inside with an anoscope or sigmoidoscope (plastic or metal tubes that permit a look at the inside of the large intestine), and perhaps take some barium X rays to be certain that there is no problem besides hemorrhoids.

This advice does not mean that each time you note spots of blood on the toilet paper you should run to the doctor. The first time, yes. See your doctor again if the amount or color of the blood changes drastically.

Prevention
The best way to prevent hemorrhoids is to change your diet. Add bran and coarse grains to your diet, building up gradually to about 30 grams per day (see chapter 11) to allow your intestines to adapt. Otherwise gas, cramps, or loose bowel movements can result. It also helps to drink eight or more glasses of fluid per day, to soften your stool, and to exercise daily, even if it is just a brisk walk around your neighborhood or in your home.

Treatment
Once hemorrhoids are inflamed, they can almost always be treated at home in this way:

1. Sit in a tub of warm water several times a day or use moist compresses with warm water and witch hazel.

2. Avoid sitting or standing for long periods of time, since these positions increase abdominal pressure on the hemorrhoids. For the same reason, avoid lifting heavy bundles.

3. Do not strain at bowel movements. If you try to eliminate without success, wait until you feel an urge. Try not to rub the rectal area hard when wiping after bowel movements.

4. If necessary, use over-the-counter hemorrhoid preparations for a short period of time. Suppositories of Anusol, with or without cortisone, can also be very helpful. If the inflammation or bleeding persists for longer than ten days, consult your physician.

The least drastic way of treating repeated hemorrhoids is the rubber band technique, usually done in the doctor's office. An elastic band is tied around the base of each hemorrhoid, cutting off the blood supply. The hemorrhoidal tissue shrivels up and drops off in a few days, and the base of the hemorrhoid closes off. The procedure is not very painful, and no anesthesia is needed. You can go about your routine business after a day's rest.

Hemorrhoids can be frozen off in the doctor's office, but this technique is more painful than the rubber band technique.

Infrared coagulation, related to laser technology, is the newest method of outpatient care for the hemorrhoid sufferer. This technique uses a special probe to clot hemorrhoids by heat and can be done safely in the doctor's office.

Occasionally, surgery in the hospital is needed for particularly bad hemorrhoids that bleed a great deal or become repeatedly inflamed despite treatment. Usually the patient needs general anesthesia and several days to a week of hospitalization. Sometimes scarring occurs after hemorrhoid surgery, causing a narrowing of the anus. It is best to use "an ounce of prevention" before resorting to the surgical cure.

Diverticulosis

Saccular outpouchings of the colon, called diverticula, increase with age (see figure 25). Nervous tension, constipation, and the low-fiber diet common in the United States play a role in increasing the number of diverticula. While diverticula in themselves are not dangerous, they are vulnerable to two serious complications: inflammation of the sac, called diverticulitis, and bleeding.

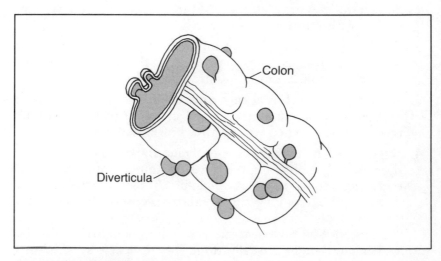

Figure 25. Diverticulosis   In diverticulosis, the wall of the intestine develops small pouches called diverticula. Inflammation of these pouches is called diverticulitis.

1. Diverticulitis. Constipation can cause hard stool to plug the sacs and irritate their walls, exposing them to attack by intestinal bacteria. Symptoms include lower abdominal pain, particularly on the left side, made worse by bowel movements; muscle spasm of the abdomen; and fever.

Mild diverticulitis is treated by resting, applying heat to the lower abdomen, eating less or fasting for a few days, taking antibiotics, and occasionally taking medications to decrease bowel spasms. More severe illness requires hospitalization, no food by mouth, intravenous fluids, and intravenous antibiotics.

Repeated bouts of severe diverticulitis can result in scarring of the bowel, leading to its possible blockage or perforation. These are medical emergencies that need a surgical solution.

2. Bleeding of the diverticula, including severe hemorrhage (which is a medical emergency). In this case, blood appears in the stool. Anemia can result if the bleeding is extensive. Severe bleeding may require removing the section of affected bowel.

COLORECTAL CANCER

Cancer of the large bowel and rectum (colorectal cancer) is a disease of affluent Western countries and is virtually nonexistent in Third World countries. About 93 percent of these cancer cases occur in people over fifty years of age. In women, it is the most common cancer after lung and breast cancers. Like breast cancer, colon cancer can be detected early through screening and can be completely cured in its early stages.

All women over fifty should be screened annually for colorectal cancer.

Risk Factors for Colorectal Cancer
Several risk factors for colorectal cancer have been identified.

1. A family history of bowel cancer increases your own risk. Hereditary factors play an important role in 10 percent to 20 percent of bowel cancers.

   A rare disease, familial polyposis, is associated with a very high rate of colon cancer among family members. If this disease is in your family, see your internist or gastroenterologist every six months.

2. Ulcerative colitis can lead to cancer of the large bowel. Your internist or gastroenterologist should see you regularly. In certain cases, the doctor may recommend surgically removing your entire large intestine as a precaution.

3. High dietary fat, especially animal fat, and high serum cholesterol levels predispose you to an increased risk of bowel cancer. Food high in fat takes longer to travel through the bowel and is converted by microorganisms in the bowel into carcinogens.

4. Gallbladder removal leaves you with a greater risk of colon cancer—close to twice the risk for other women. The reasons for this increased risk are not yet understood.

Symptoms
Bowel cancer may be indicated by any of the following symptoms.

* sudden change in bowel habits—sudden constipation, sudden loose stools, or change in the size of stools
* feeling of fullness in the rectum
* lower abdominal pain or pressure
* blood in the stools
* prolonged, unexplained fatigue or anemia

Protecting Yourself by Screening
Bowel cancer causes no symptoms for many years. During these early years, it is usually confined to a very small area (such as at the base of a polyp, as was President Reagan's bowel cancer in 1985) and is potentially completely curable.

There are five ways of identifying the early stages of bowel cancer:

1. The simplest screening test is the guaiac slide test for occult blood. This test detects stool blood that is not visible to the eye and that may originate from a precancerous growth (polyp) or from cancer. The test can be done at your doctor's office or at home by yourself. It should be performed once a year. The test can save your life by detecting colon cancer in the early, curable stage. Generally, you should test one stool sample a week for three weeks. For three days prior to the test, avoid rare red meat, vitamin C, and iron tablets, each of which can create a falsely positive test. Also, if possible, avoid aspirin and arthritis medications for those three days, since these drugs can cause microscopic bleeding in the stomach, which will result in a misleading positive test. A few drops of chemical are put on a sample of stool on a special card. Blood is diagnosed by a change in color of the chemical.

2. Digital rectal examination permits the doctor to examine the lining of the rectum to check for irregularities. This technique can detect about 10 percent of colorectal cancers; the rest are above the reach of the examining finger. This exam should be performed once a year.

3. Proctoscopic examination involves inspecting the rectum and lower part of the colon through a hollow, lighted tube. This test can be done in the doctor's office and is only minimally uncomfortable. After fifty, you should have a proctoscopic examination once each year for two years and, if both exams are normal, once every three to five years thereafter.

4. An examination with a sigmoidoscope is much like a proctoscopic examination but allows the doctor to examine about ten inches more of the colon.

5. Colonoscopic examination is done with a long, flexible tube that permits inspection of the entire length of the colon. Polyps can also be removed through the colonoscope. This test must be performed by a gastroenterologist or a doctor with special training in the procedure.

Treatment and Outcome

Cancer that is detected early and is confined to the bowel lining may be cured if the cancer is completely removed. If the cancer arises in the lower left colon, the surgery often results in a colostomy, which means that the remaining end of the bowel is brought to the surface of the lower abdomen, and stool is excreted through the opening into an attached disposable plastic bag. The other end of the cut, leading to the rectum, is sewn closed. Only small amounts of mucus then pass out of the rectum. The United Ostomy Association, with chapters in all major cities, provides information and support for colostomy patients.

Cancer that has spread through the bowel wall and to the lymph glands is treated with radiation therapy and surgery—and with chemotherapy—to prevent blockage of the intestine and to reduce the amount of cancer. About 44 percent of women treated with these techniques survive beyond five years.

Bowel cancer that is discovered after it has spread throughout the body has a poor prognosis. Treatment is aimed at comfort—preventing blockage in the intestines and controlling pain. The sad outcome only reinforces the need to be screened once a year after age fifty and to seek medical advice as soon as symptoms occur.

Prevention

Evidence suggests that certain dietary changes may dramatically decrease your risk of getting colon cancer.

Try to eat foods low in animal fat. It is best to consume sixty to eighty grams of fat per day, about one-third less fat than the average American diet. Look at the nutrition labels on foods. They give the number of grams of fat per serving. For example, one tablespoonful of butter contains eleven grams of fat, and one tablespoonful of safflower margarine contains four grams.

Try to eat more fiber, about thirty to forty grams per day (more than double what most North American diets contain). Include fruit, vegetables, and starches. For example, one cup of All-Bran cereal contains twenty-three grams of fiber, one apple has three grams, and one medium raw carrot has nearly four grams.

High-fiber food moves through the intestines more quickly than food low in fiber. This speed seems to protect the bowel from becoming cancerous. Fiber also alters fecal content and may prevent the production or absorption of carcinogens or reduce the amount of time that the bowel lining is exposed to carcinogens. Fiber increases the acid of bowel contents, which may protect against colorectal cancer. Fiber also binds with potential carcinogens and washes them out of the digestive tract.

Nutrients such as vitamin C, selenium, vitamin E, Beta-Carotene, and vitamin A may offer some protection against large bowel cancer (see chapter 11).

WHEN TO REPORT BOWEL PROBLEMS TO YOUR DOCTOR

Certain bowel symptoms can indicate a serious medical problem. Many of us postpone reporting bowel problems until quite late, when complications may have already set in. But discovering and treating problems early in such serious diseases as diverticulitis and bowel cancer can mean the difference between life and death.

The following bowel problems should be brought to your physician's attention.

1. *Blood in the stool or dark, tarry stools.* These symptoms may be caused by ulcerations in the intestines, benign polyps, large bleeding hemorrhoids, or, in rare cases, rectal cancer.

2. *Constipation that comes on suddenly.* This symptom may indicate a sudden blockage from the bowel twisting on itself, from adhesions or scar tissue following surgery, or from cancerous growths.

3. *A sudden and definite change of bowel habits.* Low thyroid activity, urinary tract disease, neurological problems, elevated calcium levels in the blood, or cancer can underlie such a change.

4. *Involuntary loss of control of bowel movements.* This embarrassing problem can be caused by impaction, or partial blockage of the bowels by a hard ball of stool. Meanwhile liquid stool, which may be mixed with mucus, oozes out. Other causes may be prolapse of the rectum; nerve damage from diabetes, dementia, or stroke; inflammation of the colon; or cancer.

SUGGESTED READINGS

Goldberg, Myron D., M.D., and Rubin, Julie. *The Inside Tract: Understanding and Preventing Digestive Disorders.* Washington, D.C.: AARP; Glenview, Ill.: Scott, Foresman & Co., 1986. (An AARP Book)

Plant, Martin E., M.D. *The Doctor's Guide to You and Your Colon.* New York: Harper & Row, 1982.

Schindler, Margaret. *Living with a Colostomy.* Wellingborough, England: Turnstone Press, 1985.

Eight

Your Genitourinary System

THE pelvis houses the organs of reproduction and elimination. Three organ systems crowd themselves onto the pelvic floor: the reproductive system, opening at the vagina; the digestive system, terminating at the anus; and the urinary system, ending at the mouth of the urethra.

THE FEMALE REPRODUCTIVE ORGANS

Within the female pelvis sit two ovaries. Suspended next to each is a fallopian tube, the funneled pathway into which—before menopause—mature eggs find their way, perhaps to become fertilized. The fallopian tubes end at the uterus—a pear-shaped, muscular organ whose lining is called the endometrium. The exit from the uterus is a slender neck, called the cervix, through whose opening—the cervical os, or mouth—mucus, menstrual flow, or a baby may pass. Beyond the cervix lies the vagina—a slender, expandable chamber about three to five inches in length composed of elastic tissues that are kept moist and soft by mucous glands just inside the vaginal opening. All these reproductive organs (see figure 26) are held in place in the pelvic cavity by a series of broad ligaments that gradually become lax, causing the pelvic organs to sag slightly as a woman ages.

On the outside of the vagina are the vulva, or outer genitals. The vulva extend in the front of the body to the mons—the soft,

185

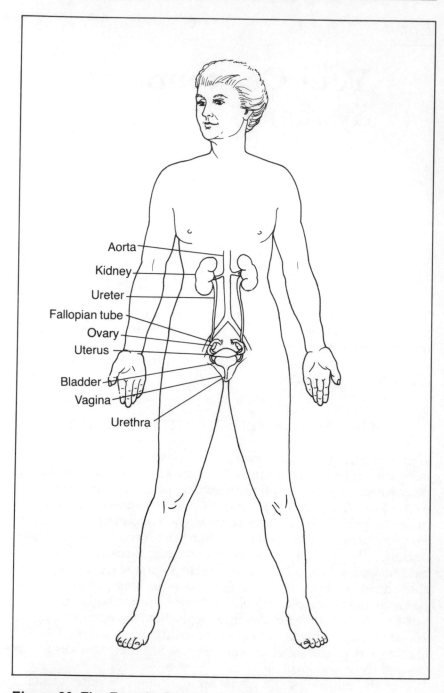

Aorta
Kidney
Ureter
Fallopian tube
Ovary
Uterus
Bladder
Vagina
Urethra

Figure 26. The Female Genitourinary System

fatty tissue over the pubic bone at the bottom of the abdomen—and extend in the back to the anus. The inner lips of the vagina are soft flaps of moist, hairless skin that swell with sexual stimulation. Where they meet in the front, the inner lips protect a delicate bud of skin known as the clitoris. The clitoris, with its shaft and glans that become erect with sexual arousal, is the most sexually sensitive part of a woman's genitals.

THE URINARY SYSTEM

About a half inch below and underneath the clitoris is the opening to the bladder, the urethra—a thin, short tube whose proximity to the sexual organs exposes it to irritation during sex; right below the urethra is the opening to the vagina (see figure 27). The muscles around the vagina are the pelvic floor muscles, which, along with ligaments, hold and support your pelvic organs.

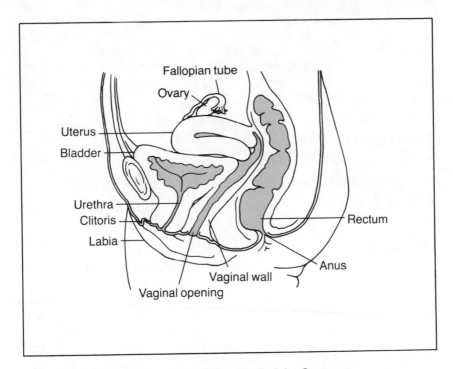

Figure 27. Side View of the Female Pelvic Organs

Bladder Infections

A woman's anatomy makes her particularly vulnerable to bladder infections. Unfortunately, bladder problems and symptoms linked to sexual activity, pregnancy, weak pelvic floor muscles, dropped bladders, irritations, poor hygiene, and stress often continue as a woman grows older and increase in her oldest years. The proximity of your urethra to your vagina and anus makes it more vulnerable to infection. In addition, the urethra is only 1½ inches long in women (as compared with 8 inches in men) and thus offers bacteria a much shorter route to the bladder. Multiple pregnancies weaken the pelvic floor muscles, causing the urethra to be even shorter than normal. Menopause, too, weakens muscles and ligaments in the pelvis, sometimes leading to a dropped bladder, a shorter urethra, and less muscle control.

Other conditions also set the stage for bladder infections. Mechanical irritation of the urethral opening from sexual activity and bicycle or horseback riding can cause inflammation of the urethra, making it more susceptible to bacterial invasion. Douches, feminine hygiene sprays, and bubble bath preparations containing perfumes can also irritate the urethra.

Symptoms

The following symptoms may be present with a bladder infection.

- pressure in the lower abdomen
- need to void suddenly and urgently
- temperatures of 100° F–101° F
- desire to void more frequently
- burning pain before, during, or after urination
- blood in the urine

Diagnosis

The only certain way to diagnose a bladder infection is to have your physician analyze a "clean" sample of your urine. He or she first examines the urine specimen under a microscope for signs of active infection: abundant bacteria; white blood cells, which combat infection; and red blood cells from bleeding infected tissues.

Next, your physician cultures the sample to identify and measure the types and quantities of bacteria causing your symptoms. If a million or more bacteria grow in the sample overnight, your urine is infected. The procedure allows your doctor to determine which antibiotics the offending bacteria are sensitive to so that he or she can tailor your treatment to the exact cause.

Natasha K., sixty, noticed lower abdominal pressure, a frequent need to void, and a sense of urgency when she urinated that brought tears to her eyes. She even noticed a bit of blood in her urine. She gave a urine specimen to her doctor, who started her on sulfa drugs while awaiting the results of the culture to determine what drugs could combat the bacteria found.

Three days later, her doctor prescribed another antibiotic. The culture had revealed an infection from bacteria that were not sensitive to sulfa drugs.

Treatment of Bladder Infections

The treatment of bladder infections varies. Usually doctors prescribe antibiotics for an average of ten days.

Sulfa drugs, such as Bactrim or Gantrisin, kill most of the common bacteria residing in the pelvic area and are therefore the antibiotics most commonly prescribed. Some women develop allergic skin rashes from sulfa drugs. In rare cases, sulfa causes a drop in blood platelets, which are needed for clotting, and makes a person bruise easily. If you should notice many new bruises on your body while or shortly after taking sulfa, stop taking the medicine and alert your doctor. A quick blood test can determine whether your platelets are low. The condition is temporary.

The drug-sensitivity analysis of your bacterial infection may suggest a number of antibiotics, such as tetracycline, ampicillin, amoxicillin, cephalexin, or cephradine.

Nitrofurantoin (Furadantin, Macrodantin), another antibiotic, is sometimes prescribed. Women with G-6-P-D deficiency of the blood (see chapter 4) should alert their doctors before taking this drug, since nitrofurantoin can cause hemolytic anemia. In rare cases, the drug can cause lung inflammation and shortness of breath. If you have breathing difficulties while on the drug, alert your doctor immediately.

Ascorbic acid (vitamin C), in doses of two grams per day, will make your urine slightly acid, which slows the growth of bacteria. You can take vitamin C regularly if you have repeated bladder infections.

The most commonly prescribed drug for pain in the bladder and urethra is Pyridium, taken three times a day. It will turn your urine bright yellow-orange and will relieve the burning sensation.

Symptoms usually subside two to three days after treatment starts, but it is important to finish taking all the prescribed medication even after your symptoms subside to avoid a recurrence of the infection.

Prevention of Bladder Infections

There is no cure like prevention. You can decrease or eliminate bladder infections if you do the following:

1. Drink fluids throughout the day—about eight glasses a day. Fluid flushes bacteria out of your urinary tract. Acidic juices (such as lemon or cranberry) suppress bacterial growth.

2. Do not hold your urine in. Voiding frequently during the day and emptying your bladder completely when you void clears out bacteria that have multiplied in your bladder.

3. Wipe yourself from the front of your pelvic area to the back so that you will not bring fecal bacteria close to the urethra.

4. Wash your pelvic area every day with warm water and mild soap, and dry yourself completely.

5. Wear cotton underpants or underpants with cotton liners. Nylon holds in heat and moisture, providing perfect conditions for bacteria to multiply. For the same reason, avoid wearing nylon panty hose for longer than you have to—take them off as soon as you get home.

6. Avoid perfumed feminine hygiene sprays, douches, or bubble bath preparations.

7. Empty your bladder before and after sexual intercourse. An empty bladder is less likely to get irritated during sex, and voiding afterward flushes out bacteria that might multiply in an irritated urethra.

8. If your pelvic area is irritated from sexual activity or horseback or bicycle riding, soak in a warm bathtub for twenty minutes. The warmth will relax your pelvic muscles and reduce inflammation.

9. If your vagina is dry and uncomfortable, try using lubricating jelly (such as K-Y jelly), available over the counter, since recurrent infections may be aggravated by atrophic vaginitis, caused by estrogen loss after menopause. If the jelly doesn't help, consider consulting your doctor about a prescription for estrogen cream (see chapter 9).

10. If your pelvic muscles are weak, do the Kegel exercises (see page 193) to strengthen them. This weakness may contribute to repeated bladder infections.

Recurrent Bladder Infections

Sometimes, despite all preventive measures, you may have

repeated bladder infections that warrant further investigation of your urinary tract by a urologist. Your doctor may prescribe an X-ray study of the kidneys and bladder, an I.V.P. (intravenous pyelogram), in which dye is injected into a vein and pictures are taken as the dye is cleared out by the kidneys. The urologist may need to look into your urethra and bladder by means of a small tube, a cystoscope, to check for narrowing of the urethra, bladder stones, or polyps.

You may need antibiotics prescribed over a long term but in lower doses than used to combat an active infection. This suppression treatment is used to prevent long-term damage to the kidneys by bladder infections that might travel upward into the kidneys.

Urinary Incontinence

Urinating is a complex act controlled by the brain, the autonomic nervous system, and a series of muscles in the bladder and urethra.

Losing control of your urine, even in small amounts, is embarrassing. Unfortunately, urinary incontinence is not rare. Women of all ages may involuntarily dribble urine during a cough, sneeze, or laugh. As many as 50 percent of women who live in nursing homes wet themselves regularly. Some women are too embarrassed to talk about this problem even with their doctors and try to hide it with absorbent pads.

The inability to control urination can be either temporary or permanent.

Maude B., seventy, suddenly required hospitalization for pneumonia. Surrounded by strange nurses prodding and poking her, she felt very uncomfortable in the hospital. She had trouble getting out of the bed to go to the bathroom because of the IV's and hated urinating on a bedpan with only a curtain between her bed and her roommate's bed. Her high fevers and fits of coughing drained her. Maude became quite confused and started to wet her bed regularly.

But as soon as her pneumonia cleared up and she was back home, Maude's bladder control returned.

Temporary Bladder Incontinence

Temporary bladder incontinence can usually be explained by one or more of the following situations.

1. Bladder infections cause inflammation that can interfere with bladder control. As soon as the infection clears up, control returns.

2. Stress incontinence occurs in women who have lax pelvic muscles from age, many pregnancies, or large babies. Bladder and urethral supporting tissues weaken, causing the loss of small amounts of urine anytime there is pressure in the lower abdomen—from straining, coughing, laughing, sneezing, or lifting.

3. Atrophic vaginitis, causing dry mucous membranes in the vaginal and urethral areas, can produce incontinence. Treatment of the vaginitis improves the urinary condition (see chapter 9).

4. Constipation can interfere with the normal exit of urine from the bladder. The bladder gets overly stretched, and urine spills out a little at a time. When the constipation is relieved, urinary control returns.

5. Drugs—particularly tranquilizers, such as Thorazine and Mellaril, and the antidepressant Sinequan—can interfere with bladder control. When the drug is no longer taken, control returns.

6. Confusion and delirium associated with illness can cause incontinence in older women, especially when they find themselves in an unfamiliar place. When the illness improves and the woman returns to her own home, the bed-wetting stops.

7. Bedridden elderly women sometimes unconsciously express their anger or frustration by bed-wetting.

8. Arthritis or stroke can cause impaired mobility, which can lead to loss of urinary control.

Usually a doctor can discover and treat the cause or causes of temporary incontinence. There are several ways to reduce the problem in the meantime.

• Try to void every two hours to cut down on the number of accidents.

• Get a bedside commode if you have difficulty getting to the bathroom.

• Do not restrict fluids. This will only make you feel weak and nauseated and will increase your chances of infection.

• Keep the skin in the genital area as dry as possible. Using Vaseline or Desitin Ointment on skin exposed to urine reduces the risk of skin rashes and bedsores.

Stress Incontinence

Most women who experience incontinence have sagging pelvic muscles and organs, which pull down the urethra and lessen muscle control. Some women have a dropped uterus, which can be felt just inside the vagina or, in some cases, pushes through to the outside. Others have a dropped bladder (cystocele), which bulges into the vagina, or a dropped rectum (rectocele), which also bulges into the vagina.

Kegel Exercises

The best way to treat these problems is to strengthen the muscles of the pelvic floor. Kegel exercises—named after Arnold Kegel, the physician who invented them—can be done daily at home, in the office, or wherever you happen to be; no one will be able to guess that you are doing them.

When you suddenly force yourself to stop urinating, the muscle that stops the urine is the pubococcygeus—a broad band that stretches from the pubic bone in front, around the vaginal opening, to the tailbone behind. Tightening this muscle is just what you want to do as a regular exercise. Make sure that you are not just tightening your buttocks but are also squeezing the pubococcygeus. You can imagine that you are pulling together the vagina and anus. You can tighten, hold for two seconds, and release. Do it a few times in succession and then relax for a few minutes. Repeat the exercise again, and work your way up to several groups of squeezes each day.

Pessary

In case the exercises do not help bring your incontinence under control or remedy your lax pelvic organs, the next step is to try a pessary. A gynecologist or nurse specialist inserts this device (made out of rubber and shaped like a doughnut, ring, square, or bent ring) into the vagina to push the pelvic organs back up from their dropped position. The pessary can stay in place for months, and usually you are unaware it is there. Every three months or so, the pessary should be removed, cleaned, and reinserted. While this is usually done by the gynecologist or nurse, you can be taught to do it yourself.

Pessaries occasionally cause problems. The most common of these is constipation. The pessary, especially if it is large, may be pressing the rectal area and narrowing the size of the passage. If you have this problem, eat foods, such as prunes or bran, that prevent constipation or hardness of stool (see chapter 7). In rare cases, a pessary will cause pain or bleeding in the pelvic area. If these symptoms occur, see your gynecologist or go to the emergency room of a hospital to be sure that you do not have an infection or irritation that needs treatment. You can also reach into your vagina and—with a slow, steady tug—pull the pessary out to get relief.

Surgery

If your stress incontinence is not cured by any of the above remedies, consider asking your doctor about surgical correction of your dropped bladder. A gynecologist or urologist can reposition your urethra by tightening up the pelvic floor. This repositioning allows you to regain control over urination. Occasionally, for a severely dropped uterus, the gynecologist will recommend a hysterectomy. Many women can have a vaginal procedure, but some may require an abdominal incision.

Permanent Incontinence

Some conditions permanently end one's bladder control. Multiple sclerosis, diabetes with nerve damage, spinal cord injury, dementia, or stroke can cause permanent damage to the nerves that control urination.

In such cases, the options for handling the condition are these:

1. Medications. Depending on the particular nerves involved, drugs, such as bethanechol chloride (Urecholine), flavoxate (Urispas), nortriptyline (Imipramine), oxybutynin chloride (Ditropan), or propantheline (Pro-Banthine), can help control urination. Diagnosis requires an X ray of the kidneys and bladder (I.V.P.) and a cystometrogram by a urologist or geriatric specialist.

2. Adult briefs or diapers. Absorbent briefs can be worn day and night and should be changed at least four or five times a day. At each changing, wash your skin, dry yourself well, and cover any irritated area with Vaseline. Rashes should be treated with Desitin Ointment or A and D Ointment.

3. Intermittent artificial drainage. You can learn to drain urine out of your bladder through a small clean or sterile plastic tube that you pass through the urethra to the bladder. This procedure is not painful and is repeated four or more times a day.

4. Catheter. The method of last resort is to leave a small, flexible plastic tube, called a catheter, in your bladder and urethra permanently.

The catheter drains into a bag, which is emptied as needed, at least twice a day. The advantage is that you will be dry. The disadvantages are that you are exposed to frequent bladder infections and that your catheter can become plugged and will need changing. Nevertheless, for many very elderly or disabled women, catheters are a blessing.

Nine

Menopause

W HEN a female infant enters the world, she brings with her between a quarter million and a half million egg follicles, each surrounding an immature egg. During each month after the beginning of her puberty, one of this legion of follicles begins to ripen. As it ripens, the follicle secretes two hormones into the bloodstream: first, estrogen, which causes the lining of the uterus to thicken; then, progesterone, which readies the lining to nourish the egg should it be fertilized. Less than 1/500 of a woman's egg follicles ripen during her lifetime; most of the rest wither and die.

Control of the body's monthly cycles and hormone levels issues from the hypothalamus—a structure in the brain acting on the pituitary gland, the master hormone factory, also in the brain. The hypothalamus is sensitive to the circulating levels of estrogen and progesterone secreted by the egg follicles. After menstruation, when the estrogen level is again low, the hypothalamus directs the pituitary gland to release FSH, or follicle-stimulating hormone, into the blood. FSH then travels to the ovaries and stimulates the ripening of another follicle.

As you slowly approach menopause, the cessation of menstruation, your ovaries become less sensitive to FSH, so follicles ripen only now and then. Consequently, your estrogen level drops, and the uterine lining does not have enough regular stimulation to thicken and shed on a monthly basis. Menstruation, therefore, may become less frequent. The hypothalamus responds by stimulating the pituitary gland to produce excessive levels of FSH, trying to cause the ovaries to

197

ripen follicles and to continue secreting estrogen and progesterone. Eventually, the ovaries can no longer respond to FSH, so they stop ripening eggs. As a result, menstrual periods cease altogether.

The waning of a woman's fertility is not necessarily smooth. For several years, the usual balance of hormones among the ovaries, hypothalamus, and pituitary is upset. Hormone levels vary widely—sometimes rising high, sometimes dropping low. Eventually a new state of equilibrium is reached, and harmony prevails.

The average age of menopause in North American women is fifty-one years. As with the onset of menstruation, there are great variations. Some women begin menopause as early as forty; others begin as late as fifty-eight. Heredity is a strong factor. If your mother had an early menopause, you are more likely to stop menstruating early too.

You are said to be postmenopausal after you have stopped menstruating for twelve consecutive months. There is a small chance of conception for a full year after your last period stops. If you have been using contraceptives, continue their use during this year.

SYMPTOMS OF MENOPAUSE

The symptoms of menopause result from the decrease in estrogen production by the ovaries. After menopause, you continue to produce a hormone, androstenedione, in your ovaries and adrenal glands, some of which is converted into estrogen in your body's fat cells. Thus, some women endowed with a generous supply of fat tissue can experience fewer symptoms of menopause than thinner women.

Irregular Monthly Flow
The most usual sign of decreasing ovarian function is lighter menstrual flow, with longer and erratic intervals between periods. A few women have shorter intervals between periods, and some women have a heavy flow. Ultimately the menstrual intervals widen, and periods cease.

A blood test for FSH can help diagnose whether you are menopausal if you are wondering why your periods are irregular. If your FSH level is very high, chances are you have begun menopause.

Hot Flashes
Your body temperature is normally kept between 97.6° F and 99.6° F by a complex system of checks and balances. The system depends to some extent on the regular ebb and flow of estrogen levels circulating in your bloodstream. During premenopause and menopause, when hormone levels are in flux, your body's temperature-regulation system is upset.

A "hot flash" is an actual surge of heat through the body that can be measured by sensitive thermometers. The body's regulatory mechanisms react quickly to reduce the sudden heat by causing you to sweat and flush. Blood flows to the skin, allowing your body to release heat. Sometimes the cooling process can result in a chill, or even shivering.

Each woman who experiences the condition has a characteristic hot flash that starts at a specific point, such as the neck, and spreads in a particular pattern. Hot flashes can occur only a few times a day or as often as twenty or more times a day and can be mild, moderate, or severe.

About 15 percent of menopausal women experience severe and frequent flashes that can interfere with work and sleep and cause emotional upsets. Some women have found relief from hot flashes by taking 800 international units (I.U.) of vitamin E complex accompanied by 2,000 milligrams of vitamin C and 1,000 milligrams of calcium from dolomite or bonemeal each day. After the severe flashes have subsided, the vitamin E can be reduced to 400 I.U. Relaxation techniques (see chapter 14) or mild tranquilizers, such as Valium or Librium, can lessen the stress caused by severe hot flashes. Estrogen replacement (see pages 202–204) can control the most severe cases.

Vaginal Changes
After menopause, the external lips of the vagina, or labia, and the clitoris may diminish in size, but the change does not affect sexual responsiveness. The vaginal walls, previously dependent on estrogen for their strength and elasticity, become thinner and more rigid over a number of years. As the vagina's stretching capacity decreases (a condition called vaginal atrophy), you may experience dryness, burning, itching, and pain on intercourse (dyspareunia), which can interfere with your sexual pleasure.

The discomfort of vaginal dryness is avoidable, however. You can lubricate the vagina with K-Y jelly or polyunsaturated vegetable oils (without preservatives) before intercourse, do pelvic exercises (see chapter 8), and maintain regular sexual activity to maintain the vitality of the vaginal walls and reduce the undesirable dryness. You can treat extreme cases of discomfort with estrogen creams applied in the vagina (see page 204).

Urinary Tract Changes

The decrease in estrogen also thins the walls of the urethra, or passage leading from the bladder to just above the vaginal opening. The thin-walled urethra is vulnerable to frequent bladder infections (see chapter 8).

Fortunately, most women do not experience uncomfortable urinary symptoms to any significant degree unless they have concurrent weak pelvic floor muscles, stress incontinence, or uterine prolapse. You can strengthen your pelvic muscles by doing Kegel exercises (see page 193) and prevent the thinning of the urethral walls by taking estrogen pills.

Bone Changes

Older women, much more than older men, are prone to osteoporosis, or thin bones. Such bones fracture easily and cause bone pain, backache, and collapsed vertebrae. Loss of height follows. Calcium from tablets or from four glasses of milk per day, vitamin D from sunshine or tablets, and regular exercise will help retard bone loss, as will estrogen taken by mouth (see chapter 2).

Other Changes

The decreased estrogen levels accompanying menopause also cause thinning of the scalp hair, growth of facial hair, weight gain, and loss of skin tone. These effects appear gradually and are mild in most women, but they can be distressing (see chapters 1 and 2). Many women, of course, experience very few difficulties with menopause and consider their period-free life a blessing.

STRESSES

As recently as twenty years ago, gynecologists thought that severe depressions of middle-aged women were inevitably related to menopause. Today, women and their doctors realize that life brings stresses that are as likely to be responsible for pain and sadness as the loss of estrogen.

There is no question that your personality can be affected by the drastic fluxes in hormonal balance during menopause as well as by the physical changes. You may experience sleeplessness, irritability, increased stress, difficulty in concentrating, and fatigue. You may feel a sense of loss in acknowledging that your childbearing years are over. Many women become insecure about their identities.

We do well to remember that the "change of life" is, after all, a change. Menopause may make us feel more vulnerable because it reminds us that we are, in fact, physical creatures with a limited number of years on earth. We may be single and feel suddenly alone; we may be childless and be forced to recognize that the door to motherhood has closed; we may have children and chafe that our door to grandmotherhood is not yet opened; we may have ambitions beyond our opportunities to fulfill them. We realize that some of our ships will be forever lost at sea.

Talking with women who have similar problems helps. If your friends' support is not enough, you may want to join women's discussion groups such as those offered through churches, synagogues, libraries, health centers, and YWCAs. Local chapters of NOW, the National Organization for Women, run groups for older women. Some women prefer getting individual counseling through hospital or community mental health facilities or from private social workers or psychiatrists (see chapter 14).

ARTIFICIAL MENOPAUSE

Hysterectomy is the second most commonly performed operation in the United States, after cataract surgery. In a total hysterectomy, the entire uterus, including the cervix, is removed; in a subtotal hysterectomy, the cervix is left intact. In a hysterectomy with salpingo-oophorectomy, the uterus and one or both tubes and ovaries are removed.

Many women are persuaded to have a hysterectomy without fully understanding whether there are other options. Contrary to popular belief, the majority of hysterectomies are not performed to cure or control cancer. They are most often performed to remove fibroids, which are benign growths of the uterine muscle, or to cure pelvic relaxation or prolapse—a condition common in women who have had multiple pregnancies, in which the uterus has loosened from its proper position and slipped into the vaginal tract.

When both ovaries are removed before you have passed through menopause, you will experience all the symptoms of estrogen withdrawal regardless of your age—unless you are prescribed estrogen pills. The usual justification given for removing the ovaries during hysterectomy is to eliminate the possibility of the patient ever getting ovarian cancer. Ovarian cancer, while less common than uterine or cervical cancer, is the leading cause of death in women with gynecologic cancer and occurs most commonly in women fifty to sixty-five years of age.

The decision whether or not to remove your ovaries must be made by you and your physician. A premenopausal woman (under forty-six) should always question the necessity of such an operation, require a detailed explanation from her physician, and feel free to obtain a second opinion.

ESTROGEN REPLACEMENT—A CAUTIOUS APPROACH

Twenty years ago, many physicians prescribed estrogen pills for women going through menopause. It was known that estrogen in high or low doses could cause cancer in animals, but not until the mid-seventies was there evidence that estrogen could also cause cancer in women. Long-term studies showed that women taking estrogen for five or more years had a 5 percent to 20 percent greater chance of getting uterine cancer than those who did not. Studies also showed that estrogen stimulates certain breast, cervical, and vaginal cancers. Physicians reacted sharply to this information, and most took their women patients off estrogen.

Doctors now appraise estrogen replacement more calmly. Estrogen therapy has definite benefits that for some women outweigh its risks.

Who Should Have Estrogen Replacement

About 15 percent of women experience menopausal symptoms of such severity that their work, sexual life, and sleep are disrupted. Even when their menopausal symptoms are not severe, some women feel that the benefits of estrogen on bone, skin, and vagina are significant enough to outweigh its risks.

Some doctors recommend that long-term (twenty or more years) estrogen replacement be used to prevent osteoporosis and feel that the risks of cancer are outweighed by the risks of fractures from osteoporosis. This idea is being debated in the medical community. If you have a strong family history of osteoporosis, it may be in your best interest to take estrogen.

Who Should *Not* Have Estrogen Replacement

Women who have or have had breast, cervical, uterine, or ovarian cancer should not take estrogen; the estrogen might stimulate the growth or spread of these cancers. Women who have migraine headaches, high blood pressure, a history of blood clots, gallbladder disease, or uterine fibroids should preferably not take estrogen, or should take it with close medical supervision.

Reasons to Take Estrogen	*Reasons Not to Take Estrogen*
1. Severe menopausal symptoms	1. Previous breast, cervical, uterine, or ovarian cancer
2. Osteoporosis or strong family history of osteoporosis	2. History of mother taking DES (diethylstilbestrol) during pregnancy
3. Desire to take estrogen despite the risks	3. Blood clots when on estrogen treatment in the past or a present blood clot
	4. History of migraines, high blood pressure, blood clots unrelated to estrogen, gallbladder disease, or uterine fibroids

The Risks of Estrogen Replacement

The chances of getting cancer of the lining of the uterus (the endometrium) increase from one per one thousand women to four to five per one thousand women when women take estrogen more than five years. The risk of breast cancer may also increase, as well as the incidence of gallbladder disease, blood clots, and high blood pressure, in women taking estrogen replacement over a long term. Some women on estrogen are bothered by side effects, such as nausea, vomiting, bloating, fluid retention, breast tenderness, headaches, dizziness, hair loss, and growth of facial hair. Estrogen also stimulates the growth of existing uterine fibroids; hence, the fibroids may become bothersome and require surgery.

Minimizing the Risks of Estrogen Treatment

The use of estrogen-progesterone combinations is now the standard way of prescribing estrogen for menopausal symptoms. Studies show that when estrogen is taken alternately with progestin (a synthetic form of the hormone progesterone that you produce naturally when you are fertile), the combination lessens the risk of endometrial cancer that taking estrogen alone may carry. In fact, women on this combination of drugs had lower endometrial cancer rates than women not taking any hormones, which suggests that progesterone may help prevent uterine cancer. This combination of drugs causes some women to menstruate—a side effect that you may or may not welcome.

The estrogen-progesterone combination is prescribed as follows:

Days 1–25. Take an estrogen pill daily.
Days 15–25. Take a progesterone pill along with the
estrogen pill.
Days 26–30. Stop all pills.
Day 31. Begin the cycle again, calling this Day 1.

Both the dose and duration of estrogen treatment affect your risks. Only the lowest dosage that relieves symptoms should be used. Except in instances where you are using estrogen to prevent osteoporosis, it is wise to limit your use to two years or less, since using estrogen for this time interval seems not to increase the risk of cancer. In case your doctor feels you should have estrogen without progesterone, interrupted use in the form of three weeks on estrogen and one week off also seems to reduce risk.

Estrogen can be used as a cream in the vagina to relieve painful intercourse and itching and burning in the vaginal walls. The cream should be used for one week out of four or according to other staggered schedules, depending on your physician's recommendations.

Women taking estrogen pills or creams should have regular gynecologic checkups—every year for the first two years, and every six months thereafter—including a pelvic examination, a Pap smear (see chapter 10), a breast examination, and a blood pressure reading.

Common Brands of Oral Estrogens and Progesterones

1. *Estrogens*

Premarin	Estrace
Estinyl	Menest
Ogen	Evex
Estratab	

2. *Progesterones*

Provera	Norlutin
Amen	Norlutate

VAGINAL BLEEDING AFTER
MENOPAUSE

Unexpected vaginal bleeding after menopause is frightening. Some women are so certain it is a sign of cancer that they delay getting a diagnosis for fear of confirmation. In fact, most postmenopausal bleeding is due to benign causes that can be treated and that are unrelated to cancer.

Causes of Vaginal Bleeding at Different Phases of Reproductive Life

1. Adolescence
     Irregularities of hormone secretion, lack of ovulation
     Inflammation or infection of the cervix
     Complications of pregnancy
2. Maturity
     Hormonal irregularities
     Complications of pregnancy
     Birth control pills, intrauterine devices
     Benign tumors—polyps of the cervix, fibroids of the uterus
     Inflammation or infection of the cervix or the uterus
     Cancer of the cervix or the uterus
3. Premenopause
     Hormonal irregularities, lack of ovulation
     Benign tumors—polyps of the cervix, fibroids of the uterus
     Inflammation or infection of the cervix or the uterus
     Cancer of the cervix or the uterus
4. Postmenopause
     Estrogen treatment
     Atrophic vaginitis
     Inflammation or infection
     Benign tumors of the cervix, the endometrium, or the uterus
     Cancer of the cervix or the uterus

Usually there are no other symptoms accompanying postmenopausal bleeding. The blood can be scanty, appearing only as stains on your underpants, or it can be as plentiful as in a period, even producing blood clots. Depending on the cause, you may feel mild cramping in the lower abdomen. There are six principal causes of postmenopausal bleeding:

1. Endometrial hyperplasia. The most common cause of unexpected bleeding in a postmenopausal woman is endometrial hyperplasia, an overgrowth of the uterine lining from excess estrogen stimulation similar to the condition of the uterus just before a menstrual period. Endometrial hyperplasia is not cancer but can progress to uterine cancer. It is treated by a dilation and curettage procedure (D and C), by discontinuing estrogen if the patient has been on estrogen treatment, and sometimes by taking progesterone.

2. Estrogen treatment. The use of estrogen alone, or in combination with progesterone, can cause estrogen withdrawal bleeding when the pills are taken in a program that involves discontinuing them for a week before starting another series. Estrogen stimulates the growth of the uterine lining, and when the hormone is stopped, the lining is shed as a bloody flow.

If you are taking estrogen or estrogen-progesterone combinations, you should not have blood flow or spotting during the days when you are taking the hormones. Some breakthrough bleeding can and sometimes does occur because the estrogen dose may be too low for you and require adjustment.

On the other hand, unexpected bleeding may have other underlying and more serious causes, and you should consult your gynecologist or physician about this sign. Your gynecologist may want you to have a D and C in the hospital in order to examine scrapings of the uterine lining for diagnosis.

3. Atrophic vaginitis.

4. Inflammation or infection. Inflammations or infections can occur on your cervix (the neck of the uterus, which protrudes into the vagina), causing the irritated tissues to bleed, particularly after intercourse. In rare instances, you can also have pain, cramping, and a low-grade fever (100° F–101° F).

You need a pelvic examination to check your cervix, a Pap smear (see chapter 10) to be certain that the inflammation is not due to cancer, and a culture to search for yeasts and bacteria that could be causing the infection. Your doctor will prescribe antibiotic pills or antibiotic vaginal creams to combat the infection. If the antibiotics fail to heal the inflammation, the gynecologist may try cauterizing or freezing the affected area to clear away the inflamed tissue and allow healthy tissue to regrow.

Occasionally, inflammation can alter cervical cells so that they appear almost precancerous on a Pap smear. Your doctor may perform a further diagnostic test in the office, a colposcopy, in which he or she examines your cervix and vagina, using a special magnifying microscope, and removes a sample of any abnormal-looking tissue for analysis for cancerous cells. Or, the doctor may decide to remove more tissue by a cone biopsy, performed in the hospital under anesthesia. The procedure removes all inflamed tissue, allowing healthy tissue to regrow in the area. The cone of excised tissue is examined under a microscope to be certain that it contains no cancer cells. Afterward, you may have a bloody discharge for a few weeks and should not have intercourse for a month because the cervix is susceptible to infection until it heals. Laser treatments are also being used to cure cervical inflammation that appears precancerous.

Women who have cone biopsies that do not show cancer—or who have a diagnosis of carcinoma in situ, an early stage of cancer—usually require Pap smears every six months thereafter to be certain that abnormalities do not recur.

5. Benign tumors of the cervix, the endometrium, or the uterus. Cervical or endometrial polyps develop out of the glands lining the cervical canal (cervical polyps) or in the uterine lining (endometrial polyps). Usually, you do not know that you have these benign, tubelike growths until they are diagnosed following an episode of abnormal bleeding or until your gynecologist remarks, during a routine pelvic examination that he or she can feel or see polyps.

Polyps are rarely cancerous. Many cervical polyps can be removed in the doctor's office and sent for analysis to be certain that they contain no malignant cells. Endometrial polyps require a D and C, performed in the hospital, to scrape them out of the uterus.

Uterine fibroids are benign tumors of the muscle of the uterus and are present in about 30 percent of women. They tend to be most noticeable during childbearing years, since their growth is stimulated by the natural supply of estrogen. During menopause, they often shrink and even disappear, but they can grow in postmenopausal women who take estrogen pills. Most women who have fibroids have more than one.

Fibroids can be large—even larger than a grapefruit—and can result in bleeding. When this occurs in a postmenopausal woman, the gynecologist often recommends hysterectomy.

6. Cancer of the cervix or the uterus. (See chapter 10 for a detailed discussion.)

SEX AND MENOPAUSE

Many women find that their postmenopausal years bring increased sexual pleasure. Freed from the fear of pregnancy, the restrictions of birth control, and the disruptions of menstruation and free to enjoy more privacy after children leave home, they feel more spontaneous sexual desire and enjoyment.

About 25 percent of women have menopausal symptoms that interfere with sex. They suffer from hot flashes, pain on intercourse from vaginal atrophy, and uncomfortable urinary symptoms and may wish to avoid sex altogether. Some women have no uncomfortable symptoms but simply feel less interested in sex after menopause.

SUGGESTED READINGS

Lettvin, Maggie. *Maggie's Woman's Book: Her Personal Plan for Fitness and Health for Women of Every Age*. Boston: Houghton Mifflin, 1980.

National Women's Health Network. *Menopause Resource Guide*. Washington, D.C.: National Women's Health Network, 1980.

Reitz, Rosetta. *Menopause: A Positive Approach*. New York: Penguin, 1977.

Ten

Women's Cancers

I N the past, cancer was a death sentence. Today, many cancers detected early are completely curable; in fact, one in three Americans with a diagnosis of cancer is cured. Even cancers found at later stages can often be treated, prolonging life and comfort.

Nevertheless, people dread thinking of cancer and may compromise their health by ignoring important symptoms. In the United States, breast cancer discovered too late is the second major cause of death in women thirty-seven to fifty-five years of age; lung cancer is now the leading cause. Many cancers unique to women can be cured if detected early by regular screening techniques—the breast self-examination, mammography, the Pap smear—and attention to critical symptoms.

Cancer is the uncontrolled growth of cells that can spread and ultimately kill their host. Mutations, or changes, in the genetic material of a cell produce cell growth that does not respond to signals that normally limit the growth and spread of cells. What causes these changes in the genetic material of the cell? Certain viruses may play a role. Sometimes heredity predisposes our cells to cancerous changes. Sometimes the man-made environment is responsible. The cancer-causing substances, or carcinogens, in our environment are part of the price we pay for the richness and variety of our food, the efficiency of our transportation, and the myriad other achievements afforded by our technology. We can no more free ourselves from all carcinogens than we can free ourselves from all the other hazards of daily life, but we should continue trying to identify and limit carcinogens in our air, in our food, and in our homes and workplaces.

REDUCING THE RISK

You will reduce your contact with carcinogens if you do the following:

1. Stop smoking.
2. Eat more fiber, less fat, and more vegetables from the cabbage family—broccoli, cauliflower, and brussels sprouts.
3. Reduce your consumption of saccharin (unless you are diabetic).
4. Cut down on the amount of food you eat that contains color additives.
5. Reduce or avoid consumption of nitrites and nitrates—found in salami, bologna, and other sausages and in luncheon meats and bacon—which may be converted in the body to nitrosamines, potent carcinogens.
6. Wash all fruits and vegetables to remove potentially carcinogenic insecticides.

One-third of all cases of cancer in the United States could be eliminated if Americans stopped smoking; an additional third could be eliminated if we improved our diets.

CANCER OF THE CERVIX

Alice T., fifty, had not had a Pap smear in years, but she finally made an appointment for one. Why at that particular time, she did not know. She had no symptoms, knew of no one who had cancer, and had no premonition of illness.

Her doctor called her a week later and said that the Pap smear was suspicious for cancer and that he wanted to do another test. Alice fell into a state of panic until her next appointment. She was certain that she had cancer and kept asking herself, "Why? Why did I wait so long? It's probably too late to cure! I'm going to die soon! I'm so stupid for waiting!"

When her doctor next examined her, he performed a colposcopy and biopsy in the office. The biopsy analysis showed persistent dysplasia in the wall of the cervix. The doctor recommended a cone biopsy in the hospital. Again Alice was scared to death. She refused all sexual overtures from her husband.

She awaited the results of the biopsy on pins and needles. Her doctor telephoned to say that, yes, he had detected a few signs of early cancer in the biopsy but felt confident that all traces had been removed with the cone biopsy.

Understandably, Alice continued to be fearful for a year and a half. After three further Pap smears were found to be completely normal, she allowed her life to begin again.

Risk Factors for Cervical Cancer

You are at greater risk for developing cervical cancer if any of the following apply:

1. You started having intercourse in your early teens.

2. You have had multiple sexual partners.

3. You have genital herpes or another sexually transmitted disease.

4. You were pregnant before the age of twenty.

5. You have genital papilloma virus (genital warts).

6. You have had little or no preventive medical care.

The Pap Smear for Diagnosis

A Pap smear—named for its inventor, Dr. George N. Papanicolaou—is a sample of cervical cells scraped from the neck of the uterus and examined for the presence of abnormal cells. Abnormal cells are not necessarily cancerous; in fact, most are simply cells altered by infection or inflammation or originating from benign tumors.

The results of the Pap smear, or Pap test, fall into one of five classes:

Class 1. *No abnormal cells* (negative Pap smear)

Class 2. *Atypical cells* caused by inflammation, infection, or benign growths.

Class 3. *Abnormal or premalignant cells*

Class 4. *Severely altered cells* that are likely to be cancer. The abnormality may suggest carcinoma in situ, which is malignant change in cells confined to one area and level of tissue. Some gynecologists believe that carcinoma in situ is not really cancer. Yet some evidence suggests that some of these cases may become invasive, or spreading, cancers within ten years.

Class 5. *Cancerous cells*

Many laboratories do not label results according to these five classes but merely describe the findings.

Prevention of Cervical Cancer
You cannot change the past, but you can develop habits that may help prevent cervical cancer.

- After menopause, have a Pap smear every year or two. Your doctor should perform, at the same visit, a pelvic examination and a rectal examination.
- Have a Pap smear every year if you have had genital herpes.
- Visit your gynecologist or family physician if you have vaginal discharges that are not normal or have irregular bleeding.
- Keep your vaginal area clean—wash it daily and dry it carefully. Don't use douches. They can introduce bacteria or irritating perfumes into the vagina.

For the past sixty years, the rate of cervical cancer has been decreasing. Whether this change is due to better standards of living, better hygiene, more circumcision, or better medical care is unknown.

CANCER OF THE UTERUS

Cancer of the uterine lining, or endometrium, is primarily a disease of postmenopausal women. Unlike the decreasing incidence of cervical cancer, the incidence of uterine cancer has increased in the past decade. Part of the explanation may be the overzealous long-term use of estrogen in the 1970s. It is possible that with the more recent decrease in estrogen use and the more careful monitoring of users, there will be a corresponding decrease in uterine cancer in the future.

Lydia V., sixty-one, noticed some bloodstains on her underpants. A mild flow of blood continued over the next few days. She remembered having had the same symptoms four years earlier before going into the hospital for a D and C, which had been negative.

This time, the bleeding stopped. But when it returned three months later, she was worried and saw her gynecologist, knowing that he would probably schedule another D and C.

Lydia's biopsy results showed cancer of the lining of the uterus. She had a complete hysterectomy along with removal of both tubes and ovaries and, luckily, seemed to have no spread of the cancer elsewhere. She is alive and well today, thankful that she finally heeded the warning signs of her cancer.

Risk Factors for Uterine Cancer

You are at greater risk for developing uterine cancer if any of the following are part of your medical status:

1. Family history of uterine cancer
2. Obesity
3. High blood pressure
4. Diabetes
5. Polycystic ovaries
6. History of irregular periods, with many skipped periods or irregular bleeding
7. Late onset of menopause (after fifty-five)
8. Childlessness or only one pregnancy
9. Long-term estrogen use (five years or more)

Diagnosis of Uterine Cancer

Several procedures help diagnose uterine cancer:

1. *Endometrial biopsy.* The doctor obtains samples of the endometrium by scraping the surface of the uterine lining with a small metal rake or suction tube.
2. *Endometrial aspiration.* The doctor extracts cells for analysis by first pushing sterile solution into the uterus to wash its surface and then suctioning the fluid into a syringe. The procedure is less painful than a biopsy.
3. *D and C.* Dilation and curettage offers the greatest chance of detecting cancer. The cervix is dilated, or stretched open, and the lining of the uterus is scraped so that uterine tissue may be analyzed under a microscope.

    If the laboratory results indicate cancer, your doctor must start treatment quickly, since uterine cancer can spread easily.

Treatment of Uterine Cancer

Cancer of the uterus that has not yet spread to the lymph glands or elsewhere is best treated by total hysterectomy and removal of both fallopian tubes and both ovaries through an abdominal incision. When the cancer has spread, it is best to have a radical hysterectomy, which includes removal of all the lymph glands in the area. In addition to surgery, the cancer specialist, or oncologist, may recommend implanting radium rods or using other types of radiation and/or drug treatment (chemotherapy).

Prevention of Uterine Cancer

Cancer of the uterus is curable in many instances *if* discovered in time. After menopause, women should consider these precautions:

- Report any vaginal bleeding, even very slight spotting, to your gynecologist or family physician. In all likelihood, you will be scheduled for a D and C to exclude the diagnosis of cancer, even though many benign conditions are more likely to be responsible for the bleeding.
- Take estrogen only after careful consideration of the risks (see chapter 9) and under close medical supervision. If you do decide to take estrogen, do the following:
  1. Ask your doctor to prescribe an estrogen-progesterone combination, unless there are reasons you should not take progesterone.
  2. Ask your doctor to prescribe the lowest dose of estrogen that will relieve your menopausal symptoms.
  3. Take estrogen for less than two years, if possible.
  4. Have a gynecologic checkup every six months.
  5. Every two to three years, ask your gynecologist if you need an endometrial aspiration or biopsy to be certain that the uterine lining is not overgrown. (A normal Pap test rules out cervical cancer; it does not rule out uterine cancer, since the Pap test does not analyze cells from the uterus.)

DES AND VAGINAL CANCER

Some middle-aged and older women were prescribed diethylstilbestrol, or DES, during their pregnancies in the 1940s, 1950s, and 1960s to prevent miscarriage. If you were prescribed the drug, you unknowingly took something that now has been shown to have exposed daughters to two potentially serious conditions, which need careful medical surveillance:

1. Adenosis of the vagina. In this benign condition, the cervical glandular cells have overgrown onto the surface of the cervix (sometimes resulting in copious mucous discharge from the vagina). This has occurred with about 80 percent of daughters exposed to DES. Because of their greater risk of developing cancer, they should have a gynecologic examination every year including Pap smears of the cervix and vagina and colposcopy or special stains of the cervix and vagina.

2. Vaginal cancer. One in four thousand DES daughters will develop vaginal cancer as a result of the DES taken by her mother. Treatment of the cancer requires hysterectomy and removal of large parts of the vagina, a devastating outcome for young women in their twenties and thirties.

CANCER OF THE OVARY

Cancer of the ovary is the leading cause of death in women who have cancer of the reproductive organs. Unfortunately, the majority of ovarian cancers are detected when the disease has spread too far to allow proper treatment. Its victims are usually between the ages of forty and eighty; the majority of cases are diagnosed when the women are in their sixties.

Risk Factors for Ovarian Cancer
Included among the risk factors for ovarian cancer are the following:

1. Ovulations. The more eggs your body has released, the greater is your risk of ovarian cancer. Women whose ovulation was suppressed for years by birth control pills may have protection lasting up to ten years after discontinuing the pill.
2. Childlessness.
3. Family history. If a blood relative has had ovarian cancer, you are at greater risk of developing the disease.
4. Postmenopausal estrogen replacement treatment.
5. Diets high in animal fats and low in vegetable fats.
6. Breast or colon cancer. These diseases are associated with a higher than normal risk of ovarian cancer.

Diagnosis of Ovarian Cancer

Ovarian cancer rarely causes symptoms until late in its development, so women must have thorough, regular gynecologic checkups. Certain signs may suggest the presence of ovarian cancer, such as enlarged ovaries or postmenopausal bleeding. In these cases, the gynecologist may recommend an ultrasound of the abdomen and, in more suspicious cases, laparoscopy (a minor surgical procedure in which the gynecologist looks into the pelvic region with a magnifying instrument).

Treatment of Ovarian Cancer

Generally, ovarian cancer is not discovered until it has spread beyond the ovary. Surgery is the first step of treatment. The surgeon attempts to remove as much of the cancer as possible, depending on the woman's general health and her ability to tolerate surgery. Chemotherapy is the second step of treatment. This therapy may cause many side effects such as nausea, hair loss, suppression of the immune system, and kidney damage; however, use of this therapy has doubled patient survival rate five years after diagnosis. No doubt treatment in the next decade will enable women to live longer with this disease.

Prevention of Ovarian Cancer

While there are no proven ways of preventing ovarian cancer, it makes sense to avoid diets high in animal fats and to avoid receiving estrogen replacement treatment for longer than two years unless you have severe osteoporosis.

BREAST CANCER

No cancer is more feared by women than breast cancer—and with good reason, for one in thirteen women develops this disease. Next to lung cancer, it is the leading cause of death in women between the ages of thirty-seven and fifty-five. The frequency of breast cancer increases with age to one in eleven for women over fifty-five. Today 50 percent of patients with breast cancer survive the disease. Early detection often makes the difference.

Until recently, a diagnosis of breast cancer meant surgical removal of the afflicted breast (mastectomy). Over the past decade, women's concerns about losing their breasts have stimulated research that has proven that mastectomy is not always necessary.

Risk Factors for Breast Cancer

All women are at high risk for breast cancer, but not all women have the same chance of getting the disease. Factors that increase risk include these:

1. *Family history.* Women whose mother, sister, or maternal aunt or niece have or have had breast cancer have twice the risk of those whose families are free of the disease.

2. *Long menstrual history.* The earlier a woman menstruates and the later she has menopause, the greater her risk of breast cancer. Women who experience menopause after fifty-five have twice the risk of those whose menopause occurs before they are forty-five.

3. *Age at first pregnancy.* Women who bear their first child after age thirty or who remain childless are more likely to develop breast cancer than women who bear children before they are thirty.

4. *Postmenopausal estrogen use.* Postmenopausal women who have used estrogen ten or more years have about twice the risk of breast cancer as nonusers.

5. *Diet high in saturated fats.* Women who eat a lot of saturated (animal) fats may have higher risk (see chapter 11).

6. *Endometrial cancer.* Women who have had endometrial cancer, even if it has been completely cured, are more likely to develop breast cancer.

7. *Fibrocystic breasts.* There is controversy about whether women who have a history of lumpy breasts, or tender breasts during menstruation, are more at risk for cancer. Fibrocystic breasts occur in about one-third of women and are not a mark of disease. Caffeine and its derivatives—found in coffee, tea, colas, chocolate, and cocoa—aggravate the swelling and tenderness of fibrocystic breasts. Although recent studies do *not* suggest a link between caffeine and cancer, as earlier studies did, it still makes sense for women with fibrocystic breasts to avoid large amounts of these compounds.

Signs and Symptoms of Breast Cancer

In its early stages, breast cancer rarely causes pain or symptoms. Usually all that is apparent is a lump or thickening in one breast but not in the other. Unfortunately, the lump may have been there for years before it could be felt. About 90 percent of breast lumps that are diagnosed as cancer are first noticed by women themselves. You can prolong your life by examining your own breasts regularly each month. (See "How to Examine Your Breasts" below.)

Following are signs that can suggest breast cancer and that should be reported to your doctor as soon as possible.

1. Any breast lump in a postmenopausal woman, and, in menstruating women, any lump that persists without change through menstrual cycles.

2. Bloody or brownish discharge or spontaneous whitish discharge from one or both nipples (as opposed to discharge that can be squeezed out, which is normal).

3. Dimpled skin, like the peel of an orange, over a portion of the breast.

4. Irregular pulling or scarring of the skin in a part of the breast.

5. Flaking or crusting around the nipple.

6. Firm lumps in the armpit area.

Breast Self-Examination

Ninety percent of breast cancers that are treated before the cancer has spread from the breast are curable. If a breast cancer is cured, a woman can have a normal life span, which underscores the importance of detecting and treating breast cancer early.

You are the most important part of the detection campaign. You cannot allow yourself to avoid feeling your breasts because you are afraid of what you will discover or because you are forgetful. You must become familiar with the way your breasts normally feel and train yourself to check them.

How to Examine Your Breasts

1. **In the shower:**
   Examine your breasts during bath or shower; hands glide easier over wet skin. Fingers flat, move gently over every part of each breast. Use right hand to examine left breast, left hand for right breast. Check for any lump, hard knot or thickening.

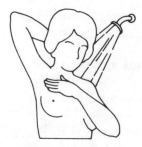

2. Before a mirror:
Inspect your breasts with arms at your sides. Next, raise your arms high overhead. Look for any changes in contour of each breast, a swelling, dimpling of skin or changes in the nipple.

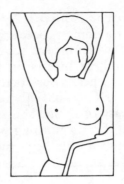
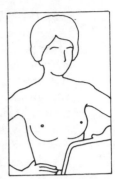

Then, rest palms on hips and press down firmly to flex your chest muscles. Left and right breast will not exactly match—few women's breasts do.

Regular inspection shows what is normal for you and will give you confidence in your examination.

3. Lying down:
To examine your right breast, put a pillow or folded towel under your right shoulder. Place right hand behind your head—this distributes breast tissue more evenly on the chest. With left hand, fingers flat, press gently in small circular motions around an imaginary clock face. Begin at outermost top of your right breast for 12 o'clock, then move to 1 o'clock, and so on around the circle back to 12. A ridge of firm tissue in the lower curve of each breast is normal. Then move in an inch, toward the nipple, keep circling to examine *every part of your breast,* including nipple. This requires at least three more circles. Now slowly repeat procedure on your left

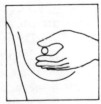

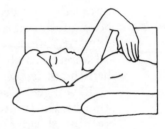

breast with a pillow under your left shoulder and left hand behind head. Notice how your breast structure feels.

Finally, squeeze the nipple of each breast gently between thumb and index finger. Any discharge, clear or bloody, should be reported to your doctor immediately.

The Best Time to Examine Your Breasts

Follow the same procedure once a month about a week after your period, when breasts are usually not tender or swollen. After menopause, check breasts on the first day of each month. After hysterectomy, check your doctor or clinic for an appropriate time of the month. Doing BSE [breast self-examination] will give you monthly peace of mind, and seeing your doctor once a year will reassure you there is nothing wrong.

Reprinted with the permission of the American Cancer Society.

Discrepancies in Breast Tissue

Often in walking your fingers around, you will feel certain areas of breast tissue that are firmer than others. These discrepancies are perfectly normal. Breast tissue is composed of fat, glands, and fibrous tissue. Very fatty breasts feel very soft. Glandular breasts feel more lumpy. Fibrous breasts are firmer. Each woman has her own individual breast type and texture, and, in general, both breasts will feel approximately the same. (Sometimes one breast is a bit larger than the other, which is normal.)

If you feel a spot about which you are uncertain, check the other breast. If the same kind of area is present on the other breast, both breasts are probably normal. Breast lumps that are cancerous are usually much harder in texture than the rest of the breast and are often the size of a walnut or peach pit when detected by palpation.

Since most breast cancers occur between the nipple and the armpit area, double-check this region.

During a regular medical checkup, ask your gynecologist or family physician to watch you do a breast exam, to be certain that you are doing it correctly. Upon request, the American Cancer Society, 219 E. 42nd Street, New York, NY 10017, will send you literature on breast self-examination, as will your local American Cancer Society chapter or breast screening clinic.

Breast X Rays

Cancerous lumps may be present for eight or ten years before they can be felt. X rays of the breast can sometimes detect such lumps as much as one to two years earlier than is possible with manual or visual exams. It is advisable for all women over fifty to have a screening X ray every year or every few years, depending on your physician's recommendation. There is currently no "best" time interval. The advantage of having yearly checks is that you are more frequently screened; the disadvantage is that you are exposed to increased radiation, however slight. High-risk women (those who have one or more risk factors for breast cancer) should have annual breast X rays.

Mammograms are usually done in the radiology department of a hospital or in special medical offices. Each breast is compressed between X-ray plates in the horizontal and vertical planes, and pictures are taken.

Since 1979, the dose of radiation from a mammogram is about 0.5 to 1 rad (the same as from a chest X ray), which is almost ten times less than when mammograms were first used. Thus, since 1979, having an annual breast X ray, even over a thirty-year period, does not amount to significant radiation exposure.

Diagnosis of a Breast Lump

Many breast lumps turn out to be benign. There are three ways for your doctor to determine whether a suspicious breast lump is benign or cancerous:

1. Needle biopsy. This procedure, usually done in the doctor's office, requires either no anesthesia or an injection of anesthetic into the area of the lump. The needle is pushed into the breast and punctures the lump. The doctor tries to draw fluid from it with a syringe. Cysts, which are benign, contain clear fluid and will collapse or shrink. If the lump does not contain fluid, it can be benign (fibroadenoma) or cancerous. The doctor will send the few cells that have been aspirated to a laboratory for analysis.

2. X rays (mammogram). These pictures allow the doctor to identify abnormal patterns of tissue that suggest cancer. These patterns include clusters of tiny calcium deposits, asymmetry of breast tissue, and lumps that are too small or too deep to be felt. If a lump is present, it must be further examined or followed over time, even if the mammogram does not show cancer.

3. Surgical biopsy. This procedure, unfortunately, is most often done under general anesthesia, which exposes older women to risks of heart, lung, and brain complications. Most surgical biopsies could be done with local anesthesia, which not only minimizes the risk of complications but also saves the patient considerable time and money. Before you agree to be hospitalized, you and your doctor should discuss the risks of general anesthesia and explore the possibility of local anesthetic.

When to Begin Treatment

Some doctors prefer to hospitalize a patient and use general anesthesia in order to be able to operate for cancer immediately after a biopsy, should the biopsy show malignancy on laboratory analysis of a frozen section. Such a course of action can spare the patient a second exposure to general anesthesia. Before 1980, physicians favored this one-step procedure.

Only recently, a committee formed by the National Institutes of Health to arrive at new guidelines for advice regarding breast cancer concluded that the treatment of breast cancer should be separated in time from its diagnosis. The two-step procedure has several advantages.

1. For most women, it is too traumatic to go into the hospital for a biopsy and wake up after anesthesia to find they have lost a breast. Separating the diagnostic biopsy from the treatment of malignancy gives a woman time to deal with the reality of her cancer and then to consider all options for treatment.

2. Since about one in four women undergoing biopsy for suspicious lumps will turn out to have breast cancer, three-quarters of the patients will be spared the unnecessary anguish of signing a breast away before knowing for certain that they have cancer.

3. Breast cancer patients may have several choices of treatment: a lumpectomy; a modified radical (simple) mastectomy; or a radical mastectomy, perhaps followed by radiation and/or chemotherapy (treatment with drugs). Each situation has to be evaluated by the woman and her physician. Women should not hesitate to seek a second opinion. There is now clear evidence that for almost all women whose breast cancer shows no sign of having spread, less extensive surgery (sometimes combined with radiation therapy) achieves the same cure rates as radical surgery.

Surgical Treatments

With a lumpectomy, or partial mastectomy, about one-quarter or less of the breast in the area around the lump is removed. Subsequent radiation treatments aim to kill any microscopic traces of cancer that might remain. Generally, the results of this approach are as good as those after simple or radical mastectomy; however, most oncologists feel that it should be restricted to removing fairly small tumors.

When a modified radical mastectomy is done, the breast and the adjacent lymph glands are removed, but all or most of the muscle tissue is preserved. This operation causes less disfigurement than a radical mastectomy, takes less time to heal, and causes less arm swelling. Breast reconstruction after this surgery produces a very good result.

With a radical mastectomy, the entire breast, all the breast (pectoral) muscles, and the associated lymph glands are removed. Today, this treatment is used only when the cancer has spread from the breast to the muscles beneath. Recovery takes a long time, and breast reconstruction is difficult.

Treatment of Disease That Has Spread

Several studies have suggested that only 25 percent of breast cancers have not spread beyond the breast at the time of diagnosis. Another 15 percent have spread to other parts of the breast and the lymph glands. The remaining 60 percent have spread further, often so microscopically as to be undetectable at the time of the original diagnosis.

These likelihoods suggest that, ideally, the diagnosis of breast cancer should be made earlier than it is now. They also suggest that surgery should be followed by radiation and/or chemotherapy. The problem is that no ideal form of these treatments is yet available; each method has risks and complications as well as benefits. Both radiation and chemotherapy cause distressing side effects such as hair loss, depression of the immune system, reduced blood cell formation, nausea, vomiting, and diarrhea—and even other cancers. Such reactions depend on the particular drug used and/or radiation dose and on the patient's particular response to these.

The best form of chemotherapy seems to be treatment with a combination of low doses of several drugs rather than with large doses of a single drug. The combination approach results both in better treatment and in fewer side effects.

Estrogen-Positive Tumors

Breast cancer in postmenopausal women is often a type that is sensitive to estrogen. This type of tumor grows more slowly than in other breast cancers, is less likely to recur soon, and, if it does recur, shrinks with the use of the antiestrogen drug tamoxifen citrate (Nolvadex). In premenopausal or menopausal women with estrogen-sensitive tumors, the cancer may shrink after removal of the ovaries, adrenal glands, or pituitary glands.

Women who need to have a breast lump examined for cancer must be certain to ask their surgeon to test the suspicious tissue for estrogen-receptor sensitivity. The tissue sample must be tested within fifteen minutes of its removal from the breast. If your local hospital is unable to perform the analysis, consider having the diagnosis made in a larger hospital, since if you have a cancer that is sensitive to estrogen, antiestrogen treatment could help prevent its spread.

Prevention of Breast Cancer

You may reduce the risk of getting breast cancer by heeding the following advice.

1. Avoid postmenopausal estrogen use for more than two years unless you have severe osteoporosis.

2. Avoid diets high in saturated fats, and substitute more vegetable fats.

3. Avoid large quantities of coffee, tea, colas, chocolate, and cocoa.

4. Exercise regularly, since recent studies show that women who have exercised vigorously from adolescence on have reduced their risk of getting breast cancer.

Psychological and Sexual Functioning After Mastectomy

To many women, the loss of a breast is a devastating experience. A Gallup poll showed that 60 percent of women felt their womanhood would be impaired by such a loss, and 9 percent said they would rather die. After a mastectomy, you may see yourself as mutilated, sexually repulsive, and facing the possibility of a lingering and painful death. You may wish to avoid any sexual or even affectionate encounters.

Your adjustment will depend upon regaining confidence in your body and in your prospects for the future. With the help of friends, family, and other women who have survived breast cancer, you can learn not to focus on your fears of cancer spreading or recurring and to try to live with some measure of assurance. Even if you are undergoing treatment for cancer that has spread, you should not postpone living actively. Optimism is still good medicine.

Women often dread their sexual partner's response to their mastectomy. Try to address your fears before you have the surgery. Consider the following:

1. Your partner should, if at all possible, be near you both before your surgery and during all stages of recovery.

2. You and your partner can grow accustomed and even indifferent to the changes in your body contour. You should remind yourself that the chance of defeating the cancer and gaining life far outweighs the shock of losing a breast.

3. Your partner should be encouraged to express love in physical ways—by touching, holding hands, and hugging. You need all of his support and reassurance.

4. You should learn to care for the incision and change the dressings with your partner's help. This contact allows both of you to accept the reality of your new shape.

5. You can usually resume sexual activity as soon as you leave the hospital. Just be sure to use positions that will not injure the wounded area.

6. Consider breast reconstruction with your surgeon and partner as soon after surgery as possible. Research has shown that women with reconstructed breasts feel less anxiety about their cancer and their sexuality and less depression and grief over the loss of their breast. The results of breast reconstruction can look and feel very natural.

7. If sexual problems arise, do not hesitate to ask for help from other women who have gone through similar operations or from a professional counselor. Your local chapter of the American Cancer Society can put you in touch with women who have had breast surgery; with support groups; and with literature on prostheses, reconstruction, and treatments. Reach for Recovery is a national support group for women who have undergone breast removal and are contemplating prostheses or breast reconstruction.

Mastectomy usually does not mar marriage or other close relationships. Sharing such a crisis can actually foster more communication and affection. The result is often an improvement in sexual relations.

Breast Reconstruction

Breast reconstruction is a recently developed surgical technique that offers mastectomy patients the chance to have a normal-looking chest (see figure 28). Age need not be a barrier to breast

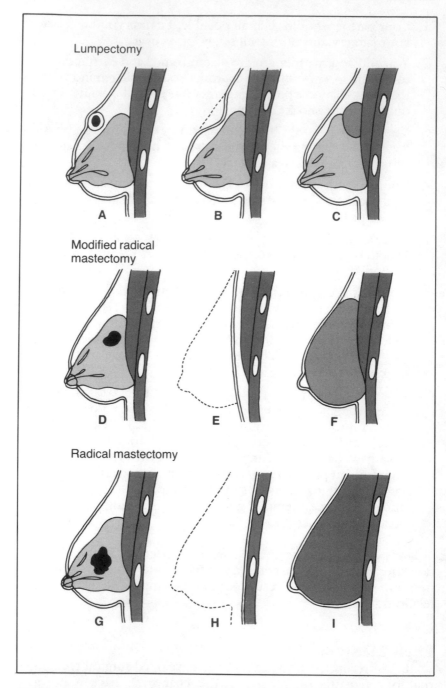

Figure 28. Breast Cancer Surgery and Reconstruction

reconstruction. Breast cancer is more frequent in women over forty, so it is older women who most frequently seek reconstruction. Sound health, not age, is the important consideration.

If you had a mastectomy many years ago, when reconstruction techniques did not exist, you may still be a candidate for reconstruction if you are in good health.

Select a plastic surgeon carefully, making sure that he or she is board certified in plastic surgery. In addition, the surgeon should have experience in all forms of breast reconstruction. A list of board-certified plastic surgeons who perform breast reconstruction may be obtained from the American Society of Plastic and Reconstructive Surgeons, Suite 1900, 233 N. Michigan Avenue, Chicago, Illinois 60601.

A general surgeon or other physicians in your community can be sources of referral. Women who have had reconstructive surgery may be located through the Reach for Recovery organization (which can be contacted through the local office of the American Cancer Society).

The timing of reconstruction will depend on the woman, her particular cancer, and the judgment of her doctors. (Breast reconstruction does not hinder further examinations for breast cancer.) Reconstruction can be done at the time of the mastectomy or after the mastectomy site heals and the tissues have had time to soften again. Some plastic surgeons believe results are better and complications fewer if they delay reconstruction. The delay also

Breast cancer surgery and breast reconstruction techniques depend on the type and location of the cancerous growth. A lumpectomy is most often done for a small growth that has not spread (**A**); all that is removed is the lump itself and a small amount of tissue (**B**). A small silicone implant may be used to restore the shape of the breast (**C**). A modified radical mastectomy is used for larger or deeper cancers (**D**); the entire breast is removed, but the chest muscle is left in place (**E**). A new breast to match its partner can be molded of silicone and covered with the patient's own skin. Sometimes the nipple can be saved; usually a substitute is created with skin from the inner thigh (**F**). A radical mastectomy, sometimes performed when the cancer has spread outside the breast (**G**), requires removal of both breast and chest muscle (**H**). A new breast can be reconstructed by transplanting tissue from the back, abdomen, or buttock (**I**).

allows the patient time to cope with the experience of having had cancer.

Some women want immediate reconstruction because they feel unable to deal with the postmastectomy defect. If a woman requires chemotherapy and/or radiation therapy as part of her treatment, however, reconstruction must be postponed until the course of the treatment is completed.

Several techniques for reconstructing a breast are now being used. Exactly which technique is used depends on the woman's expectations, the type of mastectomy she has had, whether she has undergone radiation, and the size and shape of her other breast.

In general, two procedures are required to reconstruct a breast—the first one to construct the breast mold, and a second to construct the nipple-areola area of the breast and to make any minor adjustments in contour to better match the opposite breast.

The goal of breast reconstruction is to give the mastectomy patient symmetrical, attractive breasts. The shape or size of the remaining breast may make duplication difficult or impossible. The plastic surgeon may, for this reason, also recommend enlarging, reducing, or lifting the remaining breast. If surgery is performed to alter the shape or size of the remaining breast, it is done when the breast mold of the "new" breast is constructed.

For further information and helpful photographs of the results of breast reconstruction, read *A Woman's Decision—Breast Care, Treatment, and Reconstruction* by Karen Berger and John Bustwick III, M.D. (St. Louis, Mo.: C V Mosby, 1984).

SUGGESTED READINGS

Glucksberg, Harold, M.D., and Singer, Jack W., M.D. *Cancer Care: A Personal Guide.* Baltimore: Johns Hopkins University Press, 1980.

Petrek, Jeanne A., M.D. *A Woman's Guide to the Prevention, Detection, and Treatment of Cancer.* New York: Macmillan, 1985.

Eleven

Your Nutritional Health

T HE gains in health and longevity that we have enjoyed in this century owe more to improved nutrition and sanitation than to any medical breakthroughs. Diets that supply adequate proteins, carbohydrates, and fats help us resist disease and allow us to live actively and energetically. Diets that are rich in essential vitamins and minerals have eradicated many of the deficiency diseases that were once prevalent. Sound nutrition strengthens the ability to resist disease, to cope with stress, and to preserve maximum vitality throughout the life span. The bounty of the American diet, however, carries its own hazards.

We are becoming increasingly sophisticated about the role that food plays in our lives. We understood very early that food was love. We learned a little later that food was fattening. Now we hear that food is toxic; even more recently we've read that food is preventive. We are still learning that food plays a critical part in the development of specific diseases, such as diabetes and cancer of the colon and breast, but we haven't yet fully grasped the extent of its role. Confusing and often contradictory information and ideas about what we should eat and what we mustn't eat and which foods will kill us and which foods will cure us leave us feeling queasy and vulnerable.

You cannot live in fear that every barrel is full of poisoned apples. Weighing the benefits and risks of every morsel is probably not nearly as helpful as occasionally stepping on the scales yourself. The shape and composition of your body changes with age; the proportion of muscle to fat and water decreases even though your weight may stay the same. Since fat tissue requires fewer calories to maintain itself than muscle, you will burn up less food as you age.

THE ENERGY VALUE OF FOOD

The proteins, carbohydrates, and fats in food have energy value, measured as calories. Chemical reactions in your body transform the energy in food into electrical energy for the transmission of nerve messages, into mechanical energy for your muscle movements, and into chemical energy for building or breaking down tissues.

About 60 percent of your body's energy supply is used just to keep you warm—to maintain your 98.6° F body temperature. The rest of the energy supply fuels the other physiological processes necessary to life.

Your basal metabolic rate—the amount of energy used by your body at rest to accomplish all the chemical reactions needed for respiration, circulation, and digestion—diminishes by about 10 percent to 15 percent after the age of fifty. Your body stores energy as glycogen in the liver or muscles or as fat when you take in more food than you can use. This latter state can be achieved by regularly doing your hardest work at the dinner table. Conversely, when you use up more energy than can be derived from the food you eat during stress, activity, illness, dieting, or starvation, your body has to utilize its glycogen, its fat, and, ultimately, its own muscle.

While your particular nutritional needs depend on your size, metabolic rate, state of health, and level of activity, you can follow these general caloric guidelines recommended by the National Academy of Science, keeping in mind that if you are very physically active, your needs will resemble those of younger people:

- Adults between the ages of fifty and seventy-five should eat only 90 percent of the calories that those under fifty eat, or about 1,800 (1,400–2,200) calories daily, depending on their level of activity.
- Adults above seventy-five years should eat only 75 percent to 80 percent of the calories that those under fifty eat, or about 1,600 (1,200–2,000) calories daily, depending on their level of activity.
- Older adults should divide their daily caloric intake so that it contains about 12 percent protein, 30 percent fat, and the remainder (over 50 percent) carbohydrates. (See sample menus.)

**Recommended Daily Dietary Allowance for the Maintenance
of Good Nutrition of Older Women (age 50+)**

Food Substance	Amount Recommended*	Representative Food Sources
Protein	44 g	Meat, poultry, fish, milk, cheese, eggs, soybeans
Carbohydrates (excess stored as fat)	40–70 g	Bread, sugar, cereals
Fats	No more than 30% of diet	Eggs, liver, kidney, whole milk, oils

Fat-Soluble Vitamins
(stored in the body if an excess is taken)

Vitamin A	800 µg	Liver, carrots, greens, sweet potatoes, cantaloupe, eggs
Vitamin D	5 µg	Milk, oily fish, salmon, shrimp, egg yolks
Vitamin E	8 mg	Wheat germ, vegetable oils, nuts, eggs, green vegetables

Water-Soluble Vitamins
(excreted if an excess is taken)

Vitamin C	60 mg	Citrus fruits, berries, tomatoes, liver, vegetables
Vitamin B_1 (thiamine)	1.0 mg	Yeast, wheat germ, pork, legumes, nuts, grains
Vitamin B_2 (riboflavin)	1.2 mg	Liver, almonds, wheat germ, mushrooms, egg yolks, cheese
Niacin	13 mg	Yeast, wheat germ, liver, poultry, fish, mushrooms
Vitamin B_6 (pyridoxine)	2.0 mg	Yeast, wheat germ, poultry, meat, fish, legumes, bananas
Vitamin B_{12}	3.0 µg	Clams, liver, shellfish, sardines, salmon
Folic acid	400 µg	Yeast, wheat germ, bran, liver, egg yolks

* g = gram; mg = milligram; µg = microgram

Recommended Daily Dietary Allowance for the Maintenance of Good Nutrition of Older Women (age 50+)

Food Substance	Amount Recommended	Representative Food Sources
Minerals		
Calcium	1,200–1,500 mg	Milk, yeast, almonds, fish, eggs, grains, meats, vegetables
Phosphorus	800 mg	Grains, yeast, nuts, eggs, cheese, seafood, poultry, meat
Magnesium	300 mg	Bran, wheat germ, soybeans, nuts, raisins, shellfish
Iron	10 mg	Bran, yeast, wheat germ, liver, soybeans, parsley
Zinc	15 mg	Yeast, beef, lamb, cheese, egg yolks, crabmeat
Iodine	150 µg	Iodized salt, seafood
Electrolytes		
Sodium	1,100–3,300 mg	Ham, cheese, meats, seafood, celery, spinach
Potassium	1,875–5,625 mg	Fruits, nuts, meats, seafood, vegetables, grains, seeds
Chloride	1,700–5,100 mg	Salt

It is important to realize that the Recommended Daily Allowances (RDAs) are based on healthy older adults and that nutritional needs are altered by disease, stress, drug use, and other conditions.

THE NUTRITIVE VALUE OF FOOD

In addition to energy value, food has nutritive value drawn from proteins, carbohydrates, fats, vitamins, and minerals. Your body can manufacture some of the nutrients it needs for normal growth, health, and vitality, but it depends upon food for the rest. Protein, vitamin, and mineral needs do not decrease with age; when you reduce calories, you must increase the nutrient density of your food.

Nutritionists have identified the four basic food groups necessary for a healthful and balanced diet.

**The Four Basic Food Groups and
Recommended Daily Servings**

Food Group	Recommended Daily Servings	Sample Servings (measurements are for 1 serving)
Milk	4	1 cup milk 1 cup yogurt
Meat	2	2 eggs 2 oz cheddar cheese 2 oz lean cooked meat ½ cup creamed cottage cheese
Fruits and Vegetables	4	1 medium-sized apple 1 cup raw broccoli ½ cup orange juice ½ cup cooked spinach
Grains	4	1 slice bread ½ cup cooked cereal ½ cup cooked pasta ½ cup cooked rice

Daily Menu Sample (about 1,800 calories)

Day 1	*Day 2*

Breakfast:

1/2 cup grapefruit juice	1 orange, sliced
1/2 cup oatmeal	1/2 cup unenriched grits
1/3 cup low-fat milk	2 slices bacon
1 tablespoonful brown sugar	tea
1 slice whole-wheat bread	
1 teaspoonful margarine	
coffee	

Lunch:

Grilled mozzarella cheese (1 oz) and tomato (1/8 tomato) sandwich	1 cup cream of tomato soup
	1/3 cup tuna salad in a half slice of whole-wheat pita bread
Baked apple	1/5 of a head lettuce
1 cup low-fat milk	1 cup apple juice

Snack:

tea	
2 oatmeal-raisin cookies	

Dinner or Supper:

3 1/2 oz broiled chicken, white meat	1 cup beef stew
1/2 cup mixed rice, green peas, and mushrooms	1 cup enriched rice
1/3 cup cucumbers, sliced	1/2 cup coleslaw
1 tablespoonful oil	1 slice whole-wheat bread
1 slice rye bread	1 teaspoonful margarine
1 teaspoonful margarine	1/2 cup raspberry sherbert
1/2 cup pineapple chunks	
tea	

Snack:

2 cups popcorn	six-ounce cup of cocoa
1 tablespoonful margarine	1 bran muffin, small

A BALANCED DIET

If you want to stay as healthy as possible, you cannot take your nutrition for granted. You need to know how to evaluate your diet and how to shift the balance between proteins, carbohydrates, and fats.

Proteins

Protein is essential for the growth, maintenance, and repair of body tissues. Protein contains twenty amino acids—the protein building blocks. Nine of these, the essential amino acids, cannot be manufactured by the body and must come from foods. Some foods, such as meats, eggs, and soybeans, contain all the essential amino acids. Other foods, such as beans or peas, have only some of the essential amino acids; however, when eaten with rice or wheat, the combination provides all the essential amino acids. Vegetarians need to be particularly careful to eat appropriate combinations of foods.

To handle your protein intake wisely, skin and trim your meat, fish, and poultry whenever possible. Also, broil or poach these foods. Cut down on roasted, braised, smoked, or basted meats. Limit consumption of foods high in cholesterol, such as egg yolks, cheese, whole milk, and even whole-milk cottage cheese. Eat more chicken, veal, fish, and tofu than beef, and think in terms of three-ounce servings rather than the eight-ounce servings the butcher and fish seller recommend, and the restaurants regularly serve. During illness your body uses more protein, so try to increase your protein intake when you are sick.

Carbohydrates

Carbohydrates have been touted as both the dietary heavies and the dietary heroes. The trouble with lumping all carbohydrates together is that they are not all alike. Some complex carbohydrates —vegetables, including potatoes; fruits; pastas; rice; and whole grains—are replete with vitamins and minerals. Other, simple carbohydrates—highly refined sugars and grains—are empty of anything but calories. In some forms, carbohydrates are chemically broken down more quickly than either proteins or fats and thus provide a more readily available form of energy; in other forms (fiber, for example), they are not digestible at all but provide bulk to aid in stool formation.

Under no circumstances should you go on a reducing diet that eliminates or drastically cuts down on carbohydrates. For that matter, no reducing diet should require you to eliminate an entire food group. You can cut down your portions, but don't, for example, treat grains and starches such as rice, potatoes, or pasta as enemies—they are rich in nutrients.

Fiber

The lack of fiber, or roughage, in the American diet now appalls nutritionists. Fiber means the parts of plant foods that are not absorbed by the body. People in countries where diets are high in fiber have low rates of constipation, diseases of the intestinal tract, and bowel cancer (see chapter 7). Vegetables, fruits, and grains that have not been too refined are high in fiber.

Most Americans eat about ten grams of fiber a day. To prevent bowel disease and perhaps reduce the cholesterol in your diet, you should have about twenty-five to thirty grams of fiber a day.

Fats

Fats, also known as lipids, are made up of 90 percent triglycerides, or fatty acids, and 10 percent cholesterol and phospholipids. Fats are a concentrated source of energy, the building blocks of hormones, the transporters of some of the fat-soluble vitamins, and the source of your body's insulation. Fats are also important in the manufacture of chemicals (prostaglandins) that help regulate blood pressure, heart rate, clotting mechanisms, and parts of the nervous system.

For the past seventy years, Americans have consumed about 40 percent of their diets in the form of fats. Evidence suggests a strong causal relationship between high fat intake and the incidence of cancer. It is also known that diets too rich in animal fats increase your risk for heart disease, cause obesity and indigestion, and create absorption problems in your digestive system. Each gram of fat yields nine calories, while each gram of protein or carbohydrate yields four calories. If you reduced your dietary intake of fats from 40 percent to 30 percent of your total intake, and you increased your carbohydrates by 10 percent, you would automatically cut down on your calories.

On the other hand, if you don't have enough fat in your diet, you may develop dry, scaly skin; dry hair; hormonal deficiencies; and bleeding problems. In addition, any wounds you might have would not heal readily. Also, one of the big problems with reducing the fats in your diet is that it inevitably means tampering with your protein consumption. (Most good sources of protein also contain

Fiber Content of Representative Foods

Fruits	Quantity	Fiber Content (grams)
Apples	½ medium	0 – 2
Bananas	½ medium	0 – 2
Blackberries	½ cup	4 – 6
Cranberries	½ cup	2 – 4
Grapefruit	½ medium	0 – 2
Grapes	10 – 15	0 – 2
Peaches	1 medium	2 – 4
Prunes	2 medium	2 – 4
Raspberries	½ cup	4 – 6
Vegetables		
Broccoli	½ cup (raw or cooked)	2 – 4
Cabbage	½ cup (cooked)	2 – 4
Carrots	½ cup (raw)	0 – 2
Celery	½ cup (raw or cooked)	0 – 2
Corn	½ cup (cooked)	4 – 6
Lentils	½ cup (cooked)	4 – 6
Lima beans	½ cup (cooked)	8 – 10
Peas	½ cup (raw)	6 – 8
Potatoes	½ cup (cooked)	2 – 4
Spinach	½ cup (cooked)	6 – 8
Tomatoes	½ cup (raw or cooked)	0 – 2
Cereals		
40% Bran Flakes	⅔ cup	4
Corn Flakes	1 cup	3
Grits	¼ cup	4
Oat Bran	⅓ cup	7
Grains		
Bread (white)	1 slice	less than 1
Bread (whole-wheat)	1 slice	1 – 2
Graham crackers	2	1
Rye wafers	2	2

fat and cholesterol.) Without adequate protein, your body starts to feast on itself instead of on the food you eat.

Cholesterol and Arteriosclerosis

Cholesterol is part of all animal cells and is vital in the manufacture of hormones affecting your metabolism and hormones regulating your sexual function. The liver makes cholesterol, and the rest of your body's cholesterol comes from animal sources, such as meat, eggs, dairy products, and fish.

Cholesterol globules in your blood are transported to various tissues by high-density lipoproteins (HDL). When you have high levels of cholesterol in your blood, you need large numbers of high-density lipoproteins to transport it, since the cholesterol can deposit in your arteries and result in arteriosclerosis, which, in turn, can result in heart attack or stroke. You can raise the level of HDL by exercising vigorously and also by drinking small quantities of alcohol, such as two four-ounce glasses of wine a day.

While it has not been definitively proved that you can lower the level of cholesterol in your blood by lowering the amount of saturated fats in your diet, the American Heart Association strongly recommends that you eat less saturated, or animal, fats. It also recommends that you adhere to these guidelines:

- Limit fats to 30 percent of your diet. One-half to one ounce of fat (15–28 grams) a day, half saturated and half polyunsaturated, is sufficient to meet your body's requirements. Reduce your consumption of foods that contain hidden fats, such as doughnuts or luncheon meats.

- Eat fats from plant sources rather than from animal sources (unsaturated fats, as in corn and corn oil margarine, safflower seeds or oils, and vegetables, rather than saturated fats, as in butter and fatty meats).

- Eat fats from fish sources rather than from meat sources at least three times a week. There is some evidence that such a diet can reduce the risk of heart disease.

- Eat small amounts of salad or corn oil daily and/or fresh or frozen vegetables, all of which contain essential fats that your body cannot manufacture on its own.

- Make sure your diet includes fiber-rich foods, since they can reduce your body's absorption of cholesterol from your intestines.

Vitamins
Understanding carbohydrates is a simple matter compared with sorting the facts from hopes and wishes about vitamins and minerals. It is bedeviling to try to make sense of, and choose among, the proliferating packages of vitamin and mineral supplements that appear in the pharmacy, the supermarket, and the health food store.

Vitamins are compounds needed to sustain life; they cannot be made by the body. There are two major types of vitamins—fat-soluble and water-soluble. Fat-soluble vitamins are carried in the body by fats and are responsible for regulating various metabolic processes. Water-soluble vitamins bind to proteins to form enzymes and are also needed for many vital chemical reactions. Fat-soluble vitamins can build up in your body and be toxic, whereas your body excretes any excess water-soluble vitamins. (It has been said that the richest source of vitamins in the world is the sewers of New York City.) Accordingly, the National Academy of Sciences cautions against significantly increasing consumption of the fat-soluble vitamin A even though researchers suspect that Beta-Carotene, a substance found in leafy green and yellow vegetables that in part is converted to vitamin A in the body, may offer some protection against cancer.

If you eat a balanced daily diet from the four food groups, you usually do not need vitamin supplements. Eating vegetables and fruits raw or steamed helps preserve their vitamin content. A regular daily vitamin pill is advisable if your diet is erratic or if you are suffering from a disease.

Vitamins are found naturally in many foods, and many foods manufactured in the United States are vitamin-enriched. Despite this fact, the myth of superhealth through larger and larger doses of vitamin pills enjoys great popularity.

The Food and Drug Administration plays no role in regulating vitamins and minerals in our diets other than to establish maximum limits for pregnant and lactating women and for children under twelve. Many pharmaceutical companies are therefore free to imply that more is better, though excess vitamins can, in some cases, be harmful. Many companies also falsely advertise that natural vitamins are better than synthetic ones, though most of the expensive so-called natural vitamins contain synthetic components. When you take megadoses of many vitamins, you are taking these compounds as drugs rather than as vitamins, and the same precautions should be taken as with other drugs.

Vitamin Facts

	Recommended Daily Allowance for Women 50+
Fat-Soluble Vitamins (Excess stores in body can be toxic.) Vitamin A	800 μg
Vitamin D	5 μg
Vitamin E	8 mg
Water-Soluble Vitamins (Excess is excreted.) Vitamin C	60 mg
Vitamin B$_1$ (thiamine)	1.0 mg
Vitamin B$_2$ (riboflavin)	1.2 mg
Vitamin B$_6$ (pyridoxine)	2.0 mg
Vitamin B$_{12}$	3.0 μg
Niacin	13 mg
Folic acid	400 μg

Major Body Functions	*Signs of Deficiency*
Helps form and maintain skin and mucous membrane; promotes healthy eye tissue and adaptation to dim light	Night blindness; dry, rough skin
Helps maintain bones and teeth by aiding calcium and phosphorus absorption	Rickets (a crippling bone disease), rare in adults
Not clearly understood; helps protect vitamin A in body	No symptoms known; very unlikely in adults
Maintains collagens; aids resistance to infections	Bleeding gums; degeneration of skin
The B-complex vitamins aid in metabolism of foods; are very closely related—too much or too little intake of one may affect the effectiveness of the others	Swollen limbs; edema
	Cracks at corner of mouth; eye lesions
	Irritability; convulsions; kidney stones
B$_{12}$ is needed for blood-cell formation	Pernicious anemia
	Skin lesions; mental disorders
Needed for blood-cell formation; helps break down carbon and hydrogen in body	Hair loss; depression; fatigue

Minerals

Minerals occur naturally in the environment, and about sixteen of the ninety-odd existing minerals are essential for growth and well-being. The major minerals in the body are calcium, phosphorus, potassium, sodium, iron, sulfur, and magnesium. In addition, your body needs trace quantities of zinc, copper, iodine, fluoride, manganese, cobalt, molybdenum, selenium, and chromium.

Many minerals—such as calcium, phosphorus, and fluoride—are found in the skeleton; some are found in hormones, as iodine is attached to the thyroid hormone; others, like iron, are attached to hemoglobin and circulate in the blood. These substances maintain critical balances between cells and their surroundings and between acids and bases so that the body's vital chemical reactions can occur.

Generally, a healthful diet provides adequate and balanced minerals with two notable exceptions, which are particularly important to the older woman's health: calcium and iron. Also, women with high blood pressure or those on diuretics need to limit their sodium intake and increase their potassium intake.

Mineral supplements (other than calcium, iron, or, in certain cases, potassium) are not needed, can be hazardous, and can upset delicate balances within the body. Foods are far safer and are more natural sources of nutrients than pills. A wise woman will be pill-free whenever possible.

Water

About 60 percent of your body is composed of water. Six percent of your body's store of water is lost daily in urine, stool, sweat, and breath and must be replaced each day. Drink six eight-ounce glasses of liquids each day.

Alcohol

Alcohol, consumed in moderate doses, may be more beneficial than harmful to your health. Several studies have concluded that moderate drinkers (those who have one or two drinks a day) live longer than those who abstain. Moderate drinkers have higher levels of high-density lipoproteins, or HDL, in their blood. This reduces arteriosclerosis and may help the heart by relieving stress and lessening tension in arterial wall muscles. A drink is taken to mean 1½ ounces of 80-proof distilled spirits, one 12-ounce glass of lager beer, one 5-ounce glass of French wine, one 4-ounce glass of American wine, or one 3-ounce glass of sherry.

Mineral Facts

Mineral	Recommended Daily Allowance for Women 50 +	Major Body Functions	Signs of Deficiency
Calcium	1,200– 1,500 mg	Strengthens bones and teeth; helps blood clot; maintains water balance; maintains nerve responses	Osteoporosis
Phosphorus	800 mg	Helps maintain teeth and bones; needed to promote acid-base balance in body; aids energy metabolism	Unlikely to occur
Magnesium	300 mg	Activates enzymes; helps control body temperature; helps body use proteins	Hormone or kidney problems
Iron	10 mg	Part of hemoglobin in blood—carries oxygen to blood	Anemia
Zinc	15 mg	Needed to produce insulin (hormone); helps body metabolize nutrients	Loss of taste (similar to vitamin A deficiency)
Iodine	150 μg	Needed to maintain function of thyroid gland	Enlarged thyroid (goiter)
Sodium	1,100– 3,300 mg	Helps maintain acid-base balance in body; aids water balance; needed for proper muscle and nerve activity	Unlikely to occur
Potassium	1,875– 5,625 mg	Helps maintain water balance in body; needed for proper nerve and muscle activity	Unlikely to occur
Chloride	1,700– 5,100 mg	A source for hydrochloric acid in gastric juices; helps maintain water balance; needed to maintain acid-base balance in body	Unlikely to occur

Alcoholic beverages contain calories that you must consider in your daily caloric intake. Note these amounts:
12 ounces beer or ale = 150 calories
12 ounces light beer = 95 calories
4 ounces dry table wine = about 100 calories
1½ ounces distilled spirits = 90–120 calories
1 ounce liqueur = 70–115 calories

EATING PROBLEMS OF OLDER WOMEN

Changing circumstances quite often can change eating patterns. Loneliness can lead to an unbalanced diet, especially if overeating or undereating occurs. Women who have enjoyed cooking for many may find it a chore to cook for one or two. When children leave home or particularly when a spouse dies, it is not hard to lose interest in regular meals and to let the good eating habits of a lifetime deteriorate.

Poor health can interfere with proper eating. Illnesses that keep you at home—arthritis, heart disease, or impaired respiratory conditions, for example—may prevent you from keeping perishables such as milk, fruits, and vegetables on hand. Poor teeth or lack of teeth can make eating unpleasant or leave you choosing foods with low nutritive value. The diminished sense of taste and smell that accompanies age can also decrease your interest in eating. Drugs taken for medical or psychological conditions can interfere with your ability to absorb vitamins and minerals or interfere with their role in your body's normal chemical reactions.

Research teams have found that women over fifty-five often have diets low in calcium, protein, vitamin A, thiamine (B_1), and iron and that women over sixty-six often eat too little food to meet their energy needs.

Lactose Intolerance

Many people have a complete or partial lack of an enzyme called lactase, which is needed to digest lactose, the main sugar found in milk. This problem is more common in older persons, since lactase levels decrease with age, and older people may notice gas, cramps, and diarrhea after drinking milk.

If you have problems tolerating milk, try drinking small amounts of milk at a time or, instead, buy soybean milk, available at health food stores. You can also purchase LactAid, a product that provides the deficient enzyme from yeast and can help you digest milk. You may also find that dairy products that are fermented—such as live-culture yogurt, buttermilk, or cheeses—are usually much easier to digest, since they contain less lactose than milk does.

RECOMMENDATIONS FOR GOOD NUTRITION

The following suggestions should prove helpful in maintaining good nutrition.

1. Try to keep fresh or frozen vegetables and fruits on hand, and eat them raw or steam them to prevent loss of vitamins.
2. Try to eat fewer processed fast foods to reduce empty calories.
3. Walk every day to stimulate your appetite, move your bowels, and burn calories.
4. If your appetite is poor, try drinking a small glass of wine before lunch and/or dinner to stimulate it. Add a few teaspoonfuls of dry milk or instant breakfast powder to your food to get added protein and calories.
5. Eat foods that are varied in texture, flavor, color, and temperature.
6. Eat slowly and chew thoroughly to decrease gas and indigestion.
7. Try to eat smaller meals at regular times; several small meals a day are better than one or two large ones.
8. Eat at a restaurant occasionally, or have some of your meals at a senior center.
9. Cook in large amounts and freeze several portions if you want to reduce your cooking time. Do not refreeze food that has been thawed, since refreezing poses a risk of bacterial infection.
10. Hire a shopping service or a local teenager, or apply for Meals on Wheels if you cannot get out to shop or if you have trouble cooking.
11. For accurate sources of nutrition information, ask your doctor to refer you to a registered dietician in a hospital or read books on nutrition.

SUGGESTED READINGS

Brody, Jane. *Jane Brody's Nutrition Book: A Lifetime Guide to Good Eating for Better Health and Weight Control.* New York: W. W. Norton, 1981.

Cumming, Candy, and Newman, Vicky. *Eater's Guide: Nutrition Basics for Busy People.* Englewood Cliffs, N.J.: Prentice-Hall, 1981.

White, Kristin. *Diet and Cancer: There Is a Connection.* New York: Bantam Books, 1984.

Twelve

Your Sexuality

S EX wasn't invented during the 1960s, but some of the older generation let younger people think it was. Less repressed than our Victorian parents, but sometimes floored by the outspokenness of the younger generation, as often as not we keep quiet about sex. This habit of discretion has not always been helpful; it has sometimes kept some of us in the dark about the nature and extent of sexuality in our own generation, and often it has made us less able to communicate openly about sex, limiting our sexual potential.

SEX AFTER FIFTY

The studies of sexual behavior conducted by Kinsey, Masters and Johnson, and the Consumers Union fully document that healthy men and women often have active sex lives well into old age and that they often enjoy sex more and are less inhibited about it than in their youth. A study conducted by Dr. Alexander Leaf in villages in Nepal, Soviet Georgia, and Ecuador—where some of the world's oldest people live—further revealed that even people a hundred years old or older can lead sexually vigorous lives.

Both Kinsey, in the late 1940s, and Masters and Johnson, in the 1960s, found that there was little decline in women's sexual responsiveness until very late in life, that most men over sixty were fully capable of intercourse, and that people are particularly apt to maintain their sex lives if they have been sexually active in youth and middle age.

Hormonal and Psychological Factors

Just after menopause, some women feel increased or decreased sexual desire because of the temporary instability of their hormone levels. Once the hormones restabilize, however, most older women continue to have the same level of sexual desire they had before menopause. Menopause can represent a liberation from the fear of pregnancy and from the disruptions accompanying menstruation; often it coincides with children's leaving home. All these changes can encourage more spontaneous sexual activity. Nevertheless, after fifty, women as well as men note changes in their sexual functioning that are normal but that may necessitate accommodations by each partner.

Physiological Factors

From adolescence onward, women as well as men have similar responses to sexual stimulation that can be separated into four phases, though men—particularly younger men—experience all four in a much shorter time than do women. First is the excitement phase, a response to touch or to psychological stimulation. Next is the plateau phase, an intensification of sexual excitement and tension. This is followed by the orgasmic phase, or the climax. The final phase is the resolution phase, the return to the relaxed state.

Starting around the age of fifty, physiological changes in a woman's skin, breasts, and pelvic structures affect her sexual responses. The older breast swells less with sexual stimulation. After menopause, the walls of the vagina thin and are less lubricated. The vagina is not as capable of stretching as before, so intercourse may be painful and may cause small tears in the vaginal wall. Also, because of the thinning vaginal walls, the urethra can be irritated by the thrusting of the penis, resulting in burning on urination, more frequent urination for two or three days after intercourse, and, occasionally, cramps in the lower abdomen or bloating. During orgasm, older women experience fewer pelvic spasms and return more quickly to the relaxed state than younger women. Occasionally, however, the uterine contractions that occur during orgasm can be prolonged and cause cramps.

You can compensate for the physiological changes of the vagina. The secretions that lubricate your vagina are less apt to decrease if you experience sexual stimulation at least once or twice a week. Many women have found that using a simple lubricant during intercourse such as K-Y jelly, cocoa butter, or sesame or coconut oil provides safe relief. Using an estrogen cream (such as Premarin cream) in the vagina once a week over a short period of time can reverse the dryness and thinness of the vagina and relieve painful intercourse. Some doctors prescribe estrogen pills, which relieve many of the pelvic symptoms of aging. The risks and benefits must be evaluated by you and your doctor (see chapter 9).

SEXUAL NEEDS OF OLDER MEN AND WOMEN

Medical researchers have studied female sexual physiology and clarified some of the important differences in sexual response between women and men. Most notably, the indispensable role of clitoral stimulation in producing the female orgasm is now clearly understood. This information allows both men and women to recognize that difficulties in achieving mutual satisfaction in the sex act can often be explained by problems in technique rather than by the inadequacy of either partner. If sex is to produce mutual pleasure, it requires consideration for the differences between two human beings. It may not always require words, but it does require sensitive attention to each other.

> I had difficulty reaching orgasm during inter-
> course until I read a book on female orgasm and
> realized that there was nothing wrong with me—I
> just needed a different kind of stimulation. I
> started to guide my husband's hand over my
> clitoris, exactly as I needed to intensify my sexual
> feelings. Believe it or not, he was thrilled to learn
> that he could arouse me so.
>
> —*Olga P., fifty-nine*

As women age, they will be wise to recognize and appreciate the fact that the sexual needs of the older men with whom they make love are changing also. You can be helpful to your male partner and afford both of you greater sexual pleasure if you know that after fifty the majority of men need the kind of physical attention that women have needed all their lives.

From Masters and Johnson, we know that older men are slower to become sexually aroused. Erection is delayed, the sex act must last longer for them to achieve orgasm, and the amount and force of their ejaculate decrease. Older men often require twenty-four to forty-eight hours between orgasmic experiences to be potent.

Older men do not experience psychogenic erections—erections stimulated solely by their minds—as frequently as younger men. More often, the older man needs to have his penis stimulated directly for it to become erect. When this need is something new in a couple's sex life, the woman may erroneously assume that she is no longer as attractive to her partner. In fact, a limp penis may not indicate the absence of intense desire but may merely indicate the need for more tactile stimulation. Because the older male takes so much longer to reach orgasm, the sexual pace of men and women becomes more similar, and sex can improve correspondingly.

IMPROVING SEXUAL COMMUNICATION WITH YOUR PARTNER

It is not easy to alter your sexual habits and routines. Even after years of intimacy, it can be uncomfortable and awkward to discuss your needs openly and frankly. A man and a woman do not necessarily understand each other sexually even when they do understand each other in other ways. Confusion and misinformation about both male and female sexual functioning, about what is "normal" and what is expected, can create barriers to a satisfying sex life. Self-recrimination, blame, and disappointment suffered silently slowly erode your sex life.

If you feel uncomfortable with the subject of sex or have doubts about certain practices, you may want to read about the normal range of sexual behavior. (See Suggested Readings at the end of this chapter.) You will find that this range is very broad and that sexual desire and drive vary among adults and even within the same adult from week to week and month to month. If you feel unsatisfied or unloved, try to explain what you like and teach your partner what to do; encourage him to do the same. Reassure him that you do not feel that he is inadequate if he has trouble having an erection. Try to take a more active role in making love. You may wish to encourage your partner to help you have an orgasm manually, if he is having trouble with his erection, rather than have him worry about his lack of genital performance.

Your reading may inspire you to be more creative about your sexuality and to learn new ways to express your love.

IMPAIRED HEALTH AND SEX

Chronic illness in and of itself does not diminish sexual interest, but it poses particular problems. Illness can affect your self-esteem, self-image, and sexual functioning. The partner who is ill is often fearful and insecure; he or she may feel unattractive because of a deformity caused by the disease. The healthy partner is afraid to worsen a spouse's medical illness by sexual activity.

Chronic depression, anxiety, and fatigue can interfere with sexual interest and performance even without illness. Medications used to treat these states often worsen the problem. Alcohol, too, diminishes one's ability to perform sexually.

Heart conditions, strokes, and high blood pressure frighten couples into abandoning sex. Studies show that people rarely die during intercourse and that the stress caused by restricting sex can be worse than the risks posed by continuing to enjoy it.

> Since my husband's heart attack, both he and I
> are afraid to have intercourse. We worry that
> Harry could have another heart attack if we do.
> Both of us are too embarrassed to discuss this
> question with the doctor; meanwhile, we both
> feel stressed and are missing out.
> —*Tana K., sixty-eight*

Heart attack patients and persons with heart conditions need to know that sexual intercourse puts about the same strain on the heart as climbing two flights of stairs. In most cases, when you can resume climbing two flights of stairs (usually about twelve to sixteen weeks after a heart attack), you can resume sex. If you cannot climb two flights of stairs safely without suffering cardiac pain or shortness of breath, you should take your usual dose of nitroglycerin fifteen minutes to a half hour before engaging in sex. This should enable you to enjoy sex safely and without pain.

Arthritis commonly causes sexual limitations. The affected person, usually a woman, may have swollen joints that are painful to move. She may also have hip problems that hinder her from assuming the usual positions for intercourse. But people with arthritis can actually benefit from sexual activity if they make allowances for their physical impairments. The exercise itself can be a form of physical therapy that limbers the joints; the cortisone your adrenal glands release during the excitement phase acts like aspirin to reduce the inflammation of joints.

Some simple recommendations that might increase the pleasure of sex for arthritis sufferers follow:

- warm bath prior to intercourse
- proper timing of medicines

- gentle range-of-motion exercises before starting sexual activity, or done together as a part of your lovemaking
- lying on your sides or sitting in a chair for sex, rather than lying flat

Hysterectomy, total or partial, does not change the sexual performance of women. Many women imagine, however, that they have suddenly lost their sex appeal and sexual responsiveness. Education and reassurance by physicians, nurses, or other women who have had hysterectomies can help. Your partner's support after the surgery will be the most helpful. Women who undergo mastectomies, colostomies, or other necessary surgery need great reassurance from their partners concerning their sexual attractiveness.

Diabetes rarely causes sexual problems in women but often causes impotence in men, which may disappear once the disease is better controlled. If the impotence remains, a couple can find other forms of sexual expression, or the man may consider getting a surgical implant that enables him to have erections.

Prostate surgery causes impotence in about 30 percent of cases. In these cases, sexual desire remains, but erection and/or ejaculation are difficult or impossible. If this should happen to your partner, do not deny yourselves one of life's natural pleasures. Explore other ways of enjoying sex together.

CHANGING SEXUAL ATTITUDES

We now know that masturbation, for some people, can be an appropriate sexual release and an important technique both for learning about sex and for gaining satisfaction with and without a partner. However, it is a form of sexual activity that may or may not fit in with an individual's particular value system.

SEX AND THE WOMAN ALONE

It may be affection, touching, and companionship both in and out of bed rather than sex that one longs for as an older single woman.

> Yes, I miss the sex. But what really depressses me
> is loneliness, especially in bed. I miss companion-
> ship—a person that I am close to, that I can be
> totally myself with, whom I can really depend
> on. That is what I lost when Samuel died.
> —*Priscilla Z., eighty-three*

Finding a new intimate companion is not easy at any age. Older single women too often find social functions crowded with other single women and few men. Some practical tips for never married, widowed, or divorced women interested in meeting a partner are listed below:

- Ask your friends if they can introduce you to unattached male acquaintances whom they think you might enjoy meeting.

- Look up friends from your past—even your remote past. Consider old flames, good friends, and former suitors. You may be surprised to find that some of these men are also alone and wishing for companionship.

- You may want to initiate the contact—invite a man out for a drink, dinner, or a movie. It may be difficult for you to pick up the telephone, but both of you will probably be grateful for the contact.

Increasingly, women discover that they enjoy the friendship of other women, that the intimacy, fun, and support women friends offer satisfy many of their needs for love and affection.

SUGGESTED READINGS

Barbach, Lonnie G. *For Yourself: Fulfillment of Female Sexuality—a Guide to Orgasmic Response*. New York: New American Library, 1976.

Boston Women's Health Book Collective. *The New Our Bodies, Our Selves*. Rev. ed. New York: Simon & Schuster, 1985.

Brecher, Edward M., and the editors of Consumer Report Books. *Love, Sex, and Aging: A Consumers Union Report*. Mount Vernon, N.Y.: Consumer Reports, 1984.

Butler, Robert, and Lewis, Myrna. *Love and Sex After 60: A Guide for Men and Women in Their Later Years*. New York: Harper & Row, 1977.

Comfort, Alex. *The Joy of Sex*. New York: Simon & Schuster, 1974.

Hite, Shere. *The Hite Report: A Nationwide Study on Female Sexuality.* New York: Macmillan, 1976.

————. *The Hite Report on Male Sexuality.* New York: Alfred A. Knopf, 1981.

Masters, William H.; Johnson, Virginia E.; and Kolodny, Robert C. *Masters and Johnson on Sex and Human Loving.* Boston: Little, Brown, 1986.

Vida, Ginny. *Our Right to Love—A Lesbian Resource Book.* Englewood Cliffs, N.J.: Prentice-Hall, 1978.

Westheimer, Ruth. *Dr. Ruth's Guide to Good Sex.* New York: Warner Books, 1984.

Woods, Nancy Fugate. *Human Sexuality in Health and Illness.* 3d ed. St. Louis: C V Mosby, 1984.

Thirteen

Sleep and Temperature

W E are physical creatures, and, like all animals, we exhibit both cyclical behaviors and adaptive mechanisms to ensure that our species survives.

From infancy, human beings develop patterns of sleep and wakefulness. In later years, we are apt to idealize the ease with which we used to sleep. Older people often have more trouble falling asleep and staying asleep and feel less restored after a night's sleep than do younger people.

The body's temperature also fluctuates in a predictable pattern during each twenty-four-hour period. But as we get older, the body's built-in thermostat becomes less sensitive to both internal and external conditions. Most often, we notice that we feel cold more often. But older people are also particularly vulnerable to hot weather. We may also develop fevers less readily, even when we feel quite ill.

Many of the changes the older person experiences in temperature regulation and sleep patterns are normal. They do, however, require understanding, attention, and special accommodation.

SLEEP

> Sleep that knits up the ravel'd sleave of care,
> The death of each day's life, sore labour's bath,
> Balm of hurt minds, great nature's second course,
> Chief nourisher in life's feast.
>
> —*Shakespeare*

In the last fifteen years, more than ten thousand research papers have attempted to illuminate the state in which we spend nearly

255

one-third of our lives. This research has yielded some encouraging results—people can indeed improve the quality of their sleep.

Sleep Physiology
Certain bodily events occur at about the same time during each twenty-four-hour period. This daily pattern, called the circadian rhythm, includes changes in your body temperature, the secretion of various hormones, and the times you fall asleep and wake up. You take this rhythm for granted until you abruptly cross several time zones during a long airplane trip and experience the disturbing effects of jet lag, or unbalanced circadian rhythm. After a few uncomfortable days, your bodily functions adjust to the new twenty-four-hour cycle of day and night, and your rhythm of sleeping and waking is reestablished.

Research suggests that this pattern of sleeping and waking is controlled by chemicals in your brain. Research has also shown that sleep itself has a pattern. Two major types of sleep alternate with each other all night long: the sleep during which we dream, called Rapid Eye Movement, or REM, sleep; and the sleep during which we don't dream, called Non-REM sleep, which consists of four stages. During the night, you go through roughly three to five sleep cycles, each approximately ninety minutes long and each containing both REM and non-REM sleep.

Sleep Stages

REM Sleep (dream sleep)
Rapid eye movements begin; you dream; rapid, irregular breathing occurs; blood pressure and heart rate vary; blood flow to the brain increases; muscles twitch; and talking may occur.

Non-REM Sleep
Stage 1 (the transition between wakefulness and sleep): Muscles gradually relax, awareness of surroundings decreases, and the eyes roll slowly under closed lids.

Stages 2 to 4: The body progressively relaxes; breathing slows and grows regular; awareness of surroundings diminishes; and body temperature, heart rate, and blood pressure drop.

Both REM and non-REM sleep appear to be vital to normal functioning. Experiments depriving people of REM sleep for many days at a time have left the subjects confused, disoriented, inattentive, and even delusional.

Aging and Sleep

Newborns spend most of their time asleep, and more than 50 percent of that time is REM sleep. Children decrease both their REM sleep and total sleep time as they grow. Adults until roughly age sixty sleep about 7½ hours per night, with 25 percent REM sleep in each ninety-minute cycle. With advancing age, REM sleep decreases to about 20 percent of each sleep cycle; stages 3 and 4 (deep non-REM sleep), which are 15 percent to 20 percent of the cycle in the younger adult, decrease to 1 percent to 10 percent of the sleep cycle by age seventy; and we awaken more frequently during the night and have difficulty going back to sleep. It is possible that the decrease in these deeply relaxed phases of sleep and the frequent awakenings (which may disrupt the normal sleep cycles and the circadian rhythms) account for the complaints of older people that their sleep has lost its restorative power. Studies show that older people still sleep about 7½ hours in a twenty-four-hour period, but some of this sleep occurs as catnaps or a brief closing of eyelids that may not be remembered and may not be experienced as restful.

Age	% REM per Cycle	Cycle Length (in Minutes)	Total Sleep Time per Day (in Hours)
Infants (6 months to 1 year)	50	50–60	14
Children (1 year through puberty)	40	70	11
Adults (21 years to 70 years)	25	90	7.5
Over 70 Years	20	90	7.5

Sleep Disorders

Half of all adults are dissatisfied with the quality of their sleep. Women, and especially women living alone, are more likely than men to report difficulties in falling asleep; women are also more likely to take sleeping medications, particularly as they grow older.

Sleeping difficulties can be divided into two main categories: insomnia and early morning awakening.

Insomnia

Difficulty falling asleep or remaining asleep afflicts 17 percent to 33 percent of the population and has environmental, emotional, medical, and drug-related causes.

Causes of Insomnia

1. Environmental causes	Excessive cold or dryness Excessive heat and humidity Noise
2. Emotional causes	Worries over financial difficulties, illness, loneliness, insecurity, sexual problems, troubles with family and friends Grief, depression, agitation, attacks of anxiety, manic-depressive psychosis
3. Medical (organic) causes	Painful conditions, such as arthritis, back pain, neck pain, or fever Uncomfortable, frightening problems, such as heart or lung disease or cancer Discomforts, such as dizziness, muscle cramps, or numbness Frequent urination Dementia
4. Drug- and alcohol-related causes	Alcohol abuse or withdrawal Dependence on sleeping medications Overuse of caffeine

Remedies for Environmental Causes of Insomnia

Many environments are not conducive to good sleep. Sleep occurs best in a familiar and comfortable place. Try to sleep in a quiet, dark room. If the air is too dry, use a humidifier. If the air is uncomfortably humid, consider using a dehumidifier or air conditioner. If your partner snores loudly, ask him or her to turn over, or try wearing Bilesholm cotton earplugs, available from a pharmacy or surgical supply store. If light from the outside penetrates the curtains, try installing a darker window shade or wearing a sleep shade. If total darkness makes you uneasy, try plugging a night-light into an electrical socket in your room. If your room is too hot or cold, you will sleep less well than if you maintain its temperature at 65° F to 68° F. If your feet are cold, as many older women's are, bring a hot-water bottle wrapped in a towel to bed with you or wear warm socks. Make sure that your mattress is firm and comfortable. If it sags, put some plywood boards underneath it. Or, you may need to buy a new mattress or a sturdy secondhand one—it may be the best present you can give yourself.

Remedies for Emotional Causes of Insomnia

If the details of unfinished business are keeping you awake, try tackling them, instead of worrying about them. If you are having financial difficulties, sexual problems, or trouble with family or friends, try addressing these problems. Acting, rather than brooding, will help you sleep better afterward. Exercise each day; you will sleep better at night. If you are nervous and your body feels tense, try practicing the relaxation techniques described in chapter 14. Make yourself wind down toward the end of the day. Take a luxurious bath or warm shower; drink a glass of wine, warm milk, or decaffeinated hot chocolate, coffee, or tea; listen to quiet music; or read a little. If you have a partner in bed, ask for a back rub. If you are lonely, an evening telephone conversation with a friend or relative may make you feel less so.

Depression, grief, and acute or chronic anxiety are the most common psychiatric problems leading to insomnia in older women. If you suffer from any of these conditions, you may need some form of counseling, either group or individual, and may need antidepressant medication. While the antidepressant properties of the medication may take several weeks to work, these medications have a calming action that can help you sleep when you start taking them.

Remedies for Medical Causes of Insomnia

Your medical problems need not interfere with your sleep.

If you have bone, joint, or muscle pain, you can relieve the pain with warm compresses, a heating pad, massage, or gentle exercise before you go to bed, or you can take aspirin or other pain and anti-inflammatory medications. Try propping up the affected part of your body.

For gastrointestinal discomfort, eat your largest meal at midday, and keep your supper light. Take antacids, or drink a glass of warm milk or herbal tea before retiring.

If you have hemorrhoid discomfort, you can relieve the itching by sitting in a warm bath for fifteen minutes before bedtime and by using cortisone creams or hemorrhoid preparations.

If you have heart or breathing problems, your doctor may prescribe medications to relieve these conditions at night. To ease your breathing, open your window to let a little fresh air into your bedroom. In winter, moisten the air with a humidifier or with pans of warm water in your room. If you take diuretics and wake up because you need to urinate, ask your doctor if you can take the pills at another time of day.

If you experience frequent urination, limit fluids in the two or three hours before your bedtime. Certain fluids—such as coffee, tea, and beer—are diuretics, which stimulate the need to urinate, so avoid these fluids in particular.

Remedies for Insomnia Caused by Drugs

Many drugs interfere with normal sleep. Alcohol, antihistamines, and barbiturates and other sleeping medications can help you get to sleep faster but may also cause tension, a feeling of unrest, and early morning awakening. Most of these drugs interfere with REM sleep and can cause daytime confusion.

Excessive use of caffeine (coffee, tea), asthma medications (aminophylline, Theo-Dur, Brethine, and others), thyroid pills (Thyroid, Synthroid), propranolol (a blood pressure pill), Dilantin (seizure medication), or antiparkinsonism drugs (levodopa, Sinemet) cause arousal and excitement that interfere with falling asleep and remaining asleep. Sometimes your doctor can change a drug to one that interferes less with sleep.

Rest during the day or night can compensate for lost sleep.

Early Morning Awakening

Sometimes you will have no trouble falling asleep but will wake up at 3:00 A.M., 4:00 A.M., or 5:00 A.M. and not be able to go back to sleep. The most common cause is anxiety or depression. Drugs such as reserpine, taken for high blood pressure, alcohol, antihistamines, and barbiturates can also cause you to wake up in the early hours of the morning. Ask your doctor to prescribe an alternative drug, if possible.

A quiet radio or television program often can induce you to fall back to sleep. You might also try drinking a cup of warm milk.

Sleeping Pills

Sleeping pills are overprescribed and inappropriately used. Many older women become dependent upon them because they erroneously believe that they should be having eight hours of uninterrupted sleep each night and are unable to accept even a few nights of poor sleep.

There are many types of sleeping pills, including barbiturates, antihistamines, minor tranquilizers, and other hypnotics.

Ideally, a sleeping pill should put you to sleep quickly, allow the normal stages of sleep to occur, be completely out of your system by morning, and cause no side effects or dependence. No such sleeping pill exists. All sleeping pills foster dependence; most interfere with normal sleep stages; many persist in your system hours after you awake, dulling your day; and many lose their effectiveness within weeks, making you require higher and higher doses to feel an effect. The older you are, the more likely you are to experience adverse side effects from sleeping pills.

Sleeping pills should be used for particular situations and for a short time only. You and your doctor should study the source of your sleeping difficulties to approach your problems directly—for example, sinusitis that keeps you awake should be treated with decongestants and antibiotics; depression usually requires counseling therapy and/or an antidepressant rather than a sleeping pill. When you suffer personal anxieties or grief, sleeping pills can give you some relief but will ultimately complicate your difficulties unless you resolve your troubles or adapt to your situation. For these reasons, heed the following advice.

- Try not to use sleeping pills for more than twenty days of each month and for more than three months at a stretch.

- Never mix alcohol and sleeping pills—you may become dangerously oversedated and risk coma and death.

- If you are over sixty-five, do not take barbiturates (phenobarbital, Seconal), since these drugs become more concentrated in the brains of older people than in those of younger people. The barbiturates often produce excessive grogginess, diminished respiration, and confusion, all of which expose you to the risk of falling and breaking a hip.

- Be sure that you are taking lower doses of sleeping pills than a younger person would take, since the drugs remain active in the older body for longer periods of time.

- Take your sleeping pills before bedtime rather than during the night to avoid daytime sleepiness.

- If you snore loudly, inform your doctor before you obtain any sleeping pills. You may have sleep apnea, a specific type of sleep disorder, in which case sleeping pills should not be used, since they may worsen your problem.

Types of Sleeping Pills

Sleeping pills fall into these categories:

1. Barbiturates, such as Seconal, Nembutal, Butisol, and phenobarbital. These drugs can be useful in middle-aged adults but are not recommended for older persons. They are habit-forming and can cause unexpected restlessness or daytime grogginess in older people.

2. Antihistamines, such as Benadryl. These may cause confusion and early awakening.

3. Benzodiazepines, such as Serax, Halcion, Dalmane, Valium, and Librium. The first two of these minor tranquilizers are short-acting and useful in that they do not cause hangover effects; however, they cause some people to wake up too early in the morning. The last three drugs linger in the body for twenty-four to thirty-six hours and often cause excessive daytime sleepiness, lack of coordination, and depression.

4. Other hypnotics, such as chloral hydrate. Noctec, for example, is used in doses of 250 to 1,000 milligrams. Major side effects are occasional unexpected excitement or confusion. They may be habit-forming.

TEMPERATURE

With advancing age, the body is less able to regulate its own temperature and is more susceptible to changes in air temperature. In cold weather, your body may cool down, and in hot weather, you may have trouble dissipating your body heat.

Older people respond differently to illness than do the young. They may not develop much of a fever when they have infections (even serious infections), or they may have just a few degrees of fever.

An eighty-year-old woman with pneumonia might have a temperature of only 99° F or 100° F but be every bit as sick as a twenty-four-year-old with a fever of 105° F. Often, an older woman with a fever will not feel warm or not even have a temperature much above normal, yet she may show the symptoms of fever, such as headache, dizziness, restlessness, confusion, delusions, and paranoia. This fact, combined with a decreased sensitivity to many types of pain, often makes the diagnosis of medical problems in the older person a challenge.

Any older woman who has the symptoms of fever, even with a normal temperature, needs an examination by her physician for possible infection or other disease.

Other factors that affect temperature in older age include these:

1. Thyroid. The thyroid gland produces thyroid hormone, which plays an important role in all the chemical processes of the body. Too high a level of thyroid hormone speeds up all systems, including heart rate, muscle movement, digestion, and metabolism. Women with high thyroid activity (hyperthyroidism) feel jumpy, nervous, and shaky; are hot all the time; and lose weight despite vigorous appetites. On the other hand, women with low levels of thyroid hormone slow down, as if they were going into hibernation. Their voices become low, they feel cold all the time, they get constipated, their skin and scalp become dry, and their hair begins to fall out. Low thyroid is quite common in older women and should be checked by a blood test every two to four years, since the treatment simply involves taking one dose of synthetic hormone per day.

2. Exercise. Diminished exercise makes you more vulnerable to cold, since much of the body's heat comes from muscular activity. Elderly women—especially those rendered less mobile from stroke, severe arthritis, parkinsonism, or fractures—are at greater risk of losing body heat.

3. Diet. Malnutrition can lead to impaired temperature control and coldness, even in warm climates.

4. Drugs. Certain drugs can interfere with the temperature-regulation centers in the brain, prevent shivering (a normal response to cold, which builds up body heat), or open up the arteries in the skin that allow heat to escape from the body. Alcohol is probably the drug that most commonly causes low body temperatures. Other drugs are major tranquilizers (phenothiazines such as Stelazine and Thorazine), sleeping pills (barbiturates such as Seconal and phenobarbital), minor tranquilizers (diazepam, or Valium), and antidepressants (amitriptylines such as Elavil and Triavil).

Cold Hands and Feet

Every night, Helen M., seventy, had freezing hands and feet. She envied her husband, whose hands and feet always seemed to be warm. In bed, she gratefully snuggled up to him to take advantage of his body's heat. Since her health was as good as his, she wondered what caused the temperature disparity between them. Still, she had to admit that it made for a great marriage.

Many older women complain of cold extremities even in warm weather. They wear sweaters when others are stripping and would wear socks much of the time were it not unfashionable. Some get white fingertips and toes when they go out into the cold.

Most older women probably overreact to cold in their hands and feet as their blood flow shifts from their extremities to their internal organs. As many as 20 percent, however, have a disorder called Raynaud's syndrome, which affects four or five times as many women as men. In the presence of cold, the small arteries of the fingers and toes go into spasm, turning hands and feet white and cold, and, in some cases, causing pain. Occasionally, only one hand is affected. Rubbing, warming with water, or wearing gloves and socks helps reopen the arteries, returning heat and color to fingers and toes.

Raynaud's disease is a more serious manifestation of the syndrome, causing severe pain and damage to the fingertips. Treatment includes steroids, blood vessel dilators, drugs that interfere with arterial spasms, and, in extreme cases, surgery to sever nerves that control arterial muscles. Biofeedback training has proven successful for some women suffering from this condition.

To prevent cold hands and feet, you can do the following:

1. Avoid coffee, tea, and colas, which cause constriction of small blood vessels in the extremities.

2. Quit smoking. Nicotine constricts small blood vessels and accelerates hardening of the arteries all over the body, slowing blood flow.

3. Avoid tranquilizers, sleeping pills, antidepressants, and alcohol, since all of these can diminish your body temperature.

4. Try to cope with stress rather than endure it, since emotional stress can increase your feelings of cold in the extremities.

5. When the temperature drops, do not sit still—get up, walk around, and exercise to get your circulation going. A good way

to get blood and heat into your fingertips is to whirl your arms around.

6. Wear warm clothes, and cover your hands, head, and face in very cold weather.

7. Try a hot shower, warm bath, or warm foot bath just before bed.

Heatstroke

During heat waves, people over fifty are more likely to die from all causes—particularly heart disease, brain hemorrhage, and stroke—than during moderate weather. The body's ability to dissipate heat, like its ability to fend off cold, can deteriorate in later years for these reasons:

1. The temperature-regulation centers in the brain do not work well.

2. Higher temperatures are needed to initiate sweating than in younger people.

3. Older people perspire less than younger people, so it is easier for them to get overheated.

4. The skin of older people is less sensitive to hot and cold, and the arteries in the skin do not distend as much in response to warming.

5. Older people may not drink as much fluid as they should, particularly during hot weather.

Symptoms

As a person develops heatstroke, he or she loses the ability to sweat. The victim may experience headache, vertigo, faintness, delirium, and nausea. Body temperature may climb over 106° F. Severe cases can result in hemorrhages in the brain, heart, and kidneys.

Immediate cooling is essential. Often, a person with severe heatstroke is put into an ice-water bath, which may sound drastic but is the only measure that works well. Ice-water sponge baths, rubbing with ice, or wet sheets are not effective substitutes.

Prevention

You can protect yourself from heatstroke by taking these precautions:

1. During hot weather, spend as much time as possible indoors, in an air-conditioned room. Fans help very little when the temperature is over 90° F, since they only blow hot air around. A fan *can* be useful if you sponge yourself with cold water and allow the fan to cool you by evaporating the water.

2. Take a bath in tepid water.

3. Drink ten or more glasses of fluid each day. If you are on large doses of diuretics for high blood pressure or heart failure, ask your doctor if the dosage should be reduced during hot spells.

4. Wear light-colored clothing, and avoid nylon and polyester, which hold in heat and moisture and do not allow your skin to breathe properly.

5. Wear a hat outdoors in the sun. The hat will also protect your face from sunburn.

6. If you travel to a hotter climate, remember that your body will need time and protection to get acclimatized.

Hypothermia

In December 1985, Vivienne R., an eighty-year-old woman, was discovered unconscious in her tiny Boston apartment. The heat had been turned off for lack of payment; her apartment had no storm windows.

At the hospital, her body temperature was 92° F, and her pulse was extremely slow. Luckily, the emergency room team was able to warm her up.

Each year, hundreds of elderly people are admitted to hospitals across the country for accidental cooling of their body temperatures. Many are homeless, victims of winter's hostile environment. Others—particularly elderly women on small, fixed incomes—have lost body heat in their own bedrooms from inadequate heating in the winter.

Hypothermia, or subnormal body temperature, is a medical emergency that must be treated in the hospital with careful monitoring and slow rewarming. Rapid rewarming can precipitate shock and heart problems, including cardiac arrest.

Symptoms
Body fluids can leak into all tissues, including lungs, skin, and brain. Often the individual has impaired consciousness—is apathetic or disoriented. The person may be restless and suffering from

hallucinations and paranoia. The following symptoms can be evidence of hypothermia and require immediate medical assistance.

- You feel cold, and your temperature is registering at the low end of your thermometer. You need to go to a hospital for verification with a low-temperature thermometer. Household thermometers do not read below 95° F or 35° C.

- Your skin, especially on the abdomen, feels very cold and is pale and waxy-looking.

- Your heart rate is very slow, though occasionally it may be rapid with abnormal rhythms. At temperatures below 90° F (32.2° C), the heart may stop.

- Your respiration is slow and shallow, even irregular.

- Your intestinal tract slows down, and you may vomit, which can lead to choking and lung infections.

Prevention of Hypothermia in Elderly Women

During cold months, keep your bedroom warm and your windows closed and airtight. Putting Mortite or similar clay, obtainable from hardware stores, in window cracks or covering your windows with plastic will help. Indoor temperatures during winter months should be higher for persons over sixty-five than for younger people, at least 68° F. Money to pay for fuel is available in most states for older people who need it. Wear warm clothes—such as flannel nightgowns, socks, sweatshirts, knitted hats, and long winter underwear—to bed at night, and use warm bedding. Dressing in layers will help you retain heat. Low-heat electric blankets or mattress pads may be ideal. Failing that, a hot-water bottle can help warm your feet.

Eat well, especially in winter. If you have little appetite, try supplementing your regular meals with snacks of Carnation Instant Breakfast, milk shakes, or eggnogs; you might also sprinkle powdered milk into your foods.

Avoid drugs, such as alcohol and sleeping pills, that can reduce body temperature, especially during cold months and if you live alone.

If your mobility is impaired, and particularly if you live alone, be sure you are checked on regularly during the winter by visiting nurses or other health visitors. Ask your doctor for a referral, or call the Visiting Nurse Association in your hometown.

SUGGESTED READING

American Medical Association. *Straight-Talk No-Nonsense Guide to Better Sleep*. New York: Random House, 1984.

Fourteen

Your Emotional Health

P ROBABLY the most stress-free idyll we ever enjoy occurs when we, perfectly cushioned, nourished, and oblivious, are bobbing around in utero. But how quickly we become too big for such a small pond! Its waters give way; our bubble bursts. We strain, we hurtle, we push away from our parasitical preexistence, and, with great effort, we are born.

Sensing the unfamiliarity of the environment, we noisily let our caretakers know how we long for and need safety and contentment. They try to smoothe the way for us as we slowly gain our footing during the deeply dependent years of childhood. We thrash through our teens while gathering the courage to enter adulthood, when we finally fend for ourselves. And all along, we rarely take a single step without first staring down our fears and then learning to conquer them. Nor could we continue without first ensuring, for the moment at least, some measure of our physical safety and peace of mind.

Human growth and development demand that we cope with the stresses and difficulties that befall us, not that we eliminate them.

As we meet a challenge, as we solve a problem, as we overcome a sorrow, we gain more than independence—we take possession of our selfhood. We may be floored by how long it has taken and by how much it has cost, but this hard-won ownership gives us title to something we would not willingly relinquish.

The changes in our lives and in our work and the responsibilities that we learn to shoulder not only for ourselves but also, if we have them, for our children and perhaps grandchildren, a suddenly ill spouse, and aging parents continue to provide the daily test of our mettle.

STRESS

Stress can refer to the physiological responses of an organism to forces in its environment, and, in humans, to the physical or emotional factors that cause bodily or mental tension. We readily recognize the "fight or flight" response of animals to danger. The gazelle grazing on the open plains, disturbed by the scent of its predator, has autonomic and hormonal responses that prepare it to escape or to fight: its heart rate increases, its blood pressure rises, its muscles tense, its breathing becomes shallower, and its pupils dilate. Humans have similar physiological responses to stress.

Biologists define three phases of stress: alarm, resistance, and exhaustion. Alarm is signified by the sudden release of adrenaline into the bloodstream. The hormone speeds the heartbeat, increases blood pressure and the flow of blood to muscles, tenses the muscles, gives you clammy hands and feet, and makes your breathing shallow—all the symptoms that you recognize as fear, excitement, or nervousness.

During the resistance stage, the body maintains its state of readiness to respond as its resources become depleted.

Finally exhaustion sets in. The continued increased heart rate, elevated blood pressure, and muscle tightness are all symptoms that can lead to stress-related diseases.

The complexity of human perceptions causes us to recognize and defend against danger in many situations that pose no bodily threat but to which the body responds just the same. We therefore do double sentry duty by trying to protect both our psyche and our flesh and bones from attack, as well as by trying to prevent them from attacking each other.

On whichever front we're flanking, the armor and ammunition we use must come from our organism's reserves.

Harriet S., a sixty-two-year-old real estate broker, still worked part-time in addition to caring for her ailing eighty-four-year-old father and helping her recently divorced daughter with the care of two young children. Harriet was now stuck in traffic, late for a medical appointment to which she was driving her father—and looking after her granddaughter as well. Her father could not contain his nervousness and kept telling her to change lanes. She was furious inside but only sighed deeply several times, as she felt the beginning of a throbbing headache. Gail, the little grandchild, was jumping around in the backseat.

"Gail, get back in your seat belt!" Harriet barked at the child. Gail began to cry. Harriet's father reproached Harriet. She realized that the anger she had directed at her granddaughter was really intended for her father. Her heart began to thump, and there was a terrible knot in her stomach. When a car suddenly cut her off, she pounded loud and long on the horn. The sound was like a plea for help.

Recognizing the Signs and Symptoms of Stress

Each woman has a different threshold for tolerating stress, as well as a unique way of behaving when under stress. Some women will steel themselves to keep functioning; others will openly fret. But stress produces certain common physical symptoms. Your muscle tension builds, especially in the scalp or neck, sometimes producing a pounding or bandlike headache. Muscle spasm can produce pain in the lower back and sometimes pain going down one or both legs. You may feel a racing heartbeat and have cold, clammy hands; you may experience the flare-up of eczema, hives, or other rashes; you may have a nervous tic, such as a twitch of the eyelids or cheek; you may develop high blood pressure, heart disease, ulcers, diarrhea, ulcerative colitis, spastic colitis, or migraine headaches. All these conditions can be physical signs of chronic stress, and all develop involuntarily whether or not you even realize that you are in a nervous or apprehensive state.

Stressed people may begin smoking, drinking, or using tranquilizers. Some women overeat; some women suffer poor appetites and lose weight. Many women lose sleep. The cause of these behaviors may be clearly recognized or may remain hidden. The behaviors themselves may appear but be quickly nipped or, if allowed to go unchecked, grow into habits that wreak further damage on the body and mind—even gain control of them.

Usually you are able to adapt to the stresses to which you are subjected. But when stress overwhelms you and threatens to deplete all your energy, you may react by becoming acutely ill physically or by becoming numb or depressed.

You can learn to recognize the signs of physical and emotional stress in yourself. When you become aware of the situations or people that provoke the following reactions, you can learn techniques to cope with them.

Physical Signs of Stress

Dry mouth	Pounding headache
Knot in stomach	Racing heartbeat
Rapid, shallow breathing	Cold, clammy hands
Flushed face	Nausea or vomiting
Diarrhea or constipation	Tight neck or back muscles
Shaking, tics, jumpiness	Tight feeling in chest or head
Poor or excessive appetite	Increased alcohol or drug intake

Feelings of weakness, exhaustion, lethargy, or dizziness
Numbness or tingling around the mouth, hands, and limbs

Emotional Signs of Stress

Fear of injury, disease, or death	Overwhelming guilt and worry
Intolerance of others	Unhappiness or the "blues"
Anger that flares easily	Bursts of agitation, anxiety,
Difficulty in concentrating	and panic

Phobic responses (anxiety in closed spaces, such as elevators and buses, or in any crowded place)

When several of these physical and emotional disturbances occur together, you may be experiencing what is called an anxiety attack. You may feel so terrified, nauseated, dizzy, or sweaty that you fear you are about to die or that you are having a stroke or heart attack.

An anxiety attack can be over within minutes or can last up to a half hour. Some women can talk themselves out of the attack; others are relieved by speaking with a reassuring friend; others must simply leave the place where the reaction was provoked. Women who experience many anxiety attacks, to the point of being unable to go out and function comfortably during an average day, should consult a doctor or a mental health professional. Psychotherapy, behavior modification, and/or medications may be needed to abort the attacks.

Coping with Stress

Once you have learned to recognize the signs of stress, the next step is to learn to alleviate these physical reactions. Rather than automatically responding to stress with frustration and tension, you can learn to engage in activities—both physical and mental—that will calm you down.

Using Your Body

Exercise is a way of both reducing stress and making your body less vulnerable to it. Exercise limbers your muscles, releasing tension that is often stored in your back, neck, or chest muscles. It strengthens your cardiorespiratory system, so you do not have to work as hard and expend extra energy to get through the day. If your body looks and feels trim and fit, you will automatically feel better about yourself, which in itself reduces stress. Walking briskly outdoors, dancing, swimming, taking an exercise class, or slow jogging requires enough concentration to take your mind off your troubles somewhat.

In addition, you can learn to use specific techniques to deal with stressful circumstances in your life.

Complete Natural Breathing

When you are stressed, you take short, shallow breaths. You take in too little fresh air to fully oxygenate your blood; as a result, your organs and tissues become undernourished and your digestion disturbed. Inadequate breathing in itself can add to anxiety, irritability, depression, and fatigue.

The technique described below will enable you to breathe deeply and more efficiently. You will achieve a sense of relaxation when you master the technique and practice it regularly over a period of time.

1. Begin by sitting or standing in good posture. Lightly place your hands on your abdomen.

2. Breathe in through your nose.

3. As you inhale, feel your abdomen push outward to make room for the air. Then move your lower ribs and chest forward slightly to accommodate more air. Next, raise your chest slightly and draw in your abdomen a little to support your lungs as the air fills them completely. These three steps can be performed in one smooth, continuous inhalation, which with practice can be completed in a couple of seconds.

4. Hold your breath for a few seconds.

5. As you exhale slowly, pull your abdomen in slightly and lift it up slowly as your lungs empty. When you have completely exhaled, relax your abdomen and chest.

6. Now and then at the end of inhaling, raise your shoulders and collarbone slightly so that the very tops of your lungs are sure to be replenished with fresh air.

Progressive Relaxation

Learning to relax your body helps you cope with all the stimuli that daily assault you. Relaxation can reduce or prevent many of the physical symptoms of stress and can help interrupt the vicious cycle that creates further stress.

Progressive relaxation is a technique for relaxing the different muscle groups of the body by observing the difference between their tense state and their relaxed state.

1. Find a comfortable position, either sitting with your head supported or, better yet, lying down on a firm surface.

2. Inhale very slowly, letting the breath fill your lungs, much as you did in the exercise for complete natural breathing.

3. Slowly let the breath out through your nose. During the exhalation, imagine the tension slipping away with the expelled air, draining from your body with each breath.

4. Concentrate now on each section of your body. As you inhale, tighten one particular group of muscles (for instance, those in your hand—make a fist, hold it, and observe the feeling of tightness). Then as you exhale, relax the muscles and let them loosen and become heavy and inactive. Again note what the relaxation feels like.

5. Gradually, relax the different muscles of your body, beginning with your hands, forearms, and biceps. Go on to your head (don't forget the scalp), face, throat, neck, and shoulders (pay particular attention to the forehead, eyes, cheeks, lips, tongue, mouth, and jaw). Continue with your chest, stomach, and lower back, and finish with your thighs, buttocks, calves, and feet.

You need to practice breathing while relaxing all your muscles when you are not under stress so that the skill can be automatic when you need it.

The Relaxation Response

An additional important relaxation technique (developed by Dr. Herbert Benson of Beth Israel Hospital in Boston) successfully lowers blood pressure in certain people who practice it regularly. As described in his book, *The Relaxation Response* (New York: William Morrow & Co., 1975), it is drawn from ancient techniques practiced by Indians doing yoga.

1. Sit quietly in a comfortable position.

2. Close your eyes.

3. Deeply relax all your muscles, beginning at your feet and progressing up to your face. Keep them relaxed.

4. Breathe through your nose. Become aware of your breathing. As you breathe out, say the word *one* silently to yourself. For example, breathe in, breathe out, say "one"; breathe in, breathe out, say "one"; and so on.

5. Continue for ten to twenty minutes. You may open your eyes to check the time but do not use an alarm. When you finish, sit quietly for several minutes, at first with your eyes closed and later with your eyes open. Do not stand up for a few minutes.

6. Do not worry about whether you are successful in achieving a deep level of relaxation. Maintain a passive attitude, and permit relaxation to occur at its own pace. When distracting thoughts do occur, try not dwelling upon them and return to repeating "one." With practice, the response should come with little effort. Practice the technique once or twice daily but not within two hours after any meal, since the digestive processes seem to interfere with the elicitation of the relaxation response.

Using Your Brain

It is not always easy to figure out what is bothering you. Over the years you may become so adept at hiding your furies, desires, and needs from others that you succeed in hiding them from yourself as well. But identifying the causes of your stress will help you cope. What events preceded your symptoms? Try writing down the immediate associations you have with your sensations of stress. Writing these associations down, even over a period of months, can give you insight into their causes and help you recognize repeated patterns of stimulus and response.

Some kinds of stresses are easier to identify than others, particularly environmental ones, such as poor lighting, excessive noise, air pollution, crowds, traffic jams, heat, and humidity. These stresses usually do not, by themselves, seriously impair your defenses unless those defenses have already been rattled and weakened by some other stress. Conversely, making an environmental improvement may not entirely brighten your life, but it may spare you a headache and make you less irritable.

Virginia H., sixty-one, worked as a free-lancer at home. She was competent, though frequently fretful and frazzled. She had never been a particularly careful housekeeper. But when she elected to have surgery to
remove her gallbladder, she decided to organize her cupboards, closets,
and drawers—in short, to put her house in order before she "went
under." After she recovered from the surgery, she found that her well-
ordered home had a calming effect and even helped her work more pro-
ductively. She made up her mind that the time required to pay attention
to her housekeeping was worth her new feeling of serenity.

To achieve a deeply relaxed state, you might try a relaxation
technique that requires some imagination, called guided imagery.

Guided Imagery

You cannot achieve relaxation with the technique of guided imagery unless you set aside some uninterrupted, quiet time for
yourself during which to practice it.

First, get into a comfortable position and close your eyes. You
might imagine yourself walking through a beautiful meadow or a
cool dell. You find a comfortable place to stop. As you imagine
yourself resting, take the time to examine all the tension and stress
in your life. Give the tension and stress different shapes and colors.
Look at each one carefully, and then deliberately set each one
down. When you have finished, imagine that you get up and continue to walk. Imagine that you come to a spot of great beauty and
serenity. What is it like? Become aware of the sights, smells, and
sounds of this particular spot. Be aware of the way you are feeling.
Get settled and relax. Experience being totally relaxed. Pause for
three to five minutes. Look around at your special place once more.
Remember that this is your special and private place and that you
can come here any time you want. Open your eyes and tell yourself
that you can use this imagery any time you want to feel relaxed.

You may want to make a tape of yourself describing your private
imagery. You can perfect and polish your description if you wish
until you are satisfied with it. When you feel the need for deep
relaxation, you can close your eyes and play your tape.

Finding People Who Can Help You

Unburdening yourself to someone else is often the best way of
coping with stress. Finding the right person with whom to let your
guard down can be the first step to recovering your balance.

Sometimes family members or close friends will be your best
help, your best source of sympathy and comfort. Often, however,

an experienced stranger is more helpful. Many health insurance plans will reimburse ten or more visits per year to a social worker, psychologist, psychiatrist, or other counselor.

Resisting Illness During Periods of Stress

Prolonged stress depletes your body's resources, rendering you vulnerable to illness and depression.

When you are under stress, pay special attention to nutrition. Eat regularly and do not skip meals. Try not to gulp your food, since this can cause indigestion, distension, and gas. Eat moderate portions of food; bulky meals are more difficult to digest and consume more of your energy. Avoid foods containing stimulants; the effect of coffee, tea, and alcohol, for example, is ultimately wearing.

Pay particular attention to your individual dietary needs.

- If you have a tendency to hypertension, heart disease, or fluid retention, avoid salt.
- If you have diabetic tendencies, control your sugar intake. If you need to watch your weight, eat or drink often, but in small amounts.
- If you respond to stress with peptic ulcer symptoms (pain or a knot in the stomach or excessive belching or burping), eat many small meals during the day and take antacids (see chapter 7).
- If stress causes constipation, eat more fiber and drink more fluid.
- If you have stress-related loose bowels, eat foods that bind and are rich in potassium, such as rice and bananas.
- If you get migraines, avoid chocolate and fermented cheeses.

RELATIONSHIPS WITH OTHER PEOPLE

No matter how great our talent for getting along with the individuals around us, most of us have moments or periods in our lives when we heartily agree with Sartre's famous observation "Hell is other people." The demands made by family members, associates at work, and friends; the comments that cannot be recanted; the communications that misfire or cross purposes—all can amount to an attack as surely as if people's mouths were equipped with spears instead of tongues.

No one pretends that it is easy to remain unstirred by the anger of relatives, friends, or colleagues; nevertheless, if you can detach yourself from the anger, you may discover reasons for it that stir forgiveness and sympathy for the angry person.

Ann and Jerry Z., a couple in their sixties, were visiting Jerry's eighty-five-year-old mother, as they did every other week. For some time, the elderly lady had been picking on Ann, finding fault with little things: where she put dishes away, how shabby Jerry's clothes were, or how much money Ann was spending. Today, the outburst was extreme. Ann felt her blood boil, but she took a deep breath and listened closely. Then she said, "You seem to be very upset these days, Ma. Is something bothering you that we don't know about?"

The older lady unexpectedly broke down. Ann put her arm around her and asked a few more questions. It turned out that Jerry's mother had just received a drastic rent increase and was worried about being able to keep her apartment. She was proud and hated the thought of becoming dependent. She was afraid that her son might insist that she come to live with them or that Ann might suggest a nursing home. By giving her difficult mother-in-law a chance to be other than gruff and to explain her new problem, Ann was able to lessen the stress all three of them felt. Together, the three were able to cope with the mother's dilemma.

Ann was able to detect her mother-in-law's distress, rather than simply respond to its hurtful symptoms in an angry and defensive manner. She was able to find out the reason for her mother-in-law's frustration, express genuine sympathy, gather additional information, and work with her family in solving the older woman's problem. The bad relations that had gone on for weeks eased when all three people were able to understand one another better.

Learning to Be Assertive

In general, learning to be assertive is critical to your ability to deal well with other people. Being assertive does not mean being aggressive; it means telling others your feelings in a straightforward way. Your manner will come across as confident rather than aggressive. Most important of all, being direct lessens the tensions you feel and generate in family or working life.

Learning to be assertive means respecting and valuing your own thoughts and feelings and accepting your right to express them as much as anyone else. You may be only too good at puncturing your own worthiness and self-esteem. Without praise from others, you might not feel praiseworthy. Self-accusations are often what create stress: "I'm not good enough." "I'm not the wife/mother/daughter/worker I should be." "I'm too selfish." "I did too sloppy a job." "I can't deal with my boss." Practice talking to yourself more kindly. You can begin to talk yourself out of stress.

Communication Among Family Members

In families that deal well with stress, people can tolerate differences among themselves. They recognize that other people's preferences may not be the same as their own. They can express their differences and feelings without hurting one another and listen to one another with respect. Consider the example of a large family of six children who are all concerned about their severely ill, hospitalized mother. The mother's condition has just taken a turn for the worse. Her doctor has just explained to the children that a further operation on their mother might improve her condition but carries significant risks.

One of the sisters might say, "I feel Mother should not have an operation because it will just prolong her suffering." If the sister were just to exclaim emotionally, "I will never agree to an operation!" her siblings could react with equal exaggeration: "Well, you don't care about Mother!" If one of the brothers were too quiet, other family members would be wise to ask, "John, what do you feel?" instead of lashing out, "John, you're never willing to take responsibility!"

Tense situations can lead either to mutual support and concern or to even higher tension, anger, and divisions. Such situations are best borne with great closeness and clear communication. You need to state clearly and tactfully what you feel.

Several principles foster open communication in families under stress:

1. Speak clearly.

2. Ask for clarification of others' feelings if you are uncertain of them. Listen carefully, and considerately, without making hasty assumptions about what lies in other people's minds.

3. Try not to use sweeping generalizations, and do not accept them from others.

4. Try not to injure another person by using demeaning names or by giving way to emotional outbursts.

5. If emotional tensions prevent communication, agree to stop the discussion and to resume it shortly at a specific time.

6. Try to avoid blaming others, holding grudges, and being defensive. Rather, focus on identifying problems and coming to a resolution.

7. If you consistently arrive at a stalemate, get outside help from friends or professionals.

8. Try to remember the love, not the resentment, that may exist among you.

Adult Siblings

Adult brothers and sisters are most likely to renew intense contact at times of crises: the illness, disability, or death of a parent; divorce or illness; or serious illness of or trouble with a sibling's child. Often siblings can lend one another support that even a best friend cannot match. Past rivalries may be put aside permanently or temporarily, but sometimes they remain and aggravate the problem. Siblings can have terrible fights when parents are sick, disabled, or incompetent. These emotional struggles signal the eruptions of old childhood rivalries and hurts. Adult siblings often see one another as the children they once were. Frequently, conflicts are over money and property, and a great effort must be made if family relationships are to be salvaged. Siblings need to make an effort to treat one another with the dignity and respect they reserve for people outside the family.

Psychological researchers are becoming aware that the nature and importance of sibling influence may rank second to that of parents. Given a little extra love and attention when they are needed, sibling relationships often outlast other intimate ties and become valued for the witness they bear to a lifetime of liaison.

STRESSFUL SITUATIONS IN LATER LIFE

Any important change in one's life—getting a divorce, encountering difficulties in marriage or in any other serious relationship, watching children leave home, leaving or starting a job, moving, or suffering the death of a relative or friend—or even the anniversary of a major change will bring with it significant stress.

The Empty Nest

The time that your children leave home can be one of several times in your life when the question of who you are and where you go from here arises. Your marriage may come into focus as it never did before and enter a new phase. With fewer distractions at home, you may be lucky and rediscover romance if it has gotten lost in the shuffle. But the new intensity also may cause old stresses to flare up.

Adele T., a fifty-seven-year-old vigorous and energetic mother of three, the last of whom had recently left home, had always been the initiator of activities in the family. She was the one who organized excursions, planned their details, and took responsibility for seeing that all went smoothly. She had accepted that role when the children were growing.

Now that she and Max were alone, she resented doing all the calling, planning, and packing for another adult. She was ready to be taken care of or, at the very least, to have someone share the burden of these tasks. For the first time in their marriage, she became a dissatisfied, nagging woman.

Or it may inspire you to act.

Frieda G., fifty-six, emerged from the depression that enclosed her when her children left home with the resolve to become a social worker. Her husband and friends thought she was crazy, going to classes at her age and cramming for exams. But her determination was solid. She studied hard for three years, managed to find a good job working in a hospital despite the bias against her age, and established a successful second career.

The change in your life might be an opportunity to redirect yourself regardless of what you have been doing up until this time. It takes self-knowledge, courage, and determination to find your path. You may want to consider the following:

- changing jobs if you're dissatisfied or bored
- returning to the work you did before you had children
- developing new skills or trades. If you return to school, your maturity and wisdom usually will compensate for the more facile memory and recent schooling of younger students. Your example may inspire younger women who may become your friends.
- volunteering for social, civic, medical, charitable, or educational organizations. Many public issues need passionate advocates. Every community can identify many older women who have led others and forced change. As a nation, we admire the example of women who have done so: Eleanor Roosevelt, who helped found the United Nations and who championed the civil rights of minorities; Maggie Kuhn, who founded the Grey Panthers; and Coretta Scott King, widow of Martin Luther King, Jr., who became a leader in the civil rights movement in her own right.
- planning for retirement. There are many books that can help you plan for productive use of your time and energies.

Retirement

One of the great ironies of married life is that you can spend years dreaming about the luxury of retirement, when the two of you will finally begin to do all the things for which there has never been time, only to find that retirement presents a greater shock to your marriage than anything that has come before.

Glenda B., sixty-four, had always enjoyed her days at home. Now that William was retired, he was there, every day, in "her" domain. He began to venture opinions about her cooking—about how she pared potatoes, about the types of pots she used, even about her choice of measuring devices. He drove her crazy with his comments, and she angrily let him know it.

Finally, Glenda realized that he was having trouble adjusting to his retirement and that he felt useless. His interest in housework was an attempt to feel valuable. She realized she had to share her domain now that they were both at home.

The best way to deal with this problem is to turn it into an asset. Find tasks that can be shared; clearly specify the ones you want to do alone. If your husband shares more household chores, you will have more time for other pursuits.

Some husbands insist that their wives retire when they do. You may not be ready for a life of leisure when your husband is; you may not want to travel as much as he does. You may have only recently tasted the satisfaction of regular outside work. Some women have to insist on their right to continue working or pursue volunteer interests at the risk of turbulence in their marriage.

Difficulties in Marriage

There are many measures of success in marriage. When you're running a full household and preoccupied with your career, the prosperity of your marriage is often gauged in ways that don't force you to ask, "Who's the man I'm living with now?" and, "Where's the man I married?" When you finally have more time for each other, you will also have more time to appraise your relationship.

If you've grown apart and have developed interests that are not mutually rewarding, you may have to work to rekindle your friendship and intimacy. The alternative is to ignore or deny your differences until a crisis forces you to confront them. Often you can work out these problems between you, but sometimes you may have to take the difficult step of breaching marital privacy and seeking outside help. A clergyperson, marriage counselor, or therapist can help. If privacy is not a major issue, you may even consider joining a therapy group in which one counselor works with several couples at once. The advantage of group therapy is that it gives you a chance to observe the interactions of other couples, and reflect with fresh perspective on your own relationship. It may also be worth considering attending seminars and retreats devoted to marriage enrichment.

Women, almost as much as men, may feel shy and embarrassed about consulting a therapist or psychiatrist because they feel that having marital problems implies failure, incompetence, or craziness. Mental health professionals, in fact, spend most of their time helping normal people deal with the normal problems of getting along with others and finding fulfillment.

Often the most difficult part of seeking counseling is finding a counselor. To go about it, you can speak to your doctor and ask for a referral to a marriage counselor or psychiatrist. Or, you can call your local mental health center or the psychiatric department of a local hospital and ask for a referral to an agency dealing with marriage and family counseling, or a private social worker, psychologist, or psychiatrist. Also, you can speak to your religious advisor, who may be able to help you directly or refer you to another clergyperson who specializes in marriage counseling.

Many insurance plans, including Medicare and supplementary insurance, cover a given number of visits for such therapy.

What can you do, in a distressed marriage, if your husband refuses to enter therapy with you, or even to admit his part in the need for improvement? You can still gain much from getting counseling for yourself to cope with loneliness, resentment, guilt, or insecurity. Your other most valuable recourse may be group support from other women. Sharing conflicts, fears, and suggestions with other women in similar situations can be very reassuring. Often your community center, church or synagogue, or perhaps even your place of business, if it is large enough, will sponsor such supportive groups.

Celia W., fifty-three, joined a women's group at her church. She was afraid at first to disclose any personal information and to share with others the pain of her marriage. Gradually, as other women spoke, she saw that there were aspects of their lives, hopes, and frustrations that were like hers. She found herself looking forward to the Tuesday group all week. It allowed her to be completely herself on an equal basis with other women. While the group did not alter Celia's marriage, the support it offered helped her accept her marriage's limitations and have the courage to find fulfillment in other pursuits.

There are times when couples are unable to surmount their problems. The obstacles to communication may be so great that they cannot be overcome, and you may not be able to like each other again. In such cases, as you debate whether to break up the marriage or accept its limitations, ask yourself whether you could bear the pain of its breakup, the possibility of a lowered standard of living, and the social isolation that might accompany the change and whether it would be worth it. You may conclude that there is no other road to peace. This is a good time to seek professional counseling.

Divorce

> When my marriage failed, I thought the whole world would be down on me for the rest of my life. I felt like a total failure. It's amazing that so many people accepted it well.
>
> —*Edith R., sixty-one*

The decision to separate is probably one of the most wrenching ones an adult ever makes, especially after many years of marriage.

During the early part of separation, stress is overwhelming, causing such physical symptoms as poor sleeping; enormous appetite or little interest in food; headache, stomachache, and back pain; instability of chronic illnesses such as arthritis and diabetes; excessive drinking or smoking; and general irritability.

Grief sets in, even in the spouse who initiated the divorce. A sense of failure, fear, and insecurity can accompany the grief. Single older women wonder, Can I get an apartment alone? Will I be safe? Can I find a job? Will my married friends abandon me? Will the children take sides? Can I make friends without my husband's social contacts?

Older divorcées have less opportunity to meet people of the opposite sex than do their ex-husbands. There are several times as many unattached older women than men, which leaves you to wonder how you will cope with limited affection and celibacy for the rest of your years. You may not even know how to meet unattached men. It is difficult to begin dating again in mid-life, and it is natural to be somewhat apprehensive of sexual expectations when you still only have companionship in mind (see chapter 12).

If you divorce, consider taking the following advice.

• Find yourself a good lawyer, who can advise you about protecting your financial interests. Ask friends for referrals, or call the local NOW office in your community or any other feminist organization.

- Make certain that you arrange to maintain your health benefits through your husband's health insurance policy before your divorce is final. This is a benefit most older women cannot afford to lose.

- Get together with other older single women. You will need people to talk to.

- Do not be afraid of change, whether large or small. Try traveling; change your job if it is not satisfying to you. Carefully evaluate your work skills—with the help of a professional job counselor, if need be. Can you improve your earning power? Can you allow yourself a career change? Can you take courses that will qualify you for a better-paying job? Remember, adventure and opportunities still lie ahead.

- Inquire about singles clubs sponsored by your church, synagogue, or community center. These clubs offer good ways to meet other people who also need friends.

Dating and Remarriage

You may feel shy or guilty about dating again. The first step in overcoming your awkwardness is to remain active and involved with other people. Intimacy can grow from warm and enjoyable companionship.

Your children can have a difficult time accepting a new man in your life, should you start to date again or consider remarrying. They may openly discourage the relationship. They may be offended by your affections toward a man who is a stranger and not their father. Reasonably, the prospect of a parent's remarriage may make adult children uneasy about their inheritance. These issues all need to be talked about openly, if this is possible.

Grandmotherhood—with Pitfalls

> A grandmother is a lady who has no children of
> her own, so she likes other people's little
> girls. . . . Everybody should try to have one,
> especially if you don't have television, because
> grandmas are the only grown-ups who have got
> time.
>
> —*Patsy Gray, nine*

Grandmothers offer support and love that cannot be bought. They also give grandchildren a continuity with the past and provide children with a rare intimate image of older people in our society. Grandmothers can provide kind support and invaluable reassurance for their children by helping during times of financial, emotional, or physical need or when grandchildren or their parents need extra care.

But sometimes the role of grandparents is less clear and straightforward. The conflicts remaining between themselves and their grown children and the differences in child-rearing ideas that exist between the generations can cause trouble when you least want it.

Try not to preach. Insisting that your ways were better than the current generation's will isolate you from your children and leave you ignored.

It is important not to let yourself be valued just for the presents you give. Avoid being overindulgent toward your grandchildren. On the other hand, you need not wait until after your death to give grandchildren an object of value that they cherish. Do it while you can share their joy.

Your children may find it tempting to use you as a convenient babysitter. Grandmothers find it hard to say no, for it is gratifying to be needed. You may need to remind your sons and daughters to ask for, not demand, the gift of their mother's time for child care. Be honest and say no if you find that their requests are excessive or do not come at opportune times.

Divorce in your child's marriage (particularly one that leaves bitterness or enmity between the partners) can precipitate a crisis for you. You are suddenly threatened with the loss of the precious relationship with your grandchildren.

The best way to preserve your relationship with your grandchildren is to avoid entering into the conflict between the parents. The grandchildren need you to support the good points of each parent, since they do not wish to lose either a mother or a father. You can reassure all parties that you want to continue your contact with your grandchildren and that the divorce will have no effect on these bonds.

Should one parent refuse to allow you to continue a relationship with your grandchildren, you can resort to legal action to obtain visitation rights. There are organizations (Grandparents Anonymous in Sylvan Lake, Michigan, for example) that can offer guidance in such a case. If necessary, consult an attorney or your local legal aid organization.

THE SANDWICH GENERATION

The woman over fifty is often caught in the middle, between her own children and her aging parents. By design or by default, most of the nation's dependent elderly are cared for by their offspring. The obligations encircling the middle-aged daughter—to give care, supervise, earn money, and run a home—tighten just when she is beginning to feel her own age, and they may threaten her health.

Stresses on the sandwich generation include these:

- deciding whether to institutionalize frail parents or in-laws or care for them at home

- deciding whether to give up a job to care for aged parents or in-laws

- trying to salvage time for your spouse or partner

- trying to be a mother to your own children in the face of the overwhelming needs of the oldest generation

- needing to earn money to help pay your children's college tuition

Getting Help and Protecting Yourself

When you are caught between two generations needing your care and money, you need help. Draw in other members of the family to help you give care and financial support to older parents or in-laws. Brothers, sisters, and grandchildren can contribute but may need help in knowing what to do. You may have to organize a family meeting and present a list of all the tasks that need to be done and the expenses that need to be covered. Ask others to commit themselves to doing specific jobs on specific days and/or to contribute a share of the parents' expenses.

Investigate the entitlements of the older people (see chapter 17). Your parents or in-laws may be eligible for the services of a homemaker, visiting nurse, home health aide, or social worker. Perhaps day care is an option, a few days a week. If an aging parent lives with you, you may be entitled to a week or two each year of reimbursement for respite care, which would give you a vacation with your family. Ask siblings to relieve you for a week or two. Sometimes a pair of families who are both caring for elderly members take turns helping each other out so that each family can get time to itself.

Ask your attorney how you can protect your income, which may now be drained by the care of aged parents. You may elect to have your attorney draw up documents that allow your parents to pay you for room, board, and services. Ultimately, if the parents are admitted to a nursing home, all their accumulated income will be available for payment to cover its costs. They may not be able to give you an inheritance or to reimburse you for the money you may have spent on their care.

Martyrdom is neither rewarded nor admired in our society. Try to find a way to care for your family members without sacrificing your own health and your family's well-being. Women caught in difficult straits must seek help from their families and from federal, state, and community agencies. Most of these resources do not come knocking on the door when they are needed. The effort spent in mobilizing assistance will prove valuable to all family members in the end. The book *Caregiving: Helping An Aging Loved One* by Jo Horne (Washington, D.C.: AARP; Glenview, Ill.: Scott, Foresman & Co., 1985) is highly recommended as a source of valuable information on the subject.

COPING WITH SINGLEHOOD
AS YOU GET OLDER

About 5 percent of women never marry. Women accustomed to a single life know how to enjoy their independence and harvest self-respect. Many other women join the ranks of singlehood through divorce or the death of a spouse. Statistically, older single women are more vulnerable to deteriorating health as they age, particularly if their income diminishes.

You can lessen this vulnerability by solidifying family ties and moving in with a sibling for your mutual benefit and interdependence. Sharing your apartment or house with a friend or a roomer or boarder is another way of relieving the stress of being alone. One sixty-four-year-old described her solution to solitude:

> I have very much enjoyed having a male graduate
> student at the house. I enjoy the illusion of
> "family," and within the year or so that he lives
> here we become good friends . . . having a man
> to talk with (when he has time) is a real pleasure.
> This is a strictly platonic relationship, but I
> wouldn't consider having a girl roomer, regardless
> of her conversation. I like a man's voice and his
> shoulders under the T-shirt, and I don't mind
> cleaning up after him as I would after a girl. My

daughter says, "A student at your house is
halfway between a son and a boyfriend." I don't
deny it. There are all degrees of interplay between
men and women.

Not every woman feels comfortable with the idea of a male sharing the premises. A female roomer or boarder may provide more
satisfactory and sympathetic company.

You may not want a human companion but may prefer a pet.
Many studies show that single older people who have pets remain
healthier and live longer than those who do not. Pets can give you a
reason for daily exercise, be a source of companionship, and provide
you with the satisfaction of knowing that you are needed.

If your health starts to fail, seek out formal programs designed
to help ailing single people—including the services of homemakers,
home health aides, visiting nurses, and social workers.

WIDOWHOOD

For many a woman like me, old age came early,
in my fifties, with a telephone call that jarred me
into the trauma of the death of my husband.
Widow! The very word horrified me. I was in a
whole new condition, stripped of life as I knew
it. I was instantly plunged into shock, abandon-
ment, sadness, anger, loneliness, isolation; and
then there was the inevitable restlessness. What
could I do to make that awful emptiness go
away? Where was the male in my life? Was I to
live forever in a nunnery? It's embarrassing how
quickly those agonies plague all widows.

—*Liz Carpenter*

There are five widows in the United States to every widower.
The average American wife can expect about seventeen years of
widowhood. Why? Because men not only die earlier than women,
but they also marry women who are, on the average, four years
younger than they are.

Middle-aged women need to face the possibility of their
widowhood while their husbands are alive. It is tempting to put off
thinking of losing a spouse, of being financially dependent, and of
being infirm, but the future is not kind to those who fail to plan
ahead.

Widows often find themselves poorer than before. Widows sixty and over are, however, entitled to death benefits from Social Security if their husbands were entitled to Social Security. The benefits range from 71.5 percent of the husband's benefit for a widow at age sixty to the entire benefit at age sixty-five. Disabled widows can collect 71.5 percent from age fifty on. Widows of age sixty-five or over are also eligible for Medicare health insurance if their husbands worked under Social Security. Widows whose husbands were federal employees or railroad employees are also entitled to health insurance and pensions. Even if you are divorced, if you were married at least fifteen years, you can collect.

To assure your future financial health, you need to do the following:

- Choose a financial or legal advisor whom you can consult. All aspects of your family estate need to be planned to ensure the survivor's financial security.

- Make sure you and your spouse have drawn up wills and have filed copies with your lawyer.

- Familiarize yourself with all assets that are owned separately and jointly, including insurance policies, retirement funds, stocks, bonds, IRA accounts, mutual funds, real estate, and health policies. Know the location of all records of these assets. The best way to familiarize yourself with your family's assets is to go over the family tax returns annually. Be aware of outstanding bills, loans, or debts. Know what you will be entitled to from your husband's Social Security, life insurance, pensions, or other income sources.

- Have one bank account in your name alone, since joint accounts requiring both signatures for transactions may be frozen after your husband's death until his estate is settled, which may take a year or more. Also, if your husband requires nursing home placement, the money in the joint account must be used to pay the bill, regardless of the fact that part of it is yours. Have at least one major credit card in your own name.

- Check to see whether the health coverage you have will continue after your spouse's death. If not, discuss how you will obtain similar coverage.

- Discuss what each of you would do if you were to survive the other: consider how each of you might cope alone; specify any preferences you each have for your respective funerals so that the surviving spouse will be left with fewer difficult decisions. If possible, purchase a funeral plan that is prepaid and leaves few decisions at the time of death.

An excellent reference for estate planning is *The Essential Guide to Wills, Estates, Trusts, and Death Taxes,* by Alex J. Soled (Washington, D.C.: AARP; Glenview, Ill.: Scott, Foresman & Co., 1985).

Coping with Grief and Loss

> Give sorrow words; the grief that does not speak
> Whispers the o'er-fraught heart and bids it break.
> —*Shakespeare*

People who suffer the death of someone close to them move slowly but definitely through progressive phases of bereavement until they return to "normal." Feelings of sadness and loss dominate the process, though anger, denial, and resignation as well as relief and guilt are common.

Whether the death is expected or sudden, you may experience the physical symptoms of acute grief. These can include tightness in the throat, an empty feeling in the abdomen, sobbing, shortness of breath, a feeling of unreality, and weakness of muscles. Even mention of the deceased person can trigger some of these symptoms.

There quickly follows a period of shock or numbness, during which you find yourself able to cope with the business of funeral arrangements, the will, and numerous financial details. Although rationally you know otherwise, you may feel that your husband is alive and will come home soon. You might find yourself doing "crazy" things, like shining his shoes or wearing an article of his clothing to feel closer to him. Such acts are quite normal.

The permanence of the departure is gradually felt, and with it moments of intense grief return. Women vary in their manner of grieving and in the length of time grief lasts. They may neglect their own health for a while—eating poorly, not exercising, and forgetting to take medications.

To protect your health, try to eat three meals a day, even if they are small. Try to get enough sleep. If necessary, go to a health food store and get a natural sleeping aid called L-tryptophan, or ask your doctor for a small supply of sleeping pills. Try to exercise, even if you only take brief walks outdoors. You will feel better if you have a massage or facial or get your hair done. Do not neglect medications and previously planned visits to the doctor or dentist.

You may need some sort of counseling or group support for a while. The Widowed Persons Service of AARP can provide this. Your church or synagogue or the local YWCA or community hospital may sponsor bereavement groups. Physicians, social workers, hospice programs, and other widows who have already adapted to their new lives can also be of great help.

Widows often find themselves alone shortly after the funeral if their children live far away and their married friends stop seeing them. The isolation is worse if you do not have a car or do not drive.

You may have to take the initiative to keep up with old friends if they are hesitant or fearful of calling you. You will have to get out of your house if you are to make new friends, but there are friends out there to be made—and they are of both sexes.

Some women recover in months; others take years. Some are startled by the amount of sadness they feel. With the support of family and friends, most women return to normal within a year or so.

Severe Grief Reactions

Grieving women are considered medically depressed when they show no sign of overcoming their grief. Your grief may be turning into depression if any of the following signs persist more than a month after the death.

1. neglect of personal hygiene and diet
2. frequent, uncontrollable crying
3. inability to relate to other people
4. lack of interest in any activities
5. significant or prolonged weight loss
6. inability to sleep

If you are experiencing severe grief, you should not remain alone, since the combination of great stress and neglect of health can easily lead to physical illness. In rare cases, a woman may have suicidal thoughts and act on them. A family member or friend should be with you to assist in your care—to bring food, help with dressing and bathing, and provide support and companionship. You may need to be reminded to take your regular medications, such as blood pressure pills or diabetes pills.

When severe grief persists for longer than a month, you should consult a psychiatrist to help you decide whether you need care from a visiting nurse or therapist, a course of antidepressant medication as an outpatient, or a period of hospitalization. Usually, six months to a year of outpatient treatment with a psychiatrist or other mental health professional is needed to help women with severe grief reactions.

Studies of elderly couples have shown that a surviving spouse runs a great risk of dying within a year or two after his or her loss. The loneliness and the stress of adjusting to a new life leave the surviving spouse particularly vulnerable to infection, heart attack, and stroke.

To cope with depression that accompanies grief, visit your general practitioner or internist to assure yourself that the depression is not caused by, or is not being aggravated by, a physical illness. If your doctor diagnoses the problem as psychological rather than physical, you may be referred to a psychiatrist or to a mental health center. If you are severely depressed, the psychiatrist may recommend medications and/or hospitalization. Also, consider attending meetings of a bereavement group, which can help you share problems with other people enduring similar sorrow. It is especially important to guard your health with good nutrition, exercise, and the company of family and friends.

DEPRESSION

The term *depression* covers a wide spectrum of moods and behaviors, ranging from sadness at the normal disappointments of life to the severe melancholy preceding suicide. Medically, depression refers to a group of symptoms that are pervasive, last for a long time, and amount to a disease requiring treatment. The borderline between normal depression and abnormal depression is not always clear and sometimes can be determined only as time passes.

Conventional wisdom holds that depression increases with age. But research has shown that it is women under thirty-five who have the greatest incidence of depression. In fact, the Midtown Manhattan Longitudinal Study (Srole and Fisher 1978), which observed the mental health of 700 men and women as they progressed from age fifty to age seventy, noted that the rates of mental health impairment in women dropped dramatically from a high of 26 percent in 1954 to only 11 percent in 1975, while the corresponding rates in men dropped from 11 percent to 9 percent.

Nevertheless, depression is one of the leading psychological problems for which women of all ages seek help. Research suggests that about 20 percent of all U.S. women, though only about 11 percent of older women, will suffer a major depressive episode at some point in their lives; one-third of these women will require temporary hospitalization. About half the women do not experience further depression; the other half experience recurrences.

To help themselves cope, depressed women are apt to turn to tranquilizers and sedatives; men generally turn to alcohol. But suicide rates are lower for women than for men, particularly for older women, whose rate of suicide is about one-tenth that of men.

Depression can exact an enormous toll, but, luckily, it often lifts by itself. Mental health professionals (social workers, psychologists, therapists, and psychiatrists) have not been able to define the boundaries of depression or agree upon its treatment.

Most people experience a depressed mood now and then, with feelings of sadness, heaviness, inadequacy, and pessimism and a lack of interest in people and things. This mood is often prompted by a specific cause—disappointment, loss, or exhaustion—and usually doesn't last for very long. Major blows, such as the death of a loved one or the loss of a job or home, usually prolong depression, but even then the sadness begins to ease with time, not intensify.

Symptoms
Depression, as opposed to a depressed mood, is a more pervasive state that is accompanied by additional symptoms. Often a depressed woman loses her appetite and may lose weight, though some women may overeat and gain a considerable amount of weight. The routines of life become disrupted. A person may have difficulty falling asleep or staying asleep. Or a person may feel exhausted even when she sleeps much of the day. The depressed woman often cries or feels about to. Headaches are common. Anxiety and agitation may be intense, accompanied by fear, a sense of doom, guilt, and feelings of vulnerability, and helplessness. Phobias, suicidal thoughts, and disturbing—even bizarre—physical symptoms may develop. One woman may be restless, pacing the floor, sitting and standing, and starting but not completing tasks. Another woman will slow down, speak lethargically, think and move slowly, and have a blank, staring expression.

Extremely depressed women generally neglect personal grooming; they may remain uncombed for weeks and not bathe or change their clothes. Household tasks, bills, and friendships fall by the wayside, neglected. Sexual desire usually fades. These women become preoccupied with feelings of anxiousness and worthlessness.

Certain physical symptoms commonly accompany depression. These include a dry mouth; a racing heartbeat; tingling of the fingertips, the area around the mouth, and the limbs; rapid, shallow breathing; a knot in the stomach; visual disturbances such as blurred or jumpy vision; increased frequency of urination; and constipation or diarrhea, or alternating constipation and diarrhea. Depressed women often become obsessed with physical complaints that plague them, though physicians generally cannot find much to diagnose.

Types of Depression

There are four useful categories of depression: depressed mood, mild depression, major depression, and bipolar depression.

Depressed mood includes the normal transient sadness, grief, disappointment, or "blues" that do not greatly impede work, social life, or self-esteem.

Mild depression is less severe, less prolonged than major depression. A mildly depressed woman may be able to maintain some of her activities and relationships but may also experience many of the physiological and psychological symptoms of depression.

Major depression, or melancholia, is a severe, persistent condition in which a woman loses interest and pleasure in life, lacks all self-esteem, and may contemplate suicide. Some major depressions are triggered by an event from the outside; others arise from biochemical causes, such as deficiencies of chemical brain transmitters or other as yet unidentified abnormalities.

Bipolar, or manic, depression involves severe mood swings, from total elation to total depression. It usually develops before the age of thirty, occurs equally in men and women, and can persist into older age. The manic phase can last for a long time, but inevitably a period of depression sets in. This type of depression often runs in families.

Causes of Depression

Depression is rarely caused by any single factor but rather by a confluence of events, family history, and physical conditions, such as the following:

1. Stressful events (getting divorced, losing your job, running out of money, seeing children leave home, caring for aging parents, fighting with a spouse or lover, losing a close relative or friend). Important events and their anniversaries can trigger depression. You should expect stress at these times, even when the occasion is joyful. Depression can also result from losses brought on by illness—from losing a breast to cancer, from having one's activities limited by a heart attack, or from knowing that one's intellectual ability is diminished after mild brain damage caused by a stroke.

2. Family background. The tendency to severe depression can run in families. A family predisposition to alcoholism is also associated with depression.

3. Deficiencies or excesses of certain chemical messengers or hormones in certain parts of the brain. Research has shown that a group of structures in the brain regulate moods and the ability to be attentive. These areas respond to hormones and to chemicals that transmit nerve messages (acetylcholine, dopamine, serotonin, and others). The integrity of these systems can be evaluated indirectly by a blood test, the dexamethasone suppression test. The results are abnormal in about two-thirds of severely depressed people. (It is not clear whether the imbalance causes the depression or vice versa.) Research on the brain's chemistry may yield more effective treatment than we now have for some forms of depression.

4. Illness or disability. Depression may be one of the first symptoms of a serious illness, such as hypothyroidism, an infection, or cancer. A severely depressed woman should have a thorough medical examination to be sure that there is not a physical, treatable cause for her depression.

5. Certain drugs or drugs interacting with other drugs. Certain medications for high blood pressure, such as reserpine and propranolol (Inderal); mild tranquilizers, such as diazepam (Valium) and chlordiazepoxide (Librium); and interactions between drugs, such as the reaction between alcohol and sedatives, can induce depression.

6. Other psychiatric illness. Alcoholism, drug abuse, schizophrenia, anxiety neurosis, and dementia can lead to depression.

Treatment of Depression

Many an approach is appropriate for treating depression, be it one that offers the support of peers; the care and compassion of the visiting nurse; the counseling of the social worker or clergyperson;

or the benefit of drugs and psychotherapy, exercise, or nontraditional therapies of India and the Orient.

Research suggests that participation in some form of work other than homemaking, including part-time work or volunteer work, may raise a depressed woman's spirits. Many colleges and women's counseling services have established programs to guide the middle-aged woman who is reappraising her working life.

Women who become depressed for any length of time need to overcome their feelings of helplessness. The paralysis that stems from these feelings can become habit-forming. You can recover some of your balance by getting involved in structured day-care programs or in behavior modification programs at mental health centers.

Your family and friends are vital to your psychological and physical health. Depression of older people is often linked to loneliness, and women who have intimate, confiding relationships are less susceptible to mental illness. As you age into your seventies and eighties, your web of friendships weakens through retirements, relocations, or deaths. It may take unusual effort, but you can make new friends all your life.

Psychotherapy

Psychotherapy effects change by teaching you to recognize and understand your emotional processes. A psychotherapist will use suggestion, insight, interpretation, persuasion, reassurance, emotional expression, support, confrontation, and other verbal and psychological techniques to help you gain insight into yourself and the ills you want to heal.

Who can benefit from therapy that relies upon talking rather than upon drugs? Which type of therapy and therapist is best for you? The answers depend on your personality, background, need, and financial resources.

Many kinds and forms of therapy—based on many different theories—are available. The training of therapists also varies widely. Some therapists are psychologists or social workers; some are medical doctors (psychiatrists and most psychoanalysts); some are trained clergy; some are psychiatric nurses; some may not have a specific degree but have met state requirements for licensing. You should make sure that the person you are seeing is licensed in your state and is recommended by someone whose judgment you respect.

Many people assume that the most helpful mental health professional is the person with the most advanced or prestigious degrees. While advanced training is desirable, and while it is true that the therapist who has an M.D. can also provide medical supervision and prescribe drugs, do not assume that an M.D. is a prerequisite in a therapist. The ability to be a successful therapist depends on a person's talents, personal characteristics, and training. To work well with your therapist, you should like and trust her or him and feel comfortable and supported during your sessions.

If you are unsure about entering psychotherapy, discuss the matter with your family doctor, or have one-hour consultations with one or two psychotherapists to whom you have been referred by a friend or doctor. Most mental health centers can also evaluate you to determine whether psychotherapy will be of value.

Psychotherapy is not instant treatment. It requires commitment on your part to attend sessions regularly and to change.

Drugs

Four major classes of drugs are currently used to treat depression: tricyclic antidepressants, lithium, monoamine oxidase inhibitors, and some more rapid-acting antidepressants. New drugs are being added to the number constantly.

Tricyclic Antidepressants

For depressions that arise from biochemical derangements or that are triggered by life's events, tricyclic antidepressants are used. This class of drug affects many parts of the brain through its blocking activity at sites that receive messages. The first symptoms alleviated are fitful sleep or sleeplessness, nervousness, and poor appetite. Mood improves over weeks, and when it does, the doses of tricyclics may slowly be decreased. If you are experiencing your first major episode of depression, you may be able to taper off the drug completely as you improve; your physician will watch for the return of symptoms. If you have had prior attacks of depression, you are best treated for longer periods of time, such as six months.

The side effects of the tricyclic drugs are troubling, especially at the beginning of treatment, but usually these symptoms abate. The drugs can cause drowsiness, dry mouth, sweating, constipation, and urinary hesitancy. Since the doses required to treat depression are quite large, small doses are gradually increased over a two- to three-week period to minimize unpleasant side effects. A few women get hand tremors, which can persist for a long time. The most serious side effects are increased heart rate and serious rhythm disturbances of the heart. If you have a heart condition, you should not be treated with tricyclics unless you are carefully supervised by your family doctor or internist.

Lithium Carbonate

Lithium carbonate effectively treats manic-depressive psychosis. Its continuous use can prevent recurrence of depression. Dosages must be carefully controlled, since the therapeutic level is very close to the toxic level. To tailor the dosage, frequent blood tests are given at the beginning; they later taper off to one a month.

Side effects include hand tremors, nausea, vomiting, and diarrhea, which diminish as the dosage is decreased. If you have kidney failure, you cannot take lithium.

Monoamine Oxidase Inhibitors

When depression is accompanied by phobias and extreme anxiety or when tricyclic drugs fail to work, monoamine oxidase (MAO) inhibitors are often prescribed. Like the tricyclics, MAO inhibitors take a few weeks to have an antidepressant effect.

The MAO inhibitors are useful drugs when taken with the proper precautions; however, they are potentially dangerous drugs. You can get extremely high blood pressure if you combine the medication with foods containing tyramine or tryptophan, such as broad beans (fava and lima), fermented cheese, beers, wines, pickled herring, chicken livers, yeast extract, and caffeine, or with certain other drugs, such as amphetamines, Aldomet, levodopa, dopamine, epinephrine, and anesthetics.

If you take MAO inhibitors, you and your family must know the precautions necessary to reduce the risk of these drugs. You should carry with you at all times a card stating the name of your drug and listing the foods and drugs that can be harmful to you.

Fast-acting Antidepressants

Other antidepressants, such as tetracyclics, maprotiline hydrochloride, and triazolopyridines, are more rapid-acting than tricyclic antidepressants and are useful in treating depressions accompanied by anxiety.

Electroconvulsive Therapy

Known popularly as shock treatment, electroconvulsive therapy (ECT) has been used in psychiatry since the early 1940s and has proven very useful in the treatment of severe depression. A small amount of electric current is delivered to the brain through wires placed on the outside of the head, usually for one second, to induce a convulsion, or seizure. Ten or more treatments are given over a two-week period. Depression usually clears, as well as most of its symptoms.

ECT is preferable to chemical antidepressants for people who have heart disease, for suicidal older people, and for very frail, malnourished depressed older people, where time is of the essence. The major disadvantage of ECT is a period of amnesia for a few days to weeks after the shock treatments. This amnesia is almost always gone after thirty days. Electroconvulsive therapy is not painful.

SUGGESTED READINGS

Stress and Mental Health

Benson, Herbert, and Klipper, Miriam. *The Relaxation Response.* New York: William Morrow, 1975.

Benson, Herbert, and Procter, William. *Beyond the Relaxation Response.* New York: Berkeley Books, 1985.

Butler, Robert N., and Lewis, Myrna. *Aging and Mental Health.* 3d ed. St. Louis: C V Mosby, 1982.

Friedman, Susan. *A Woman's Guide to Psychotherapy.* Englewood Cliffs, N.J.: Prentice-Hall, 1979.

Kleiman, Carol. *Women's Networks: The Complete Guide to Getting a Better Job, Advancing Your Career, and Feeling Great as a Woman Through Networking.* New York: Ballantine Books, 1980.

Porcino, Jane. *Growing Older, Getting Better: A Handbook for Women in the Second Half of Life.* Reading, Mass.: Addison-Wesley, 1983.

Finances and Work

Kleiman, Carol. *Women's Networks: The Complete Guide to Getting a Better Job, Advancing Your Career, and Feeling Great as a Woman Through Networking.* New York: Ballantine Books, 1980.

Divorce

Baker, Nancy. *New Lives for Former Wives.* Garden City, N.Y.: Doubleday, Anchor Books, 1980.

Remarriage

Jacobs, Ruth, and Vinick, Barbara. *Reengagement in Later Life.* Stamford, Conn.: Greylock Press, 1979.

Peterson, James, and Payne, Barbara. *Love in the Later Years.* New York: Association Press, 1975.

Grandparenting

Cohler, Bertram. *Mothers, Grandmothers and Daughters: Personality and Child-Care in Three-Generation Families.* New York: Wiley, 1981.

Cohn, Stephen Z., and Gans, Bruce Michael. *The Other Generation Gap: You and Your Aging Parents.* New York: Warner Books, 1978.

Goode, Ruth. *A Book for Grandmothers*. New York: McGraw-Hill, 1982.

Horne, Jo. *Caregiving: Helping An Aging Loved One*. Washington, D.C.: AARP; Glenview, Ill.: Scott, Foresman & Co., 1985. (An AARP Book)

Kornhaber, Arthur, and Woodward, Kenneth. *Grandparents/Grandchildren: The Vital Connection*. New York: Transaction Books, 1981.

Women Alone

Peterson, Nancy. *Lives for Ourselves: Women Who Have Never Married*. New York: Putnam, 1981.

Seskin, Jane. *Alone—Not Lonely: Independent Living for Women over Fifty*. Washington, D.C.: AARP; Glenview, Ill.: Scott, Foresman & Co., 1985. (An AARP Book)

Shahan, Lynn. *Living Alone and Liking It!* Los Angeles: Stratford Press, 1981.

Widowhood

Loewinsohn, Ruth Jean. *Survival Handbook for Widows*. Washington, D.C.: AARP; Glenview, Ill.: Scott, Foresman & Co., 1984. (An AARP Book)

Temes, Roberta. *Living with an Empty Chair: A Guide Through Grief*. New York: Irvington Publishers, 1980.

Fifteen

Drug Use, Alcoholism, and Drug Dependence

FIFTY years ago, Americans took few drugs. Pharmacies held perhaps fifty large, dark jars of powders, pills, and elixirs. Today, pharmacies, supermarkets, and convenience stores sell over twenty thousand different kinds of tablets, capsules, powders, syrups, ointments, creams, and salves to Americans each year. The pharmaceutical industry includes over a hundred multimillion-dollar companies.

The United States is a nation of doers, who look for "quick fixes" for their problems and grow impatient waiting for the healing effect of time. A person who walks out of the doctor's office with a prescription in hand tends to feel better treated than one who walks out empty-handed after ten minutes of sound, practical advice.

Sometimes our faith in quick solutions is shaken, as in 1961, when the world was shocked by the thalidomide disaster. Thousands of families had babies who suffered the consequences of a medication that, like many medications in those days, had not been properly tested. Patients, doctors, pharmacists, and researchers were forced to recognize that drugs could do harm.

We need not return to a life without pills. But we must remember that each drug, including aspirin, has good and harmful effects. Time itself is an able healer, and there are often alternatives to drugs, which, in the long run, may provide more relief.

WHAT YOU SHOULD KNOW
ABOUT DRUGS

The National Council on Patient Information and Education recommends that all patients ask, and all health professionals answer, five questions when medication is prescribed:

1. What is the name of the medication, and what is it supposed to do?
2. How do I take it, and for how long?
3. What foods, drinks, other medicines, and activities should I avoid while taking this medicine?
4. What are the side effects, and what should I do if they occur?
5. Is there any written information available about this medication?

Purpose of Medication

Ask the generic name of any drug you are taking, what the drug is supposed to do for you, and how long it takes for the drug to start working. If improvement does not occur within the approximate expected time, call your doctor for futher recommendations.

Taking Medications

Find out how each medication should be taken. Should it be taken before or after meals? How many hours apart should it be taken? Should it be taken with or in the absence of certain foods? (Tetracycline, for example, should not be taken with milk.) Can the capsule be opened and the contents mixed with something easy to swallow? Ask how long you will need to take the drug.

Take your medications as prescribed. Too often, we take medications for a few days and, as soon as we feel better, stop. With some drugs, stopping early or abruptly can be harmful, for example with antibiotics or certain drugs taken for blood pressure or for the heart. Do not hide the truth from your doctor. If you have not taken your blood pressure pills, admit it; otherwise, you may be prescribed a stronger pill, when what you really need is to be more reliable about taking the less powerful drug.

Each drug you take should apply to a particular disease or problem. When you see your doctor, review all your current drugs to determine whether any can be discontinued or decreased in dosage. If a drug you are taking has not proven helpful in a reasonable period of time, ask your doctor about discontinuing it or changing to another drug.

If you are asked to stop taking a drug, ask whether you should keep what is left for the future or throw the drug down the toilet. Do not give your discarded drugs to friends—you may do harm.

Ursula A., seventy-six, had been an army nurse during World War II, and the other people in her building respected her medical experience. She often found herself recommending treatments to other women and, in fact, would usually have a partly full bottle of pills to give them. Her advice was, for the most part, reasonable and helpful, and, of course, she was very accessible.

One day, an older woman, to whom Ursula had given some arthritis pills, developed serious intestinal bleeding from the pills. They had interacted with a blood thinner the woman was taking for another problem and had caused bruising and bleeding all over her body. As a result, she was in the hospital for ten days. Ursula felt terrible and realized that there were many things she did not know about drugs and their interactions.

She called a visiting nurse and asked her to come to the house to help her sort through the pharmacy in her drawer. Many pills were outdated and potentially harmful. Many could cause serious side effects in people taking other medications. Frightened by the harm she had unwittingly done to her neighbor, Ursula was relieved to give up a medical role for which she was not really qualified.

Precautions with Medications

Ask if there are likely to be any untoward interactions (such as reducing or increasing the effect of a drug) with other drugs you are taking or with alcohol. Also ask whether you must limit any of your activities while taking the medication. (If taking tetracycline, for example, it is advisable to avoid direct exposure to the sun.)

Side Effects of Drugs

Find out what side effects you can expect and which ones are serious and should be reported to your doctor, which ones might persist, and which ones will usually go away in time.

The older you are, the more sensitive your system is to drugs. This is in part because your body now metabolizes them more slowly and in part because your liver and kidneys do not clear drugs out of your system as fast as they used to. Drugs tend to remain in your body for a longer time, and a drug overdose is more likely to result. Therefore, in older age, the margin of safety between a helpful dose and a toxic dose of many drugs is reduced.

Women are more likely than men to suffer from drug complications simply because they consume more prescribed and over-the-counter drugs than men. The women most likely to experience adverse reactions from drugs are women over seventy-five who are small and thin; women with a history of drug allergies; women who have had many side effects with different classes of drugs; women with several chronic illnesses (kidney failure, diabetes, and heart disease or other combinations of diseases); women with kidney, liver, or mental impairment; and women taking many prescriptions at a time.

Written Information

For further information about drugs, you can consult the *Physicians' Desk Reference,* or PDR (Oradell, N.J.: Medical Economics Company Inc., 1986) or *About Your Medicines* by the United States Pharmacopeial Convention, Inc. (Kingsport, Tenn.: Kingsport Press, 1981). These books describe drug actions, side effects, and appropriate warnings. The PDR lists even the rarest effects, so do not become too frightened by what you read.

For information in a readily understandable format, you may wish to obtain AARP Pharmacy Service Medication Information Leaflets for Seniors (MILS). Write to AARP Pharmacy, One Prince Street, Alexandria, VA 22314, and state the prescription drugs you are taking.

YOUR DRUG HISTORY

Your drug history is part of your medical history. Your drug history includes any allergic reactions or any unpleasant side effects you have had with specific medications, as well as an up-to-date list of the particular drugs, including vitamins and over-the-counter medications, you are currently taking. Keep a written record of your drug history. Always tell a new doctor the details of your drug history, and ask that this record be put on file.

GENERIC EQUIVALENTS OF DRUGS

Ask your doctor about the generic equivalent of the drug prescribed. Generic drugs are equally good and far cheaper. Do not hesitate to ask your doctor how much a prescription is likely to cost. If he or she is unaware of the price, have the doctor check with your pharmacist. If the price is exorbitant, ask if there is a less expensive alternative. Sometimes doctors are unaware of the price of medications they prescribe, and of the financial burden this can mean. If need be, ask your pharmacist if you can pay in two or three installments.

Rita Q., sixty, took the prescription she had received from her doctor to the pharmacy. The cashier rang up sixty-five dollars for a hundred pills. Rita was floored and decided to buy only twenty to start. After finishing the twenty pills, she decided not to pick up the remainder of the prescription because of the cost.

Two weeks later, the infection in her foot was slightly better but still present. The doctor ordered another round of treatment. When Rita told him how much the pills cost, he was amazed and apologetic. He prescribed a less costly alternative, which she took faithfully. Her foot healed.

Find a pharmacy that has reasonable prices and where you can get to know your pharmacist. Pharmacists have extensive knowledge about drugs, side effects of drugs, and alternative drugs and can give you sound advice about selecting over-the-counter drugs as well.

ALTERNATIVES TO DRUG TREATMENT

Ask your doctor about alternatives to medication. Often diet, exercise, relaxation techniques, yoga, or other therapies can alleviate your problem and perhaps substitute for drugs.

ALCOHOLISM

Alcoholism is a silent epidemic among women. Prior to 1970, it was considered a man's disease. The increase in alcoholism among females has been so dramatic during the past fifteen years that it is now a woman's disease as well.

> I never thought of myself as an alcoholic. While Sam was alive, we always had a few drinks in the evening and wine with supper. After he died, I found myself drinking to forget my loneliness. Often I drank into the small hours of the night. I never drank in the daytime.
> But those long nights alone were tough. It seemed that only alcohol could put me to sleep. I started to be concerned about my drinking when I began waking up with a headache. Who could I talk to? I certainly didn't want my children to know how many bottles of whiskey I drank a week—in fact, I couldn't face it myself. I knew that my friends would only think the less of me.

I began to isolate myself even from the people I loved, out of shame of being discovered.

Finally, thank God, I got pneumonia. I was quite sick and ended up in the hospital for two weeks. A wonderful nurse, bless her soul, noticed my shakiness, and I confessed all to her.

Now I'm a member of Alcoholics Anonymous. I go to meetings three times a week. I've met other women who have been lonely, "closet" drinkers, just like me. I will never have another drink in my life, and that's a very serious commitment.

—Sandra, fifty-nine

Alcoholism is not something that can be measured by a laboratory, and there is no universal standard of reasonable alcoholic consumption. What is considered normal drinking in one part of the world may be considered excessive in other regions. Alcoholism is a level of alcohol consumption that interferes with a person's health and social and economic functioning.

The distinction between "heavy drinking" and alcoholism is as follows:

- A nonalcoholic can stop drinking and, in fact, will stop from time to time. An alcoholic has a compulsion to drink, and although she might also feel that she can stop, she will never actually terminate her drinking until she starts to admit she is an alcoholic.

- A nonalcoholic uses other palliatives as well as alcohol to feel better. An alcoholic relies only on alcohol to relieve problems.

- A nonalcoholic is unlikely to miss work because of drinking or a hangover. An alcoholic periodically is unable to show up at work or perform normal household tasks because of drinking or a hangover.

- A nonalcoholic is unlikely to forget events that occur when she drinks. An alcoholic sometimes cannot remember the events of the night(s) before because she is drunk so often that she loses her sense of time and forgets the sequence of events.

- A nonalcoholic rarely gets involved with the law or the medical system as a result of drinking. An alcoholic may find herself at the police station for speeding while drunk or in the emergency room for treatment after a fall because her frequent drinking impairs her judgment.

If drinking is a regular ritual in your life, it is not difficult to slip over the line and become dependent on it. If you drink alcohol habitually, it is a good idea to think seriously when someone close to you expresses concern about your drinking. If you find yourself reacting defensively to the comment, or if you absolutely refuse to consider its truth, you should begin to worry and start talking about your drinking habit with someone neutral.

Harmful Effects of Alcohol

Some of the dangers of excessive alcohol consumption for women include the following:

- Heavy drinkers are more prone than moderate drinkers to cirrhosis (liver disease), cancer of the respiratory and digestive tracts, accidents, and suicide. The alcoholic woman seems to develop cirrhosis quicker and at an earlier age than does the alcoholic man. She is more likely than the alcoholic man to die from the disease.

- Given the same dose of alcohol, women get more intoxicated than men. This is because women usually weigh less and have a greater proportion of fat to muscle than men, which causes women to metabolize alcohol more slowly.

- Alcohol disrupts the normal sleep cycle.

- Alcoholism is often associated with poor nutrition, which exposes the alcoholic to vitamin, protein, and iron deficiencies and to anemia.

- Alcohol and depression are closely associated in women; whether the depression leads to alcoholism or vice versa is not yet known. Women alcoholics have an extraordinarily high rate of suicide attempts (the estimate is 30 percent to 40 percent) and also a high rate of suicide.

Women Who Are Vulnerable to Alcoholism

Some women are particularly vulnerable to alcoholism. They include women who have a family background of alcoholism; women with alcoholic husbands; women who face severe emotional strains such as an adulterous spouse, divorce, strife with an employer, loss of a job, death of a spouse or child, or difficult relationships with children; women who are depressed before or after drinking; women taking tranquilizers, sleeping pills, or diet pills; and women whose social lives always include alcohol.

What to Do If You Think You Have a Drinking Problem

If you are already willing to consider that you have a drinking problem, you have gone at least halfway in helping yourself. Unfortunately, the very nature of alcoholism, especially in women, fosters self-deception and self-delusion. This may be because you didn't have a problem when you first started social drinking. You simply cannot see that now you have a problem or that it has made you sick and lacking in self-judgment.

The next step is to find help. It can come from your physician, a therapist, a social worker, a spouse, or a recovered alcoholic. You might choose to go to a local branch of Alcoholics Anonymous (AA), or you can simply telephone them. One of their volunteers will probably meet you to discuss ways of dealing with the drinking. Or, you can call Women for Sobriety (WFS), a national organization that works with alcoholic women.

Women who have been very heavy drinkers for a long time may need a period of alcohol withdrawal in a hospital. Some hospitals have units that specialize in treating alcohol withdrawal.

During the withdrawal period, a drug, such as Serax or Librium, is given temporarily to ease the symptoms of tremors, anxiety, agitation, and delirium, which often accompany alcohol withdrawal. Counseling is also an important part of this first stage of rehabilitation. Counseling usually starts in the hospital and includes counseling from former, rehabilitated alcoholics and group and individual therapy utilizing a variety of behavior modification techniques.

The next stage of rehabilitation focuses on your home situation and the problems or crises that have fueled the alcoholism. You are helped to see that change is possible—that you do not have to accept the present terms of your life but can actively work to change them.

> I could not imagine leaving Jack, even though he abused me and made me share his drunkenness. But my counselors and other reformed women alcoholics showed me that I need not share his habit. They helped me to see that it was not necessary to be dragged down with him. They taught me that I would be showing him more love by taking a hard line, refusing to live with him if he did not get help. I had to help him by helping and respecting myself.
>
> —*Judy, sixty-one*

Individual or group psychotherapy can continue on an outpatient basis once you leave the hospital. Family members are often included in the counseling sessions, since their attitudes toward your alcoholism are major influences in your recovery.

> It was hard for me to look my children in the
> eye. I had abused myself and them for years
> when I was an alcoholic. Now, I felt desperately
> guilty for having failed them. But I needed them
> for my recovery—needed their love and support,
> and their forgiveness. And they needed the
> counseling too.
>
> —*Brina, sixty-three*

Rehabilitation is a lifelong effort. Never can an alcoholic let down her guard and begin drinking again. The women most likely to succeed at recovering are those who aim to never have a drink again. The relapse rate for recovered alcoholics is extremely high.

Alcoholics Anonymous

One of the groups most successful in permanently reforming both men and women alcoholics, AA uses the simple but effective therapy of group discussion and support. Men and women openly admit their alcoholism to one another and, as they begin to feel comfortable, discuss the impact of their drinking problems on their lives and relationships. They are amazed and reassured when they discover how parallel their lives and problems are. With peer support, they find the strength to fight the alcohol "one day at a time."

> I never thought of myself as a joiner of groups. I
> never thought I could share intimate details of
> my despair and destructiveness with a roomful of
> people. I was certain that there would be no one
> at the AA meetings whom I could relate to and
> no one who cared as much about the pain I had
> inflicted on those I loved the most.
>
> I found myself accepted, empathized with,
> and understood by many people at the meetings,
> old and young. We were all there, desperate,
> needing the help and support that we had finally
> found.
>
> —*Harriet, fifty-six*

**Helping Yourself If Your Spouse or
Companion Drinks Heavily**

Al-Anon is a program established by Alcoholics Anonymous to
help and support spouses of alcoholics or other family members.
Whether or not your spouse is getting help, you should find support for yourself. The stress, financial burdens, guilt, anger, and insecurity that come from living with an alcoholic are overwhelming
and difficult to handle alone.

> I found myself hating my husband. When he was
> drunk, he was just intolerable to me and the
> kids. I wished I could throw him out of the
> house. Then when I'd see him vomiting and los-
> ing weight, losing self-respect yet unable to con-
> trol himself, I'd feel terribly guilty.
>   At Al-Anon, I met other women in the same
> situation. I saw that my roller-coaster emotions
> toward Albert were perfectly normal. I saw that I
> did not have to give up my whole life because he
> was destroying his own. Al-Anon gave me the
> courage to confront him, and if you can believe
> it, he finally went for help. We are all struggling
> together now. My kids attend Alateen meetings,
> are facing their own fears about alcohol, and are
> dealing with their anger toward their father.
>   —*Joan, fifty-two*

Alcohol, in Moderation, Can Improve Your Health

Many recent studies have suggested the benefit of moderate
amounts (two four-ounce glasses of wine or one shot of whiskey per
day) of alcohol to the heart. People who drink moderately have
higher blood levels of HDL, or high-density lipoproteins, than
teetotalers. HDL protects against arteriosclerosis.

If you can tolerate it, small amounts of alcohol can be relaxing
after a stressful day.

DRUG ABUSE AND DRUG DEPENDENCE

More than half the patients treated in emergency rooms for drug-
related problems are women. Among older women, the most commonly abused classes of drugs are tranquilizers, sedatives (especially
barbiturates), and amphetamines—all of which are legal. Two-thirds

of all prescriptions for tranquilizers are written for women. Men's drug-abuse problems are more likely to involve illegal drugs.

Use of Mood-affecting Drugs in America

Drugs	Have Used	Number of People Who Use Regularly	Use Occasionally
Barbiturates (Seconal, Nembutal)	24 million	4.5 million	9 million
Other sedatives (Chloral hydrate)	4.5 million	350,000	1 million
Tranquilizers (Valium, Serax, Librium)	20 million	5 million	13.5 million
Antidepressants (Elavil, Imipramine, Sinequan)	3 million	500,000	1 million
Amphetamines (Dexedrine, Ritalin)	12 million	1.5 million	3 million
Pain pills (Codeine, Sulfate Tablets, Percodan)	36 million	3.75 million	12 million
Alcohol	120 million	18 million	12 million

GUIDELINES FOR USING MOOD-AFFECTING DRUGS SAFELY

Tranquilizers, sedatives, painkillers, and antidepressants are valuable classes of drugs that help millions of women cope with stress. To use them safely and effectively, you should heed the following advice.

1. Consider these drugs as short-term treatments that accompany other help, such as counseling, behavior modification, and/or support groups. After one or two months, you and your doctor should reevaluate your need for the drugs.

2. With your doctor's guidance, terminate your use of the drug slowly, tapering doses over time, so that your body has a chance to recover from the physical and psychological habituation.

3. Have regular checkups, since the drugs can produce side effects that should be monitored.

4. Ask your doctor whether there are alternatives and complements to drug treatment. Remember that mood-affecting drugs are generally prescribed for women too easily and too often.

SUGGESTED READINGS

Long, James W., M.D. *The Essential Guide to Prescription Drugs*. 4th ed. New York: Harper & Row, 1985.

Meryman, Richard. *Broken Promises, Mended Dreams: An Alcoholic Woman Fights for Her Life*. Boston: Little, Brown, 1984.

Physicians' Desk Reference. 40th ed. Oradell, N.J.: Medical Economics Co., 1986.

Physicians' Desk Reference for Nonprescription Drugs. 7th ed. Oradell, N.J.: Medical Economics Co., 1986.

Youcha, Geraldine. *Women and Alcohol: A Dangerous Pleasure*. New York: Crown, 1986.

Sixteen

Your Relationship with the Health Care System

B ERNICE W., a fifty-six-year-old supervisor of a department store, had not seen a doctor in years. In fact, she did not have a regular doctor; it was her style to see a specialist when a particular problem arose.

Recently she had noted changes in her bowel habits. She also felt more tired than usual. People commented on how pale Bernice looked. She attributed all this to stress and the long winter.

One day, Bernice fainted at work. She realized that she needed a medical checkup, but where would she find a doctor at a moment's notice? She called friends to get the names of their doctors and tried to get an appointment to be seen quickly. But none of the doctors could see a new patient for months.

Finally, she found a doctor who could see her that week. During the office visit, he intimidated her by his stern appearance, the rapidity of his questions as he took her history, and the brusque way he examined her.

Without much explanation, he sent her to the hospital for a series of bowel X rays. He asked her to make another appointment and ushered her out the door before she had a chance to digest what he had recommended.

Bernice was too overwhelmed to call back for explanations. She alternated between thinking she had cancer and feeling that there was nothing wrong. She desperately wished she had a doctor she could talk to and trust.

THE DOCTOR-PATIENT RELATIONSHIP

After the age of fifty, one of the most important things you can do for your health is choose a good doctor. Having a trusted doctor is like having money in the bank. At a time of crisis, you need a doctor you can count on, who knows your medical history and has these important qualifications:

1. Training in family practice or internal medicine. A doctor with these credentials (or an old-fashioned GP) will be able to treat most of your medical problems. He or she will also be able to refer you to specialists for complex problems and will interpret their findings for you.

2. Affiliation with a reputable hospital, to which he or she can admit you privately should you need hospital care. For very complex medical problems (those that present diagnostic dilemmas or require very specialized medical or surgical techniques), the doctor should be able to obtain for you knowledgeable consultants and the use of the most up-to-date technologies.

3. Participation in an on-call system with a group of doctors who can answer important questions or see you in case of emergency on a twenty-four-hour, seven-day-a-week basis. This coverage is important so that your care after 5:00 P.M. is not left to emergency room doctors who are not familiar with your case.

4. An accessible manner. You need a doctor who doesn't make you feel self-conscious about discussing your health problems. Your doctor should also answer your telephone calls within a twenty-four-hour period and be able to give you an appointment within a reasonable time or see you the same day for an emergency. If you find it difficult to get to the doctor's office or are housebound, it can make a big difference if the doctor makes house calls, but such doctors are hard to find.

5. Reasonable fees and willingness to accept Medicare assignment. If a doctor has exorbitant fees, you may not wish to consult him or her for any but the most extreme problems. Conversely, a physician who accepts Medicare assignment relieves you of some cumbersome paperwork and financial burdens that may inhibit you from seeking care.

6. Board credentials. A doctor who has specialty training in family practice or internal medicine and who has passed specialty examinations (is board certified) or is eligible to take them (is board eligible) is more likely to have a stronger background in medicine than one who has not. The credentials can be reviewed in the *American Medical Directory,* found in the reference room of any public library, or you can obtain such information from your local medical society.

How to Find a Good Doctor

The best time to look for a good doctor is while you are healthy and have the energy and time to do some investigating. Start by asking people you respect for the names of doctors with whom they are satisfied. Call your local medical society to check on the doctors' credentials, or look them up yourself in the *American Medical Directory.* Or ask the Department of Medicine of one of the better hospitals in your town for the names of three family doctors or internists. You might also call your local medical society for names of doctors and then call any large, reputable hospital, or hospitals, in your city or region to see whether these doctors are affiliated with them.

Narrow down your list to two or three qualified physicians and, if you wish, make appointments to interview them. You will be charged a consultation fee, but the process may well be worth it. How quickly can you get an appointment? How easy is it to get to the office? How friendly and welcoming is the doctor's staff? Does the doctor seem warm and have time to talk with you? Is the doctor respectful of you? Does it seem that the two of you could be effective "partners" in your care? Is the doctor willing to discuss on-call systems, coverage during vacations, hospital affiliations, specialists the doctor works with, and second opinions?

Communicating with Your Doctor

Communication with your physician requires effort from both of you. Ask yourself the following questions to determine whether your physician communicates effectively with you.

- If you are unhappy with your doctor's approach to a certain problem, will he or she discuss alternatives with you?
- If there is no reasonable alternative to a prescribed treatment, is your physician willing to explain why?
- If you refuse to accept a particular treatment (for religious, financial, cultural, or individual reasons), is your physician still willing to work with you and accept your refusal as your right?

- When investigating a particular problem, does your doctor explain the procedures necessary for a diagnosis and the risks they carry?
- When prescribing medications, does your doctor describe all their side effects and their possible toxicities?
- Does your doctor tell you what a prescription is likely to cost and discuss cheaper alternatives?
- Is your doctor able to offer you support despite the fact that he or she disapproves of some of your habits or some aspects of the way you choose to live? Some of the more "touchy" issues might be obesity, alcoholism, drug dependence, lesbianism, vegetarianism, and belief in Eastern medicine.
- Does your doctor give you enough time to present your concerns and ask questions?

When a doctor truly encourages communication, and rapport, the answers to the preceding questions will be yes. As a patient, you should expect this level of communication.

How well do you communicate with your doctor? The major hurdle in establishing rapport with your physician is to learn to speak up, to take responsibility for asking questions. Prepare yourself before going to the doctor. Make a list of your current medications, their doses, and their schedule. Know what you expect to find out as a result of the visit. Know what you wish to ask, and write down your questions, if necessary. Ask your doctor questions when you don't understand something or if you are unsure about what to do. Discuss any aspects of your doctor's advice that you feel you cannot or will not follow. Mention alternatives if you know of ones you would prefer. Tell your doctor you would like a second opinion if you are uncertain about the proposed treatment or follow-up.

A book, *Managing Your Doctor: How to Get the Best Possible Medical Care,* by Arthur S. Freese (Briarcliff Manor, N.Y.: Stein & Day, 1977), helps dispel the myth of the doctor as God. It aims to help you communicate with your doctor without being intimidated and without feeling guilt or embarrassment about expressing your ideas and fears.

Physicians are human, with human frailties. You won't be able to find a perfect physician, but you should be able to find a competent one with whom you can talk openly.

The Annual Physical Examination

Healthy women over fifty should have a general physical checkup each year. During a checkup, your doctor should do the following:

1. evaluate your risk for various diseases, such as hypertension and arteriosclerosis, and advise you about preventing these risks
2. screen you for cancer—check your breasts for lumps, perform a pelvic exam and Pap smear to exclude gynecologic cancer, give you a rectal exam and ask you to complete tests at home for occult blood in your stools to check for intestinal cancer, and order periodic blood tests
3. update your medical history and review your current medications and your need for them

The examination should last between half an hour and an hour. An electrocardiogram is usually obtained only every two to five years, but more frequently after you are seventy. (For a complete list of examinations the woman over fifty needs at regular intervals, see Appendix A.)

Staying healthy requires your active participation; the very energy you put into staying healthy can help you feel more alive.

> I am a woman of eighty-one years. I count on my own efforts to help the physicians help me, knowing that in a healthy body the mind will flourish. As a result, I slowed down the progress of arthritis, took control of my weight and reduced considerably, and limbered up my body.
>
> My enthusiasm for all facets of life is greater than ever.
>
> —*Carmen Y., eighty-one*

YOUR RELATIONSHIP WITH OTHER HEALTH PROFESSIONALS

More and more, the nurse practitioner and the physician's assistant are providing primary medical care. These health professionals have proven themselves competent to evaluate and treat many common medical problems, such as persistent colds, bladder infections, and back spasms, as well as to provide care during many chronic illnesses, such as hypertension, diabetes, heart disease, and lung disease. Their training and availability to teach about nutrition, exercise, and prevention of disease are necessary services that a doctor may be too busy to provide.

Olivia T., fifty-seven, called her doctor to try to get help for her aching back. She was asked to come in and see the nurse practitioner. "Why not the doctor?" she wondered somewhat angrily, feeling brushed off.

As it turned out, she was very pleased with her visit to the nurse practitioner. The nurse made a thorough evaluation of Olivia's back, legs, and spine—in fact, it was the most complete evaluation Olivia had ever had.

Nurse practitioners have a master's degree in nursing, which requires two years of training beyond that required for a bachelor's degree in nursing. Often the practitioner specializes in a certain area, such as family medicine, pediatrics, geriatrics, adult health, rehabilitation, or surgery. In sixteen states in the United States, the nurse practitioner can write prescriptions for most classes of medications.

A physician's assistant completes two years of intensive medical study after college, which includes training side by side with a physician. In many settings, such as nursing homes and health centers, the physician's assistant functions much as does the nurse practitioner, and with a similar broad focus.

YOUR RELATIONSHIP WITH HOSPITALS

Hospitals are the most expensive component of our health care system. They epitomize the best and sometimes the worst of modern medicine. On the one hand, they house sophisticated medical technologies that allow us to replace hearts, kidneys, joints, and corneas; pass tiny tubes into arteries to visualize the circulation of blood; dissolve stones in gallbladders; bypass blockages of arteries in legs and hearts; and prolong living—or dying, as the case may be—with ventilators and tubes that keep the body breathing. On the other hand, hospitals can be dehumanizing and impersonal, exhausting rather than restful, and efficient but inhospitable.

With Medicare costs rising sharply, and with 70 percent of Medicare benefits being used on hospital care, federal policy is trying to limit the public expenditure for medical care. For Medicare patients, hospitals are now reimbursed in fixed amounts, according to Diagnostic Related Groups, or DRGs. This practice means that hospitals are reimbursed for a specific number of days for a given diagnosis. For example, an uncomplicated appendectomy is authorized for an average of 5.3 hospital days, and a heart attack is authorized for 8.8 hospital days. Hospital stays that are longer must be approved by reviewing agencies; if not approved, the extra days are billed to the patient. The expense of the additional days can be staggering, since most hospitals charge $300 or more per day!

The ceiling on what the government ordinarily will pay for your illness means that the role of hospitals has changed radically in the past ten years. More and more, hospitals provide care during only the most critical periods of illness. There is little room for recuperating patients; they are sent home (and prescribed home services as needed), to specialized rehabilitation facilities, or to nursing homes, some of which have excellent rehabilitation services.

Many hospitals have set up ambulatory-surgery units, in which the less complex operations and procedures (such as removal of intestinal polyps through colonoscopy) can be done during the day, eliminating the overnight hospital stay and allowing the patient to recover at home.

Reducing the length of hospital stays offers certain advantages to patients. Patients who are encouraged to walk and to care for themselves as soon as they are able seem to recover more quickly from illness or surgery than those who stay in bed for a long time. Hospitalization itself creates risks for the patient, such as contracting a hospital infection, a greater likelihood of experiencing hazardous side effects from drugs or drug interactions, receiving the wrong treatment or the wrong medicine by mistake, and possibly being investigated for problems that often have no consequence for the patient.

Today, the following situations exist for any potential hospital patient.

- Most larger hospitals cannot admit you unless you have a medical problem that requires complex diagnosis and treatment.

- Most hospitals will discharge you before you feel ready to leave.

- Your hospital bill will be enormous, in terms of both the cost and the size of the computer printout that itemizes your expenses.

- Your insurance may not cover all of your hospital bill.

- The nurses may take fifteen to twenty minutes to answer your calls because they have many sick patients to care for.

- You may feel constantly exhausted because you are ill and undergoing frequent testing and surveillance.

Teaching Hospitals

Teaching hospitals have two missions: the care of patients and the training of young doctors. Such hospitals have excellent staff physicians and the most up-to-date technologies and offer the most modern medical treatment. You are cared for by medical students, interns, residents, and specialists-in-training, who are supervised by staff physicians, and your private doctor. With many doctors involved in your care, it can be hard to know who is in charge. Each may examine you at different times, which can be fatiguing and seem overwhelming, but such examination means that few of your problems are likely to be missed. You should ask what the status is of those caring for you and find out who is in charge. Generally, the person in charge will be your private doctor. Do not hesitate to ask the staff about procedures and treatments or about any confusing or conflicting information you may have been given. If you feel uncertain about your treatment by the staff, ask that your private physician be consulted about particular issues. Preferably, also discuss these issues with your doctor in person.

A teaching hospital's young doctors and medical students often offer compassion and attention that patients do not soon forget. Teaching hospitals require interns and residents to staff the patient floors at all times of the day and night—unlike many smaller hospitals, which may only have an emergency room doctor on call at night. The extra coverage can be invaluable if you suddenly develop serious medical problems during the night.

Rights of Patients in the Hospital

George Annas, chief of the health law section at Boston University School of Public Health, has developed a model patient's bill of rights. It includes all of your statutory rights, as well as other desirable rights that are not yet recognized by case law or statute. (See Appendix B.)

Preparing for Your Discharge from the Hospital

Contact the discharge planning nurse or the hospital social worker either prior to admission or once admitted. If possible, find out early how long your stay in the hospital will be. Ask your doctor what kind of care you are likely to need on discharge, what your level of disability will be, and how much time you will take to recuperate. Have the doctor consult with the discharge nurse or the social worker so that this person can help assess your needs and arrange the proper home assistance or appropriate institutional care on discharge. If necessary, the social worker can help you make the most beneficial financial arrangements.

POSTHOSPITAL CARE FOR
OLDER PERSONS

Christine D., sixty-three, had severely deformed hands, wrists, and knees from rheumatoid arthritis, a disease she had had for fifteen years. She walked with extreme difficulty, and, although her balance was precarious, she would not give in to using a cane or walker. Not at sixty-three! Canes and walkers were for old people!

One night, when getting out of bed, Christine fell onto the floor, breaking her left shoulder. She required surgical correction of the break. During her recovery, she had difficulties. Her cast was heavy, and, with only one good arm, her balance was worse than usual. She had trouble getting out of a chair; she wobbled badly trying to walk and often came close to losing her balance.

It was obvious that Christine could not manage at home alone because she needed rehabilitation and supervision. The screening departments of local rehabilitation hospitals refused to admit her because rehabilitative care for upper-extremity fractures was not reimbursable by Medicare under the system's guidelines. Christine could not afford the private rate of $165 per day.

The only option seemed to be moving to a nursing home temporarily, at a rate of $65 per day. She could not bear the thought of spending a month or two with such aged people. But she did go, since there was really very little choice.

Eleanor H., eighty-two, had been managing independently at home until one day she suffered a sudden severe brain hemorrhage. She spent two weeks in a hospital in a coma. She was kept alive by a small feeding tube that went directly into her stomach. She was not expected to regain consciousness.

Her family was devastated. In addition, none of her children lived close by or was in a position to give her the round-the-clock care she needed.

Applications to several long-term-care hospitals in the area were turned down because Eleanor needed more nursing attention than medical attention. She was also refused by several nursing homes because her needs for care were too great, and the homes were short-staffed. Meanwhile, the hospital was putting great pressure on the family members to get Eleanor out, since her severe stroke was permanent, and there was nothing new to diagnose or treat.

Finally, Eleanor was accepted by a nursing home in a distant town. Her family felt compelled to agree to moving her there.

In spite of these two examples, the stories of patients who are accepted at rehabilitation hospitals are usually ones of success. But the rehabilitation and chronic-care hospitals sometimes fail people when they can least afford such failure. Transfers of patients to the wrong place can occur. Families may blame themselves, each other, the person who is ill, or the medical staff when, in fact, it is the impersonal system that is to blame.

Admission guidelines to rehabilitation hospitals are fairly stringent and need to be adhered to if the facility is to receive Medicare or other insurance monies. However, many people fail to "fit" the needed categories of any facility and yet are not ready to be cared for at home, even with home health services.

Special Problems

If you or a family member do not "fit" the system's categories for posthospital placement, you might consider the following:

1. Ask the physician, someone in the physical therapy or other rehabilitation department, and/or the social worker to clearly identify your medical, rehabilitative, and social needs.

2. Find some advocates. Social workers can be exceptionally helpful, and, at your request, they will come to your bedside to discuss problems with you.

3. Be prepared to convince the screening team that you belong in the particular facility you desire; however, realize that you may be turned down because of strict requirements for admission.

4. If you are turned down for admission to a facility, ask to be rescreened if your condition alters and you believe you are more acceptable for admission.

5. If you feel discriminated against because of age, sex, race, or other cause, speak to the hospital lawyer or to your own lawyer. You have a right to know all the reasons you or your family member is being denied admission to a given facility.

6. Be willing to accept alternative care arrangements that may not be your first choice but that still may meet your needs.

7. Do not hesitate to call your local or state Agency on Aging or your local AARP office or write your congressional representative if you have been treated in a way that seems unfair to you.

YOU AND THE HEALTH
MAINTENANCE ORGANIZATION (HMO)

One of the models of organization for health care is the Health Maintenance Organization, a health insurance system in which you or Medicare pays a monthly premium, and the HMO's doctors and staff provide your medical care. Each HMO differs in terms of its costs and the package of medical services that it provides; for example, each may or may not include hospital or nursing home benefits, home care, drugs, or supplies. Each HMO has its own physicians, contracts for its hospital beds, and does not permit you to use outside resources unless you pay for them out of your own pocket.

HMOs are organized to do the following:

1. Deliver health services that attempt to meet your needs in the most appropriate, efficient, and least costly way.

2. Provide easy access to doctors, nurses, and other professionals so that health problems can be detected and treated early.

3. Use new services, such as home care, outpatient surgery, day care, and home monitoring, to substitute for services ordinarily performed in the expensive hospital setting. The HMO may also cover services such as mental health, dental and eye care, provision of equipment, and drugs that are often not covered under Medicare or private or group insurance.

4. Centralize and coordinate in one organization all the medical services that you might need.

5. Include preventive or wellness programs.

The federal government encourages HMOs to actively solicit members over sixty-five years of age. The government hopes to be able to purchase more services for older people at lower costs from HMOs than from the usual Medicare system.

Once you join an HMO, you abandon certain choices that were yours under regular Medicare. You agree to accept medical care provided by the HMO's doctors, laboratories, and hospitals. You must pay extra for any consultations or second opinions you seek outside the HMO plan.

In making a decision whether to join an HMO, you should do the following:

• Examine the range of services offered by the HMO and see if they offer advantages over those covered by Medicare.

• Compare your out-of-pocket expenses in each system, adding costs of the deductibles, the uncovered services that you might require, drugs, eyeglasses, equipment, dental care, and so on.

- Investigate the quality and types of doctors and nurses in the HMO. Does it have specialists on its staff? Can you choose a physician from the panel of doctors belonging to the HMO that you can call "your" doctor? Are other clients of the HMO satisfied with the services?
- Find out whether the hospitals used by the HMO are reputable.
- Find out whether the HMO has a grievance procedure that allows you to appeal certain choices or decisions made by the HMO staff. Ask what types of grievances have been brought forth and how they were resolved. If you have conflicts with the HMO, you should have ways of dealing with the problems other than withdrawing.

YOUR RELATIONSHIP WITH MEDICARE

The enactment of Title XIX of the Older Americans Act in 1965 (Medicare) was a major victory for older people. The majority of Americans over the age of sixty-five became eligible for health insurance benefits administered by the federal Health Care Financing Administration.

Medicare was not intended as a comprehensive medical insurance program for people over sixty-five; rather, it is an insurance policy for medical and hospital care. In fact, Medicare benefits cover only about 44.3 percent of total health care costs for its beneficiaries. The remaining costs are borne by other health insurance carriers, assuming that you carry supplemental health insurance or even full coverage; are paid for directly by you; or are paid by Medicaid assistance for those in low income brackets.

Medicare is a two-part program. Medicare A automatically provides hospital insurance, skilled nursing facility coverage, home health services, and hospice care, if you fit eligibility requirements. Medicare B is voluntary health insurance (for which you pay monthly premiums) that helps pay for doctors' services both inside and outside the hospital, outpatient hospital care, physical therapy, speech pathology services, home health care, medically necessary ambulance transportation, laboratory services, and equipment costs. Except in very rare instances, neither Medicare A nor B pays for nursing home care, and it offers limited home health benefits.

The particulars of Medicare A and B coverage are available on request from the Social Security office in your area or from AARP's excellent booklet *Information on Medicare & Health Insurance for Older People.*

SUPPLEMENTAL HEALTH INSURANCE

Each insurance carrier offers different health insurance benefit packages and has different costs. Which carrier you choose depends on how you perceive your needs and how much money you are willing to spend. Call various health insurance companies in your area and ask what they offer persons over sixty-five or what they offer as Medicare supplementation. Group plans, such as that offered through AARP, may offer broad coverage at low prices. Your insurance agent can help you decide among different policies. The Department of Health and Human Services can also send you its guide for Medicare supplemental insurance.

Be particularly careful to note whether the insurance carrier you choose has the following limitations.

- limits or excludes your coverage for medical problems that you have had before starting your insurance term. The uncovered period should not be any longer than six months.
- imposes waiting periods lasting up to a year for reimbursement for treatment of particular diseases, such as cancer and heart disease
- includes benefit waiting periods that do not cover the first few days of hospitalization
- limits the duration of benefits
- offers conditional renewability. Under conditional renewability, the insurance company can end your policy when the next premium is due.

MEDICAID

Medicaid provides health insurance coverage to people who are on limited incomes. Eligibility and services covered vary widely from state to state. You should call your local Department of Public Welfare to find out which services are reimbursed in your state. You should also be aware that Medicaid reimbursement in many states is below standard medical fees. For this reason, many health providers are reluctant to accept Medicaid patients, so your choice of physicians may be limited. Medicaid is the major payor for nursing home care, once people have depleted their personal resources, and, again, reimburses nursing homes at fairly low fees. Thus your choice of nursing home, should you need one, may be limited.

SUGGESTED READINGS

Robin, Eugene D. *Medical Care Can Be Dangerous to Your Health: A Guide to the Risks and Benefits*. New York: Harper & Row, Perennial Library, 1986.

Sobel, David S., M.D., and Ferguson, Tom, M.D. *The People's Book of Medical Tests*. New York: Summit Books, 1985.

Vickery, Donald M., M.D., and Fries, James F., M.D. *Take Care of Yourself: The Consumer's Guide to Medical Care*. Reading, Mass.: Addison–Wesley, 1986.

Seventeen

Slowing Down

ADVANCING age is a shadowy demon. No sooner do we glimpse the spectre than it seems to disappear, and we find ourselves again in the sunlight. Like all demons, this one harms us the most when we empower it with our own fear and resignation. Unquestionably, we slow physically as the days race by. Some days our machinery feels less limber, our joints less oiled, and our step less quick. But we are not outwitted. Our years have made us resourceful. We are good at coping and can find ways of maintaining as much independence as possible in the face of physical and mental impairments. Old brains are clever devils themselves.

Bertrand Russell was a mathematician as a young man. As he grew older, he thought he could no longer be as creative in mathematics, so he turned to philosophy, a field that he felt was intellectually less rigorous. Yet philosophy was the field in which he made his finest contributions to the human race.

Your ability to perceive and use abstract patterns and relationships, necessary for such activities as playing chess and solving complicated mathematical problems, declines from early adulthood onward. Your memory, too, loses its edge, surprising and sometimes dismaying you with its lapses. But new research challenges the long-held belief that overall intelligence diminishes with age. With continued stimulation, the aging brain responds to its natural loss of nerve cells by forging new connections to remaining cells. Researchers have found that people who have healthy brains (free of stroke or diseases that affect the brain) continue to increase their ability to use accumulated information to make judgments and evaluate complex issues.

Your brain is more likely to stay nimble through old age if you keep involved with people of all ages, keep working, continue to learn and be intellectually curious, and continue to enjoy new experiences and different perspectives.

LIVING INDEPENDENTLY—WITH HELP

One of the great fears of older women and men is not being able to maintain their own homes or apartments and being "put away" somewhere. If you lose some of your physical abilities, if you retire, or if your husband dies and your closest friends die, your home assumes more importance. It is a familiar place in which you retain a measure of security and control. What happens to you when you can no longer manage entirely on your own?

The process by which federal- or state-subsidized help at home is allocated is complex and sometimes arbitrary. Some older women struggle with too little help for years and are brought to the attention of social service agencies only by a major crisis. Other older women who can afford to buy help for themselves do not do so because (1) their ingrained frugal habits inhibit them from such spending, (2) they may regard home assistance as an open admission of failure to manage their household, or (3) they are afraid of spending money now that they feel they may need even more later.

It behooves women to recognize that accepting help does not diminish their dignity and that payment for help is money well spent. Help can mean freedom from the fear of not being able to cope alone.

Services You Can Get at Home

Most social service agencies that work with older persons can acquaint you with the home services for which you may be eligible. The Area Agency on Aging can provide the names and telephone numbers of such social service agencies. Social service departments of hospitals and the Social Security office or the welfare office of your city or town can refer you to agencies that can help you at home. The types of services available include the following:

1. **Homemaking services.** You may need someone who will shop and cook, do housework and laundry, and escort you to appointments. If you are disabled by age or disease, and if your in-

come qualifies you, you may be able to get a homemaker whose fees are subsidized by federal or state agencies one or more times per week. If your income exceeds the financial guidelines, you may be able to pay a sliding fee, or you can hire homemaking help privately.

2. Chore services. You can get someone to do heavy chores, such as washing windows, scrubbing floors, and cleaning the basement. Depending on your disability, age, and income, these services may be subsidized.

3. Home-delivered meals. Older women who have difficulty shopping or cooking can get up to one hot meal a day, five days a week, for a nominal fee.

In most cities or towns, you can go to senior meal sites that provide hot lunches and a chance to enjoy the companionship of others. You and your friends could also join forces and either hire a catering agency that delivers hot meals or hire someone to come in and cook one meal a day or even two or three meals a week for the group.

4. Visiting nurses. Nurses can monitor you at home and report findings to your doctor. They advise you about medications, treatments, exercises, and equipment and act as the link between you and your doctor. Their fees can be reimbursed under Medicare and Medicaid, provided you are getting posthospital care or have a documented need for "skilled nursing" services that have been prescribed by your physician. You can also hire visiting nurses yourself.

5. Home health aides. These workers assist you with personal needs, such as bathing, dressing, feeding, toileting, and transferring from bed to chair. Sometimes they also help with your homemaking tasks. You may be eligible for this service through Medicare if you are getting posthospital care or require "skilled nursing" services. Medicaid also subsidizes home health aides. If you do not qualify for subsidized help, you can hire home health aides privately.

6. Physical, occupational, and/or speech therapists. Therapists can come to the house to help you with rehabilitation. They can also recommend and order equipment and safety devices that simplify your life, such as a tub seat, bathroom grab bars, a bedside commode, a cane, a walker, a wheelchair, steps or a ramp, breathing apparatus, and an amplified telephone.

7. Home laboratory services. Technicians can spare you the inconvenience of going to the doctor's office or hospital for laboratory tests, ECGs, or X rays by doing these procedures in your home. These services may be reimbursed by Medicare or Medicaid.

8. Escort services. Transportation assistance and protection can be provided for errands, outings, and appointments.

9. Day care. This service often provides 9:00 A.M. to 5:00 P.M. supervision in a group setting and can also offer nursing care, health aides, social services, therapy, recreation, and companionship. Medicaid reimburses this service if your income is low enough; otherwise you can pay for it privately. Transportation to and from the center is often included, but sometimes you must arrange for it separately.

10. Religious service. Churches and synagogues will send someone to visit you if you have trouble getting to their services. Some will help you sell homemade crafts at their bazaars or gift shops, and they may provide transportation to and from worship or social events.

11. Alcoholics Anonymous. Under special circumstances, AA will send volunteers to the home of an older person who needs counseling and who cannot get out of the house to meetings.

12. Hospice care. Trained counselors and/or social services are available to persons who have chosen to die in their homes and to their families. Often hospice care is reimbursed by Medicare or Medicaid in the last six months of a person's life.

In addition, social services are available in most communities to help you with financial problems, such as getting fuel assistance; to coordinate services that you might need at home; and to provide social and emotional support if you are stressed by disease, family problems, or psychological problems. Some agencies can call you daily to check that you are doing well at home. Some agencies provide friendly visitors, such as college students or older volunteers, to do odd jobs or be companions.

DIFFERENT HOUSING OPTIONS

In your later years, you will probably face the question of keeping or selling a home you have lived in for years. If you feel insecure about your financial future, you may sell your home too hastily, only to regret the loss later. On the other hand, you may decide that moving into a condominium or apartment presents more social opportunities and fewer burdens than staying in your home does.

You have many housing options to consider:

1. Special housing for older people. Some modern apartment buildings have been specially designed for persons over sixty-two years of age. They are usually clean and well-maintained and have sunny public rooms, recreational facilities, and security at the door. Neighborhood service suppliers sometimes come to the building, for example, grocers with fresh vegetables and fruits, public health nurses offering free flu shots, and podiatrists offering foot care. There are always people around for company.

Many buildings have some financially subsidized units. In addition, many have apartments adapted for the handicapped with low sinks and counters, wide doorways to accommodate a wheelchair, and a large bathroom with grab bars near the toilet and tub.

If you are considering such housing, visit several of these housing complexes. Attend their community meetings or educational programs to see who lives there. Check the security and cleanliness of the building. Ask the residents whether the management willingly attends to maintenance problems (plumbing, heating, air-conditioning, and so on) and human problems (medical emergencies and financial difficulties, for example). Find out what programs and services the facility offers. Check the accessibility of stores, movie theaters, restaurants, and doctors' offices, hospitals, and nursing or rest home facilities. Find out whether some of the units are financially subsidized and whether you meet the eligibility requirements. Make sure you understand all the costs involved.

Many housing units have long waiting lists. It is best to start your investigations and applications as early as five years before you plan to move.

2. Sharing a house. It is not unreasonable for older women to consider living together. There are economic advantages in sharing a home. The social possibilities may also be rewarding.

3. Congregate housing. This kind of housing is organized to provide certain services, such as hot meals, to its tenants, in addition to the apartments. Some buildings also offer homemaker services to clean apartments, shop, do laundry, and cook; social and medical services; grocery services; hairdressing; and educational programs.

A very limited number of congregate buildings offer apartments to be shared by several residents, with a common kitchen, bathroom, and living room and shared homemaker help.

Women living in congregate housing can choose to utilize the services their building provides or do things on their own.

4. Retirement/life care communities. Planned communities provide an alternative living situation for retired persons. Usually set outside city limits, they combine housing, services, and recreation in one location.

The community may provide health and social services, beauty and barber shops, a variety store, a drugstore, a grocery store, and athletic facilities such as tennis courts and golf courses. Often, the residents staff the stores themselves on a volunteer or payment basis.

The retirement community may have separate dwellings for able-bodied couples who wish privacy and independence, apartments for people who wish a more social environment, congregate units for more disabled people, and nursing home facilities for residents who need round-the-clock care. Having such options and services within the community gives you the advantage of not having to leave if your needs change or if you become more dependent.

Become familiar with the financial requirements of each community you consider. Pay particular attention to entrance fees (which can be substantial) and monthly maintenance fees and to the disposition of your property and your investment in the community after your death—whether they will return to your estate or belong to the community.

5. Foster care. Some states have foster-care programs for older people who have no family or friends with whom they can live and who cannot or do not want to live on their own. The older person generally has his or her own room and receives meals, companionship, and limited services from the foster family. The foster family receives a monthly fee for the older person's room and board. This program is usually state-funded.

NURSING HOMES AND REST HOMES

There are 1.2 million nursing home beds in the United States. Contrary to many claims, the vast majority of people in nursing homes are appropriately placed. They have reached a point at which care at home would be too demanding and even hazardous, and they and their families are better off using the nursing home rather than struggling on at home.

The decision to place oneself, a spouse, or a parent in a nursing home is always painful and difficult. The most common reason that brings a woman to a nursing home is her inability to care for herself, usually because she is mentally impaired from senile dementia. About 60 percent to 70 percent of all people in nursing homes have significant dementia or have had strokes that have left them mentally impaired. The remainder are there because of physical impairments requiring care that no relative is able to give. Only rarely do women enter nursing homes because they have been pressured into it by their families.

When she first reached the nursing home, Katherine S., seventy, felt totally alienated from the severely disabled people she saw. She did not feel at all like one of them. Some were sitting in chairs, blankly staring at a TV and not communicating with anyone. Some were babbling and nodding. Others were shuffling around with walkers.

For a week, Katherine kept to herself. But pretty soon she caught a smile here and there; then she spoke to another frustrated woman. She began to make a few friends and to appreciate the community she had entered.

Nursing homes are classified according to levels of care. A skilled nursing facility (SNF) serves persons who require the skills of professionals such as registered nurses, physical therapists, occupational therapists, speech pathologists, and audiologists. Medicare will pay for some short-term SNF care for certain categories of illness (such as rehabilitation after a stroke or a hip fracture). Persons whose rehabilitation needs do not fit the Medicare categories must bear the cost of SNF care privately. Medicaid reimburses both short-term and long-term SNF care for people who need the intensive professional care and who are also indigent. The usual costs of SNF care range from fifty dollars to one hundred dollars per day, or up to $3,000 per month, and there may be additional charges for medications, doctors' visits, and other services

An intermediate care facility (ICF) is appropriate for people who have some ability to feed and dress themselves and to walk. Medicare does not pay for this care, and the costs are somewhat lower than for SNF care.

Rest homes do not offer nursing care but rather offer a socially supportive environment. The home provides three meals a day and usually keeps a nurse on its staff to dispense medications.

In most states, neither Medicare nor Medicaid pays for rest home care, but in many states, welfare does. The usual cost of rest homes ranges from twenty dollars to forty dollars per day, but there are usually additional charges for medications and medical services.

Classifying nursing homes according to these levels of care does serve most people most of the time and provides a convenient way to compute reimbursement charges. The problem is that people's needs change over time, but this system makes it impossible for them to "age in place." The system moves them from one floor to another or from one facility to another to get the appropriate level of care.

How to Select a Nursing Home

If you or a loved one are in the hospital and in need of a nursing home, you should realize that you do not have to accept a choice of nursing home made by others. As much as possible, participate in the selection even if you cannot personally inspect the facility. Consider the following:

- Find a nursing home that is accessible to your family and close friends and one that allows you weekend or day passes to visit family and friends.

- Ask someone you know well to visit the home several times before you agree to go there. No verbal description can convey what an actual visit will.

- The home should be clean, smell fresh, be bright and airy, and have windows in the bedrooms. The home should have ready access to the outside so that you can go outdoors even if you are in a wheelchair.

- How many people are in a bedroom? Four is maximum and two is preferable. Are single rooms available?

- Does the home have common rooms for dining, sharing activities, and watching TV? People should be able to eat with others rather than alone in their own rooms.

- Are the meals varied, well-balanced, and served warm, and are there opportunities for snacks and beverages between meals?

- What activities are organized for the residents? Can residents enjoy card games, bingo, movies, crafts, writing, singing, gardening, reading, exercise, day trips, dances, cooking, or educational programs? Ask especially about offerings that actively involve the residents.

- Does the home's staff include social workers and physical and occupational therapists to help with social problems and to offer rehabilitation programs?

- Do the nurses seem kind, responsive to suggestions, and willing to spend time with you and your family?

- Are podiatry and beauty-care services available?

- How responsive can the nursing home be to possible emergencies? Can the staff give CPR (cardiopulmonary resuscitation)? first aid? Can the nursing home reach your doctor or the doctor's substitute twenty-four hours a day? Is the home affiliated with a good hospital?

- Study the attitude of the staff toward residents of the home. Are staff members respectful? Do they encourage independence rather than dependence? Do they respect a person's need for both social life and privacy? Are they kind and interested in the residents, or are they just putting in a day's work? Are they responsive to the suggestions of family? Are they willing to alert the family early if things are not going well with a particular resident? You will have to speak to relatives of people in the home to find out these things.

- Do the other residents appear content? Do they talk to one another? Do they looked drugged? Are their clothes clean and attractive? Do they have some of their belongings in their own rooms (pictures, books, afghans, furniture, and TV)? Ask your friend to talk to one or two residents about their feelings about the nursing home—its food, activities, and staff.

Cost of Nursing Home Care

It is axiomatic that the quality of care that is bought depends on the price. Sadly, nowhere is this more true than in nursing home care. Many nursing homes accept private patients only—that is, residents who will pay a daily rate of sixty to one hundred dollars out of pocket. Only after residents have spent so much of their own money that they are eligible for Medicaid reimbursement (for the indigent) will these nursing homes accept Medicaid fees.

In most states, the Medicaid rate for a nursing home bed is about half the rate paid privately by individuals. As a consequence, nursing homes that are exclusively reimbursed by Medicaid are able to adhere only to minimum standards of quality and care, rather than to the higher standards that the homes that charge more can afford to maintain.

Therefore, if you are fortunate enough to be able to pay for private nursing home care for at least six months ($15,000 to $18,000 in assets), you should try to get into a nursing home that has at least 20 percent of its ongoing reimbursement from private patients. This percentage is generally accepted as the yardstick to insure higher quality of services and care. If Medicaid is, from the onset, your only source of payment, your options are unfairly diminished. For potential residents who only have Medicaid reimbursement, there is often little recourse but to accept the nursing home bed that is available.

As a society, we could afford to give good nursing home care to all who require it. It has been estimated that this goal would cost about a 15 percent increase in state taxes and about a 2 percent increase in federal taxes. The question is, Are we willing to pay for such equity?

UNDERSTANDING DEMENTIA

Accelerated memory loss, intellectual impairment, and mental confusion that lasts months or years is described by the general term *dementia*. Only about 5 percent of people over sixty-five are disabled by dementia. The majority of them, however, are women. Sometimes older people are mislabeled "senile" and their physical and emotional complaints dismissed as hopeless when, in fact, they are not hopeless. The future for victims of all forms of dementia looks more promising than it did ten years ago. Many gerontologists believe that by the mid 1990s, the secrets of Alzheimer's disease and related afflictions will be unlocked, offering hope of treatment or prevention.

Dementia is not one disease but many disorders with different causes and treatments. While 90 percent of dementia cases are untreatable and irreversible, 10 percent have treatable causes, such as liver or kidney failure; vitamin B_{12} deficiency; brain tumor; brain infection; lupus erythematosus; hydrocephalus; blood clot on the brain; inflammation of brain arteries; thyroid, parathyroid, or adrenal gland problems; lead, mercury, and copper poisoning; psychiatric disorders, notably depression and schizophrenia; and drug reactions or toxicities.

About 50 percent of the people with untreatable dementia have Alzheimer's disease, and 20 percent have multi-infarct disease. The remaining 30 percent of irreversible dementias display a combination of Alzheimer's disease and multi-infarct disease.

Multi-Infarct Dementia

In multi-infarct dementia, the disordered thinking and memory loss result from many successive small strokes that occur in the brain, affecting 50 percent or more of the brain by the time the dementia shows itself. This disorder is more common in males than females; however, women with hypertension and/or diabetes are at risk for multi-infarct dementia. Both these conditions hasten arteriosclerosis (which clogs the arteries of the brain) when they are not properly treated (see chapters 4 and 5).

Alzheimer's Disease

At first, the term *Alzheimer's disease* was used to describe dementia in younger people, but we now know that the dementia found in older persons is the same one. Intensive research is under way to identify the causes of the disease. Possible culprits are chemical toxicities, viruses, deficiencies of chemicals in the brain, and heredity.

In Alzheimer's dementia, memory loss and impaired functioning progress slowly, over years. For a long time, the patient can compensate for these losses, so others are barely aware of the degree of the deterioration. Gradually the person abandons interests that require memory and concentration.

> I know that my memory is failing, but I
> desperately want to hide it from my husband and
> children. I make myself countless little notes to
> remember dates and conversations. I find excuses
> for not reading the papers or books they give me.
> It is becoming harder and harder to live this lie.
> —*Sophia, seventy-five*

As language impairment increases, the patient has trouble finding the right word or may use the wrong word in a conversation. He or she becomes quickly frustrated and cannot concentrate on long explanations. Self-awareness of the deficiencies can lead to agitation or depression. Later, judgment noticeably falters. The patient may forget to pay bills or overpay them. He or she may unwittingly sell prized possessions far too cheaply. Cleanliness, dress, and nutrition deteriorate. The person may forget to take needed medications or may take extra doses during the day. The individual may leave the door open at night or wander, not knowing where he or she is.

Late in the course of the illness, the patient may be very weak; live mostly in the past; suffer delusions about people stealing possessions; be suspicious of and unable to recognize close friends or family; and be unable to bathe, dress, or feed himself or herself. Ultimately the person loses control of bladder, bowels, and behavior.

> My mother accused my father of stealing her under-
> pants and slips. She thought he gave them as
> presents to the homemaker. She also was sure that
> he was having an affair with the homemaker, who
> was fifty years his junior. My mother claimed he
> was sending the homemaker messages by hanging

the underpants in the window. My father denies everything. I sometimes don't know whom to believe!

—*Annabelle B., daughter of an eighty-two-year-old Alzheimer's victim*

Alzheimer's disease leads to death. Women who have had Alzheimer's disease for years weaken mentally and physically to the point where they may not eat, may get repeated pneumonias, or may lie curled up in a fetal position. Generally the disease lasts about ten years, though some cases progress rapidly to death in less than four or five years, and others develop very slowly over twenty years.

Diagnosis

There is no simple laboratory test for Alzheimer's disease. The diagnosis is made after taking a medical history, giving a thorough medical examination, and, most important, after excluding treatable causes of dementia by laboratory tests and X rays.

The treatable dementias are usually excluded by the following tests.

1. a blood analysis for kidney, liver, thyroid, calcium, or adrenal problems; for B_{12} deficiency; for chronic infections; and for poisoning
2. a CAT scan for evidence of a stroke, brain tumor, blood clot on the brain, or hydrocephalus
3. a medical or psychiatric evaluation for serious depression or psychosis
4. a careful review of all drugs taken to be sure that the dementia is not caused by an unusual drug reaction

The only definitive way to diagnose Alzheimer's is by finding certain changes in a microscopic section of the brain. These changes show twisted nerve cell fibers that represent a degeneration of cells. A brain biopsy is rarely done to determine Alzheimer's because it is a difficult and risky procedure that usually only confirms a diagnosis that is already fairly certain.

Treatment

As of 1986 there is no effective treatment for Alzheimer's disease. National and international studies of the following medications have not shown consistent benefit.

- Hydergine. European studies have shown that patients taking four to eight milligrams of Hydergine per day for several months showed some mental improvement over people not taking the drug. Studies in the United States have not been so encouraging, but these studies used lower doses. Tests of Hydergine are not yet conclusive.

- Gerovital-H3. Magazine advertisements still tout it, but it has not been found to help dementia.

- Neuropeptides. These chemicals are being tested on animals only but may hold some promise for humans in the future.

- Neurotransmitter enhancers. Some Alzheimer's patients have been fed large quantities of lecithin, which is found to increase brain acetylcholine (the chemical transmitter that is low in Alzheimer's patients). Results have been mixed—some people show improvement, and others do not. Women who want to buy lecithin in health food stores should know that only the variety that is phosphatidyl choline, not phosphatidyl serine, helps. Read labels carefully. Most lecithin sold in these stores is of the latter, nonuseful type.

Caring for Yourself When You Care for a Relative with Alzheimer's

Any woman who cares for a relative with Alzheimer's is performing a heroic act of love. The work is constant, stressful, draining, and sad. Tending a severely mentally impaired person who years ago was a forceful, intelligent mother or a tender, strong husband is a heavy burden. You may find yourself grieving for the past, feeling depressed, and crying. You may feel angry and wish the person dead and then feel guilty afterward.

As caretaker of an Alzheimer's patient, you must take time out to restore your energies, both physical and mental. You must find time to care for yourself, and your emotional needs, in order to avoid exhaustion, depression, and burnout. Consider the following suggestions.

1. Try to involve other family members in the care of the demented member.

2. Do not isolate yourself from friends and family. Make plans to meet them, and get an adult "sitter" for an evening out.

3. Each day, plan at least an hour or two that are all your own.

4. Eat properly and try to exercise at least three times a week.

5. It may be helpful to you, as well as to your disabled relative, to arrange day care a few days a week. Your local Area Agency on Aging can refer you to the appropriate places.

6. Try to hire a homemaker–home health aide to help you with the housework, laundry, and baths for the Alzheimer's patient.

7. Plan to take a vacation of a week to ten days every six months. Some medical insurance plans will pay for occasional respite care for you while the patient is in a nursing home or in a hospital that specializes in chronic care. Some nurses or nurse's aides may be willing to live in your home and care for the patient while you go on vacation. Other people may have the capacity to take care of your relative for a brief period of time. Ask your physician or social worker to assist you with the details of getting respite care.

8. Meet with other caretakers of Alzheimer's patients. Many cities have organized Alzheimer's support groups, which can be a great source of encouragement for you. To find a group that is close to you, write to the national headquarters of the Alzheimer's Disease and Related Disorders Association (ADRDA), 360 North Michigan Avenue, Chicago, IL 60601.

DEATH AND DYING

> Some people try to achieve immortality through their offspring or their works. I prefer to achieve immortality by not dying.
> —*Woody Allen*

> I would like to die as young as possible and as late as possible!
> —*Francois, Duc de La Rochefoucauld*

When the advances of medical science kept infants, children, and women in labor from dying as a matter of course, we began to feel that we were entitled to long life. We became so unused to witnessing death in the first half of our lives that we grew unprepared for its intrusion in the second.

We live longer and in better health than ever before. We have experienced a steady increase in life expectancy from improved nutrition, housing, and sanitation and from antibiotic treatments of infections. We have raised effective barriers to most epidemic infections through vaccination. Our faith in technology has given us an illusory hope of conquering all limitations of nature, and the habit of considering death itself only a failure of the medical system.

Because our own anxieties about and unfamiliarity with death make it difficult for us to face it squarely, dying people often find themselves alone with their fears. They perceive our silence as indifference or terror, both of which hurt and frighten them even more. Death is still an inevitable part of life, and facing this reality together is the only way we can help each other transcend our dread of having life end.

Aging and Awareness of Death

We like to convince ourselves that older people lose their fear of death and welcome its arrival. Rarely is this the case. Our will to live may be as strong in older years as in youth. A seventy-five-year-old who still takes vacations with her grandchildren may feel that she's in the middle of life. An eighty-two-year-old woman marrying again may have trouble perceiving an end to it all.

But sometimes life causes enough pain that it injures our will to survive. A seventy-nine-year-old who had lost her husband, her two older sisters, and her oldest son asked, "What's the use of going on? Soon I'll be the only one left."

Loss of loved ones, chronic physical discomfort or pain, dependence upon others for personal hygiene—these accompaniments of old age may overshadow the pleasure of living and, for some, make the prospect of death less disturbing.

Definition of Death

Death is now difficult to define medically. Our technological genius facilely ignores its presence when our good sense begs its embrace. A respirator can keep a brain-dead person breathing for months, though there is no hope of consciousness returning. The medical profession has responded to such paradoxes by defining death according to four specific criteria:

1. inability to receive or respond to signals
2. absence of spontaneous breathing
3. absence of reflexes
4. an electroencephalogram (EEG, or brain wave test) that shows no activity

Needs of the Dying Person

The dying person is confronted with many fears and anxieties. In order to relieve some of the burdens of this experience, the following needs should be addressed.

Confirmation

If you are sick and suspect that you are dying, your first need is medical confirmation of the fact. Usually a doctor can confirm the fact after hospital tests or after ordinary treatments have failed. All subsequent decisions must meet your needs and improve your quality of life. For example, an operation may be totally unnecessary when cure is impossible. Or, an operation may be the only and best way to stop your pain.

Control of Pain and Symptoms

A dying person who is uncomfortable or in pain has a right to get relief and not be overwhelmed by intense and frightening symptoms. He or she may be unable to eat and may experience nausea, constipation, incontinence, stiffness and muscle aches, insomnia, fears, and agitation. In each of these instances, simple remedies can help the individual feel much better. A dying person should expect to receive pain medications, including narcotics or alcohol, as needed and not worry about addiction. If the person has always smoked, he or she should not be deprived of cigarettes even if the person has lung cancer. The most important consideration is the physical and mental well-being, and the person's own tastes and desires, not the considerations that are medically "right" for those who are not dying.

Choice of Where to Die

A person may prefer to die at home but fear being too much of a burden on the family. The dying person's family should seek assistance and may find that their relative is entitled to the services of a visiting nurse, a homemaker–home health aide, a physical therapist, a social worker, and a hospice program. These services are usually covered by Medicare, in part, or Medicaid.

If an individual has chosen to die in the hospital, the family can arrange to have visiting hours extended. A husband, another relative, or a friend may be able to stay overnight on a cot. Nurses, social workers, physical therapists, a member of the clergy, or a psychiatrist are all available for support.

Completion of Unfinished Business

Many people have put off making wills or have neglected to patch up long-standing differences and misunderstandings with relatives. The final months and days of one's life are not too late to resolve gnawing practical and emotional business. People are then free to feel more peaceful about death.

If you want to donate your organs or have a preference about cremation or burial, where you wish to be buried, or the disposition of your special belongings, express these desires clearly if you haven't already done so in your will.

Companionship

Nobody wants to die alone. A person needs the comfort and company of family and friends as well as understanding and supportive nurses, doctors, and aides. Some people may need regular visits from their minister, priest, or rabbi. Some may need their pet nearby.

Sense of Security

Preparing for death is like planning to go to another galaxy, not as a human being but in some unknown form. It means taking leave of everyone and everything familiar. Sometimes a person fears being abandoned or fears pain and suffering. He or she may want to know every detail of what is going on or may deny that anything is seriously wrong.

Most people, when asked whether they would want to know if they had a fatal illness, say yes. But many of these same people, faced with a relative who is dying, want to hide the fact. Their intentions are noble—they want to spare the person pain and suffering. They are afraid that the truth will make the relative lose hope. They may also have a need to protect themselves from facing the person's despair and sadness so that they can better control their own. There are few people for whom the knowledge of the truth is too devastating. Only in those unusual cases may it be better to give minimal information about the fatal illness.

The fact is that truth is one of the most therapeutic tools of caring that we possess—not truth coldly and insensitively stated but truth handled delicately by appropriate people who respect your nature. The process of telling the truth can take days or weeks as one becomes prepared to hear more and more. Sometimes the family doctor is the one who tells the person of the terminal illness; sometimes it is a husband, a close relative, a best friend, or a family member together with the doctor.

When a person is dying, he or she probably knows more than people suspect. The patient will be aware of increasing debility, weakness, inability to eat, and loss of weight. He or she will perceive the signs of gravity and sadness that are written all over the faces of those who visit.

Denial of the truth increases the burden and anger of the dying person. The person feels isolated from those who are desperately trying to hide information and feelings, who try to appear optimistic and happy when they feel hopeless inside. Physicians are often asked by a dying cancer patient, "Please don't tell my husband that I have cancer. He can't handle it." Minutes later, in another room, the husband will plead with the doctor, "Please don't tell my wife that she has cancer. She can't bear it." The very people who need to communicate at this time of crisis erect barriers that keep them from helping one another. Honesty should be given, along with hope—not of survival but of comfort, dignity, and companionship.

No one knows for certain what happens after death. Some hold a strong belief in reincarnation, others believe in immortality as a soul that will be reunited with those who have died before them, and still others see death as a return to elemental form. Death is the inevitable end of life, and we will summon the courage to meet it when the hour comes.

SUGGESTED READINGS

Glucksberg, Harold, M.D., and Singer, Jack W., M.D. *Cancer Care: A Personal Guide.* Baltimore: Johns Hopkins University Press, 1980.

Horne, Jo. *Caregiving: Helping An Aging Loved One.* Washington, D.C.: AARP; Glenview, Ill.: Scott, Foresman & Co., 1985. (An AARP Book)

Kubler-Ross, Elisabeth, M.D. *Living with Death and Dying.* New York: Macmillan, 1981.

———. *Questions and Answers on Death and Dying.* New York: Macmillan, 1974.

———, ed. *Death: The Final Stage of Growth.* Englewood Cliffs, N.J.: Prentice-Hall, 1975.

Mace, Nancy L., and Rabins, Peter V., M.D. *The Thirty-Six-Hour Day: A Family Guide to Caring for Persons with Alzheimer's Disease, Related Dementing Illnesses, and Memory Loss in Later Life.* Baltimore: Warner Books, 1984.

Appendix A

Health Maintenance Procedures
Recommended for Older Women

1. Physical examination including blood pressure reading, manual breast check, pelvic exam, and digital rectal exam

   Once a year.

2. Pap test (see chapter 10)

   Once a year for 2 years; if both are normal, every 2–3 years thereafter.

3. Screen for colorectal cancer (see chapter 7)

   Stool samples (3) for blood

   Once a year.

   Proctoscopic exam

   Once a year for 2 years; if both are normal, every 3–5 years thereafter.

4. Mammogram (see chapter 10)

   Once a year.

5. Blood tests

   Hematocrit (see chapter 4)

   Once a year.

   Fasting blood sugar (see chapter 5)

   Once; and if normal, every 2–4 years thereafter.

   Fasting cholesterol, HDL (see chapter 4)

   Once; and if normal, every 2–4 years thereafter.

   Thyroid test (see chapter 5)

   Once; and if normal, every 2–4 years thereafter.

6. Electrocardiogram (see chapter 4) — Every 3–5 years after initial one; if you have stable heart disease, every 1–2 years.

7. Glaucoma check (see chapter 3) — Every 2 years, or every year if you have risk factors; every 6 months to 1 year if you have glaucoma.

8. Dental exam (see chapter 3) — Once a year.

   Dental X rays — Every 2–3 years.

   Dental hygiene — Every 6 months.

9. Vaccines

   Pneumococcal (see chapter 6) — One time only.

   Influenza — Once a year.

   Tetanus booster — Every 10 years.

Appendix B

A MODEL PATIENTS' BILL OF RIGHTS

Preamble: As you enter this health care facility, it is our duty to remind you that your health care is a cooperative effort between you as a patient and the doctors and hospital staff. During your stay a patients' rights advocate will be available to you. The duty of the advocate is to assist you in all the decisions you must make and in all situations in which your health and welfare are at stake. The advocate's first responsibility is to help you understand the role of all who will be working with you, and to help you understand what your rights as a patient are. Your advocate can be reached at any time of the day by dialing _____. The following is a list of your rights as a patient. Your advocate's duty is to see to it that you are afforded these rights. You should call your advocate whenever you have any questions or concerns about any of these rights.

1. The patient has a legal right to informed participation in all decisions involving his/her health care program.

2. We recognize the right of all potential patients to know what research and experimental protocols are being used in our facility and what alternatives are available in the community.

3. The patient has a legal right to privacy regarding the source of payment for treatment and care. This right includes access to the highest degree of care without regard to the source of payment for that treatment and care.

4. We recognize the right of a potential patient to complete and accurate information concerning medical care and procedures.

5. The patient has a legal right to prompt attention, especially in an emergency situation.

6. The patient has a legal right to a clear, concise explanation in layperson's terms of all proposed procedures, including the possibilities of any risk of mortality or serious side effects, problems related to recuperation, and probability of success,

and will not be subjected to any procedure without his/her voluntary, competent and understanding consent. The specifics of such consent shall be set out in a written consent form, signed by the patient.

7. The patient has a legal right to a clear, complete, and accurate evaluation of his/her condition and prognosis without treatment before being asked to consent to any test or procedure.

8. We recognize the right of the patient to know the identity and professional status of all those providing service. All personnel have been instructed to introduce themselves, state their status, and explain their role in the health care of the patient. Part of this right is the right of the patient to know the identity of the physician responsible for his/her care.

9. We recognize the right of any patient who does not speak English to have access to an interpreter.

10. The patient has a right to all the information contained in his/her medical record while in the health care facility, and to examine the record on request.

11. We recognize the right of a patient to discuss his/her condition with a consultant specialist, at the patient's request and expense.

12. The patient has a legal right not to have any test or procedure, designed for educational purposes rather than his/her direct personal benefit, performed on him/her.

13. The patient has a legal right to refuse any particular drug, test, procedure, or treatment.

14. The patient has a legal right to privacy of both person and information with respect to: the hospital staff, other doctors, residents, interns and medical students, researchers, nurses, other hospital personnel, and other patients.

15. We recognize the patient's right of access to people outside the health care facility by means of visitors and the telephone. Parents may stay with their children and relatives with terminally ill patients 24 hours a day.

16. The patient has a legal right to leave the health care facility regardless of his/her physical condition or financial status, although the patient may be requested to sign a release stating

that he/she is leaving against the medical judgment of his/her doctor or the hospital.

17. The patient has a right not to be transferred to another facility unless he/she has received a complete explanation of the desirability and need for the transfer, the other facility has accepted the patient for transfer, and the patient has agreed to transfer. If the patient does not agree to transfer, the patient has the right to a consultant's opinion on the desirability of transfer.

18. A patient has a right to be notified of his/her impending discharge at least one day before it is accomplished, to insist on a consultation by an expert on the desirability of discharge, and to have a person of the patient's choice notified in advance.

19. The patient has a right, regardless of the source of payment, to examine and receive an itemized and detailed explanation of the total bill for services rendered in the facility.

20. The patient has a right to competent counseling from the hospital staff to help in obtaining financial assistance from public or private sources to meet the expense of services received in the institution.

21. The patient has a right to timely prior notice of the termination of his/her eligibility for reimbursement by any third-party payor for the expense of hospital care.

22. At the termination of his/her stay at the health care facility we recognize the right of a patient to a complete copy of the information contained in his/her medical record.

23. We recognize the right of all patients to have 24-hour-a-day access to a patients' rights advocate who may act on behalf of the patient to assert or protect the rights set out in this document.

Index

About the Author

Marie Feltin is a physician with the Urban Medical Group in Boston and medical director of the Independent Living Primary Care Program. She is an assistant professor at Boston University School of Public Health.

Since 1976, Dr. Feltin has lectured on the care of older people and on women's health at both Boston University School of Public Health and Harvard Medical School.

A native of France, Dr. Feltin grew up in Canada and holds an undergraduate degree from McGill University, an M.D. from the University of California at San Francisco, and an M.S. in epidemiology from Harvard School of Public Health. She is a founding member of a nonprofit group medical practice (The Urban Medical Group) that treats adults, disabled persons, and the frail elderly and that has reestablished the importance of house calls.

Dr. Feltin lives in Boston with her husband and five children.